DISORDERS OF THE PLACENTA, FETUS, AND NEONATE: DIAGNOSIS AND CLINICAL SIGNIFICANCE

Disorders of the Placenta, Fetus, and Neonate: Diagnosis and Clinical Significance

Richard L. Naeye, M.D.
University Professor of Pathology
Chairman, Department of Pathology
The Milton S. Hershey Medical Center
The Pennsylvania State University
Hershey, Pennsylvania

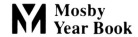
Mosby
Year Book

St. Louis   Baltimore   Boston   Chicago   London   Philadelphia   Sydney   Toronto

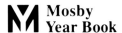
Mosby
Year Book

Dedicated to Publishing Excellence

Sponsoring Editor: Susan Gay
Assistant Editor: Sandra Clark
Associate Managing Editor, Manuscript Services: Deborah Thorp
Production Project Coordinator: Karen Halm
Proofroom Manager: Barbara Kelly

Mosby–Year Book, Inc.
11830 Westline Industrial Drive
St. Louis, MO 63146

1 2 3 4 5 6 7 8 9 0 GW MV 96   95   94   93   92

Library of Congress Cataloging-in-Publication Data

Naeye, Richard L., 1929–
    Disorders of the placenta, fetus, and neonate : diagnosis
and clinical significance / Richard L. Naeye.
      p.   cm.
    Includes bibliographical references and index.
    ISBN 0-8016-3352-4
    1. Obstetrics – Diagnosis.   2. Fetus – Diseases – Diagnosis.
  3. Infants (Newborn) – Diseases – Diagnosis.   4. Placenta – Diseases –
-Diagnosis. I. Title.
    [DNLM: 1. Fetal Diseases – diagnosis.   2. Infant, Newborn,
Diseases – diagnosis.   3. Placenta Diseases – diagnosis. WQ 212
N145d]
RG527.N34   1991   91–23580
618.3 – dc20   CIP
DNLM/DLC
for Library of Congress

PREFACE

This book was written to help physicians and other health care professionals diagnose and interpret the clinical significance of common placental and fetal disorders. To help achieve these objectives, the information is presented in a format that is quick and easy to understand. This should facilitate the use of the information in the workplace, where diagnostic and therapeutic decisions are made. The information is frequently presented in a quantitative format to help readers identify the most likely antecedents and the most probable outcomes of disorders. Finally, information on the genesis of many maternal, fetal, intrapartum, and neonatal clinical findings is presented. As will be seen, the disorder that initiates a clinical finding, rather than the finding itself, often determines the clinical outcome.

RICHARD L. NAEYE, M.D.

ACKNOWLEDGMENTS

The author wishes to recognize the contribution of the many dedicated professionals who collected the information in the Collaborative Perinatal Study (CPS). They contributed without much hope of recognition and without knowing if their efforts would bear fruit. Joseph S. Drage, M.D., was the administrator of the CPS data bank for many years. His help was essential in making this data base available and usable to us.

Nebiat Tafari, M.D., chairman of the Department of Pediatrics at the Addis Ababa University Faculty of Medicine, Addis Ababa, Ethiopia, was both the co-investigator and the administrator of many of the African projects whose information about pregnancy in stressful settings appears throughout this book. Samuel Ross, professor of Community Obstetrics and Gynaecology at the University of Natal in the Republic of South Africa, provided similar leadership for most of the projects that were carried out in that nation. I also feel a great debt to the midwives and nurses of the Kwa Mashu Polyclinic in Natal, South Africa, and to the midwives and nurses of the Lidetta, Gallele, Yeka MCH, St. Paul's, and Tikur Ambessa hospital clinics in Addis Ababa, Ethiopia, for their enthusiasm, dedication, and skill in collecting information for our studies.

The neonatologists and obstetricians at my home medical center, the M.S. Hershey Medical Center, Hershey, Penn., have provided me with many years of education about pregnancy and its outcome. Those who have provided the most help are Keith H. Marks, M.B., B.Ch., M. Jeffrey Maisels, M.B., B.Ch., and Joseph J. Botti, M.D. J. Richard Landis, Ph.D., director of the Center for Biostatistics and Epidemiology at our medical center, directed the development of several of the statistical methods employed in this book. Ellen C. Peters performed the statistical analyses and undertook many other tasks during the two decades it took to collect the information for this book.

RICHARD L. NAEYE, M.D.

INTRODUCTION

ANALYTICAL METHODS USED IN THE BOOK

The Collaborative Perinatal Study

Data from the Collaborative Perinatal Study (CPS) of the National Institute of Neurological and Communicative Disorders and Stroke were utilized for many of the analyses in this book.[2,8,9,10] The CPS was undertaken to determine if there are preventable causes of antenatal, intrapartum, and neonatal disorders that injure the central nervous system. The data are also valuable for studying the pathogenesis of non-CNS disorders. The CPS followed the course of more than 56,000 pregnancies in 12 medical school–affiliated hospitals in different regions of the United States between 1959 and 1966. Events of gestation, labor, delivery, and the neonatal periods were recorded, as were children's psychomotor, sensory, and physical development to 7 years of age. Detailed descriptions of the sampling methods, definitions, and study procedures have been published.[2,4,8–10] The last evaluation of a child's development was conducted in 1974, and several years later all of the data became available for analysis on computer tapes. These data are still being analyzed today, because they are the largest and most complete set of prospectively collected information ever gathered to study the genesis of disorders that originate before birth.

Of the original 58,957 children in the study, 2,865 could not be analyzed because their mothers delivered at a non-CPS hospital. Of the remaining 56,092 children, not all of their data sets are complete. As they grew older, an increasing number moved away from the CPS center where they were born, so follow-up information on their growth and development was sometimes not collected. Information on the placenta is missing in about a quarter of the cases, mostly because placentas were not always saved for examination, particularly from births that took place at night and on weekends.

During visits to the prenatal clinic, the gravida provided interviewers with her medical history and socioeconomic and genetic information about herself, her family, and the baby's father and his family.[2] Family and social history was again obtained from the mother at the time of the 7-year examination of her child. Obstetricians and specially selected CPS staff recorded the results of physical examinations, histories, and laboratory tests. Prenatal clinic visits were scheduled every month during the first seven months of pregnancy, every two weeks during the eighth month, and every week thereafter. At admission for delivery, the mother's physical status was reevaluated, and the events of labor and delivery were recorded by a trained observer. A summary of labor and delivery was completed by the obstetrician in charge.

The neonate was observed initially in the delivery room and examined by a pediatrician at 24-hour intervals in the newborn nursery.[4] Neurologic examinations were undertaken at 2 days, 1 year, and 7 years of age. Psychological examinations were undertaken at 8 months, 4 years, and 7 years of age.[2] Speech, language, and hearing examinations were conducted at 3 and 8 years of age.[6] Efforts were made to insure that the test results were reliable by setting high standards for the selection of examiners. At each hospital all examination results were reviewed by a second examiner who checked for scoring errors and tabulation accuracy. The results were reviewed and edited a second time at the central office of the project.

At each participating institution the placenta was initially examined by CPS pathologists who also conducted postmortem examinations on children who were stillborn or who died in the newborn period. I reviewed all of the gross descriptions of organs and conducted a microscopic reexamination of the slides made from these organs, after which I recorded the appropriate diagnoses using standardized diagnostic criteria.[9] I supervised a team of technicians who microscopically reviewed slides from all of the available placentas in the study.

Risk Factors

We included more than 300 risk factors in analyses designed to evaluate their relationship to various antenatal, intrapartum, and childhood disorders and to children's growth and mental, motor, and behavioral development. Most of these risk factors are self-explanatory, but others need to be described because they are included in consolidated categories. Risk factors were placed in consolidated categories when their individual frequencies were too low for separate analysis but they shared a presumed common mode of acting on the placenta, the embryo, the fetus, the gravida, or the child after birth.[8] For example, both cerebral palsy and individual birth asphyxial disorders have low frequencies in the general population, so if birth asphyxia is responsible for only a small proportion of cerebral palsy cases, many more children than are included in the CPS would be needed to identify a correlation between individual asphyxial disorders and cerebral palsy. To deal with this problem, we consolidated all of the disorders that cause birth asphyxia into a single composite category, which we termed *risk factors for birth asphyxia* (Table 1). Disorders and conditions that can cause antenatal hypoxia or ischemia for several days or longer were consolidated into a category that we termed *chronic antenatal hypoxia disorders* (see Table 1). Such hypoxia is most often the result of disorders that produce chronic low blood flow from the uterus to the placenta, maternal anemia, or a continuation of pregnancy beyond 42 weeks of gestation.[9] This last condition is designated "postterm" in some of the analyses.[9]

In some analyses, children who had *major CNS malformations* were put into a single consolidated category.[8] Still another occasionally used consolidated category included all children who had major *non-CNS malformations.* Another consolidated category included children who had **minor congenital malformations.** Major malformations were those that had the potential to shorten life span and minor malformations were those that did not have this potential. Another consolidated category, termed *congenital syndromes,* included children who had recognized combinations of phenotypic findings that have been given names and have an antenatal origin. Two other consolidated categories employed in some of our analyses were *symptomatic intoxications* and *CNS infections.* Symptomatic intoxications were the result of children accidentally ingesting drugs or chemicals. The most frequent of these drugs and chemicals were salicylates, kerosene, gasoline, and lead. CNS infections included encephalitis and meningitis. All of these consolidated categories were used only when there were not enough cases of individual disorders or syndromes in the CPS to undertake needed analyses.

TABLE 1.

Disorders Included in Two of the Most Frequently Used Consolidated Categories in the Analyses*

a. Birth asphyxial factors (47 children were exposed to ≥1 of the following antenatal disorders and had
    seizures in the neonatal period)†
      Abruptio placentae (2)
      Tight knot in umbilical cord (1)
      Active labor lasted >20 hr (10)
      Tumultuous labor (1)
      Maternal shock (4)
      Severe fetal hemorrhage (3)
      Umbilical cord tight around neck or body (11)
      Umbilical cord prolapse (4)
      Arrested progress of active labor (8)
      Persistent high uterine tone during labor (3)
      Maternal anesthesia accident (4)
      Severe vaginal bleeding at delivery (11)
b. Chronic antenatal hypoxic disorders (16,689 children were exposed to ≥1 of the following antenatal
    disorders)
      Maternal anemia: (3rd trimester hemoglobin level <9 g/dL) (3,059)
      Mid-pregnancy maternal hemoglobin value ≥12.5 g/dL (low 1st trimester blood volume expansion (5,740)
      Disorders that produce low uteroplacental blood flow
        Preeclampsia and chronic gestational hypertension (2,164)
        Unexpected drop in 3rd trimester maternal blood pressure (3,985)
        Postterm delivery (2,968)
        Multiple births (537)

*The number of cases with a disorder are in parentheses. There were 43,437 full-term born children in the study as a whole.
 Brain damage due to any of the above disorders could have been the result of ischemia, as well as the consequence of
 asphyxia or hypoxia.
†Neonatal seizures also had to be present for a case to be included in the birth asphyxia category.

Many possible risk factors were analyzed individually rather than in consolidated categories. Among these many risk factors were unexplained gestational proteinuria, defined as gravidas who had 2 + or greater proteinuria that was unexplained by hypertension or urinary tract infections. Other analyzed factors were cigarette smoking, maternal pregnancy weight gain, and diabetes mellitus.[9] Data on cigarette smoking were collected at each clinic visit throughout pregnancy and were usually analyzed by the average number of cigarettes smoked per day. Addiction to illicit drugs was included in only a few analyses because no detailed information was collected on the drugs used, their amounts, or the timing of their use.

Among the many delivery factors analyzed were the use of oxytocin to start or to potentiate labor, the use of gas anesthesia, and breech delivery. Oxytocin was not included in the composite birth asphyxia category because it was administered so frequently (6,723 gravidas) that it could be individually analyzed as a risk factor.

The results of a nonverbal intelligence test (SRA test) given to each gravida was included in some analyses.[4] Noneclamptic maternal seizure disorders were were also analyzed as a risk factor. Such seizures had a somewhat higher frequency in the CPS than in the general population.[10] Demographic factors that were analyzed individually included race (46% white, 46% black, 8% other), years of maternal education, family income, and the type of employment of the head of household.[4,10] Years of maternal education, family income and the type of employment of the head of household were individually scored and the total score appears in many analyses under the designation "socioeconomic status."[7]

Statistical Methods

Cross tabulations and multiple logistic regression were the methods most often used to determine if risk factors had a significant association with an outcome being analysed.[5] Factors not significantly associated with an outcome are not reported, as reporting them would make the tables too long. A method for estimating population attributable risks from logistic regression models was utilized to estimate the contribution of each risk factor to an outcome when adjusted for all of the other risk factors in the model.[3] The recently developed methods of Benichou and Gail[1] were employed to construct 95% confidence intervals for the relative risk and attributable risk estimates. Up to five risk factors were included in each analysis for attributable risk. When more than five risk factors were involved, the combined risk of the first five factors were included as a single risk factor with four new risk factors in the model. Using these methods made it possible to represent many findings quantitatively in easy to understand tables.

Limitations of the Collaborative Perinatal Study

The CPS data were collected before many currently employed obstetric and medical diagnostic and management techniques were available. Does this make the findings of the CPS obsolete? The answer is "yes" if the frame of reference is the management of very prematurely born infants, the recognition and management of diabetes mellitus, and some other maternal disorders during pregnancy. In most instances, analyses that might be heavily influenced by changed obstetrical and medical practices have not been included in the book. Most of the findings that are in the book relate to disorders and outcomes that have not changed very much since the CPS data were collected. This includes preterm delivery, whose frequency has not changed significantly in recent decades. It also includes most cases of antenatal brain maldevelopment and damage, fetal growth retardation, stillbirth, and neonatal death, which have their origins in events that are still outside of the control of the health care system. It therefore appears that the biggest limitation of the CPS data is not its obsolescence but rather its lack of information about a number of pregnancy disorders whose nature was not understood during the years of the CPS. In addition, some pregnancy risk factors are now present that were absent or rare during the CPS. Some obvious examples include the current use of cocaine by some pregnant women, the appearance of the HIV virus in pregnancy, and a fuller understanding of the effects of ethanol on the embryo and fetus. Despite these limitations, the large volume of prospective data in the CPS offers a better opportunity to explore the antenatal origins of many neonatal and childhood disorders than is possible with any other data set that is currently available.

Finally, some might think the findings from the CPS might have limited value because the CPS population was mainly urban and included many low-income and poorly educated participants. Bias that might be related to income, education, religion, type of community where born, type of employment outside of the home, degree of crowding in housing, and race was taken into consideration in every appropriate analysis by including these factors as independent variables in the analyses.

RICHARD L. NAEYE, M.D.

REFERENCES

1. Benichou J, Gail MH: Variance calculations and confidence intervals for estimates of the attributable risk based on logistic models. *Biometrics* 1990; 46:991–1003.

2. Broman SH, Nichols PL, Kennedy WA: *Preschool IQ, Prenatal and Early Developmental Correlates.* New York, John Wiley & Sons, 1975.

3. Bruzzi P, Green SB, Byar DP, et al: Estimating the population attributable risk for multiple risk factors using case-control data. *Am J Epidemiol* 1985; 122:904–914.

4. *The Collaborative Study on Cerebral Palsy, Mental Retardation and Other Neurological and Sensory Disorders of Infancy and Childhood*

Manual. Bethesda, Md, US Dept of Health, Education and Welfare, 1966.

5. Hastings RP (ed): *SUGI Supplemental Library User's Guide*, ed. 5. Cary, NC, SAS Institute, 1986.

6. Lassman FM, Fisch RO, Vetter DK, et al: *Early Correlates of Speech, Language, and Hearing.* Littleton, Mass, PSG, 1980.

7. Myrianthopolous NC, French KS: An application of the US Bureau of the Census socioeco-

nomic index to a large, diversified patient population. *Soc Sci Med* 1968; 2:283–299.

8. Naeye RL, Peters EC, Bartholomew MS, et al: Origins of cerebral palsy. *Am J Dis Child* 1989; 143:1154–1161.

9. Naeye RL, Tafari N: *Risk Factors in Pregnancy and Diseases of the Fetus and Newborn.* Baltimore, Williams & Wilkins, 1983.

10. Niswander KR, Gordon M: *The Women and Their Pregnancies.* Philadelphia, WB Saunders Co, 1972.

CONTENTS

CHAPTER 1

The Ancient Mechanisms That Regulate Human Reproductive Performance

Findings reported in this book disclose that a relatively small number of disorders are responsible for most preterm deliveries, perinatal morbidity, and mortality. Links between these disorders make it clear that a relatively small number of physiologic processes may be responsible for most of their clinical diversity. Most of these physiologic processes are the expression of homeostatic mechanisms that developed during the course of human evolution to improve the chances that women and their fetuses would survive pregnancy and the neonatal period in the face of fluctuations in available food and the need for strenuous work or walking long distances during pregnancy. When food is scarce and physical activity is required, these homeostatic mechanisms protect women by preventing many pregnancies, by limiting the transfer of maternal nutrients to the fetus, and by predisposing to a shortened gestation. Other homeostatic mechanisms appear to protect the fetal brain and accelerate fetal lung and liver maturation so that neonates born preterm from undernourished gravidas have a reasonable chance to survive and develop normally. Certain types of maternal work also appear to accelerate fetal lung and liver maturation.

How did these maternal fetal homeostatic mechanisms develop? Before the advent of agriculture about 8,000 years ago, maternal diets had a high content of meat from wild animals with added nutrients from roots, insects, and fruits.[2,6] Such diets are currently eaten by Bushmen living in the Kalihari Desert and by some of the primitive tribes of the Amazon basin. Primitive people ate most of the animals they killed, including the bone marrow and brains. This diet is low in bulk, low in carbohydrates, and relatively complete in essential amino acids, vitamins, and the minerals needed by pregnant women and their fetuses. It has been postulated that such a diet made possible the accelerated expansion of brain size that first started in our ancestors about 2 million years ago.[4]

Homeostatic mechanisms to cope with nutritional adversity and physical work are particularly important for human beings because, unlike lower animals, women do not regulate their ovulation by the season. As a result, human births are not confined to times of the year when the food supply is adequate for the nurture of fetuses and young infants. Fortunately, humans have developed compensatory protective mechanisms. Ovulation ceases when women become severely undernourished or engage in very protracted, strenuous physical activity. This occurs in undernourished populations and in athletes when the relative mass of adipose tissue to other body constituents decreases below a critical level.[1,3] Breast-feeding is responsible for another protective mechanism. Primitive women continue breast-feeding for several years after birth. This suppresses ovulation so that women's nutritional stores are spared by the resulting spacing of pregnancies. Unlike modern women, many primitive women apparently delivered from the squatting position. This spared their fetuses from some of the complications of prolonged labor.

THE ADVENT OF AGRICULTURE

With the advent of agriculture, some important changes took place in the environment of pregnancy. Meat diets were largely replaced by grain. Grain can be stored, which made it possible for many women to avoid fasting during pregnancy. This no doubt permitted many women to survive who would have died during the preagricultural millenia. Unfortunately, grain diets are much higher in bulk than are meat diets and are often deficient in protein, branched amino acids, calcium, zinc, iron, and several vitamins. In addition, the excessive phytates in some grain diets lead to zinc deficiency by interfering with zinc absorption.[5] All of these dietary changes presented women with nutritional problems for which they were not biologically prepared.

We do not know if any significant genetic adaptations took place during the agricultural era but some important cultural practices developed which pro-

tect women and their fetuses from the full consequences of the shift to grain diets. Many agricultural-based societies throughout the world provide pregnant women with special foods which have a higher protein and vitamin content than do the foods which are normally eaten in the daily diet. Some populations developed taboos against coitus during pregnancy, which protected women against coitus-induced infections that result from zinc deficiency.

THE MODERN ERA

In the modern era, a host of new environmental factors which influence fetuses and neonates have appeared. The most important appears to be the introduction of diets high in carbohydrate and calories which retard fetal lung maturation (see Chapter 3). Another notable change is employment outside of the home that often requires continuous work in the same body position throughout the day. This sometimes retards fetal growth, leads to large placental infarcts in late gestation, and markedly increases fetal mortality when mothers are hypertensive (see Chapters 3 and 4).

The effects of tobacco, alcohol, and a wide range of modern drugs were not anticipated by the homeostatic mechanisms of the preagricultural era and are often poorly controlled by current cultural practices. Cigarette smoking, for example, has both detrimental and beneficial effects. It causes both a number of life-threatening disorders and accelerates fetal lung maturation (see Chapter 5). Coitus during pregnancy, which was taboo in many primitive agricultural communities, has been resumed in most urban societies despite the fact that it sometimes leads to preterm labor and delivery, particularly in zinc-deficient populations (see Chapter 7).

The following chapters describe in detail many of the homeostatic mechanisms that developed during the course of human evolution to protect women and their fetuses. They also detail the effects of various environmental changes that entered with the agricultural revolution and with the urbanization of populations.

REFERENCES

1. Bates GW, Bates SR, Whitworth NS: Reproductive failure in women who practice weight control. *Fertil Steril* 1982; 37:373–378.

2. Bisel SLC: *A Pilot Study of Aspects of Human Nutrition in the Ancient East Mediterranean, With Particular Attention to Trace Minerals in Several Populations From Different Time Periods.* (thesis) University of Minnesota, Minneapolis, 1980.

3. Frisch RE, McArthur JW: Menstrual cycles: Fatness as a determinant of minimum weight for height necessary for their maintenance or onset. *Science* 1974; 185:949–951.

4. Martin RD: Relative brain size and basal metabolic rate in terrestrial vertebrates. *Nature* 1981; 293:57–60.

5. Reinhold JG: High phytate content of rural Iranian bread: A possible cause of human zinc deficiency. *Am J Clin Nutr* 1971; 24:1204–1206.

6. Schoeninger MJ: The agricultural revolution: Its effects on human diet in the Middle East. *Am J Phys Anthropol* 1981; 54:275.

CHAPTER 2

Environmental Influences on the Embryo and Early Fetus

Before 1941, almost no attention was given to the possibility that environmental factors might produce malformations in the human embryo. In 1941 Gregg demonstrated that maternal rubella was teratogenic.[34] Since then it has become clear that the protection of the embryo against various environmental factors is breached with surprising frequency.

PRINCIPLES OF TERATOGENESIS

There are several critical periods during which toxic insults can cause congenital malformations. These periods include spermatogenesis, the formation and survival of ova, and the early and late stages of embryogenesis.

Spermatogenesis

Spermatogonia develop during the fetal period and then remain dormant until they begin to divide at puberty. The process of transformation from primitive germ cells to mature sperm takes about 64 days. Damage to sperm can presumably take place at any stage, but evidence for such damage has only rarely been recognized. One evidence of such damage is the higher proportion of morphologically abnormal sperm in cigarette smokers than in nonsmokers.[24] A number of teratogenic or potentially teratogenic agents have been identified in semen, which raises the possibility that such agents might damage the fertilized ova. These agents include thalidomide, phenytoin, methadone, and caffeine.[31]

Development of Ova

A woman's ova enter the first division of meiosis, the process by which the number of chromosomes is reduced from 46 to 23, before she is born. Ova then remain in late prophase of the first meiotic division until just before ovulation, which can occur as early as puberty or as late as menopause. It has been suggested that this period, which can last for as long as 30 years, accounts for the relatively high frequency of meiotic nondysjunction abnormalities in the offspring of mothers over 35 years of age.[31] It is a formidable task to identify specific environmental agents that might have damaged ova over a span of so many years. Therefore, direct evidence of damage to eggs by environmental agents is sparse. Among the few examples are chromosomal breaks in meiotic cells that appear after high doses of lysergic acid diethylamide (LSD) and one report of an increased frequency of trisomies after maternal abdominal radiation.[98,102]

The Embryo

Between 25% and 75% of conceptions appear to end with an early or late spontaneous abortion of which only 15% are clinically recognized (Figs 2–1 and 2–2).[9,10] About half of the abortuses have chromosomal abnormalities which produce fatal malformations. Many other malformed abortuses have a normal karyotype. Brent and Beckman have estimated that about 3% of fetuses that reach term have major malformations and another 1% have serious genetic disorders such as diabetes mellitus and cystic fibrosis.[9]

Early Embryos. – Many drugs and chemicals that damage older embryos and fetuses do not seem to affect the early embryo, raising the possibility that the

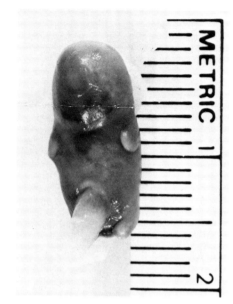

FIG 2–1.
Grossly abnormal "cylindrical" embryo from a spontaneous abortion at 9 weeks' gestation. (Courtesy of Kurt Benirschke, M.D., University of California, San Diego.)

first 3 weeks of life are a relatively protected period. A more likely explanation is that damage during this period is usually fatal, with a consequent unrecognized spontaneous abortion. However, not all early damaged embryos die. Malformed neonates have been reported after mothers ingested the known teratogenic drugs actinomycin D and cyclophosphamide very early in pregnancy. It is also widely known that implantation of the fertilized egg or embryo can be prevented by the administration of a sizable dose of estrogen.

Older Embryos. – The period from the fourth to the ninth weeks of pregnancy is the time when malformations are most apt to originate. The complex story of teratogenicity during this period is most easily understood within the context of the embryo's developmental program, a series of genetically preprogrammed instructions carried in the structure of the fertilized ovum's DNA. In humans this program appears to have more than 100 million

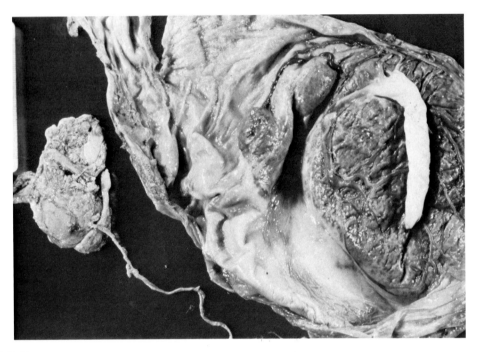

FIG 2–2.
Spontaneous abortion at 26 weeks' gestation.

pieces of information.[10] Considering this complexity, it is remarkable that recognized errors in the developmental program appear in less than 5% of newborns.

The exact means by which most teratogenic agents affect the embryo are not known, but such information is available in a few instances. Goldman has proposed plausible explanations for some of the disorders in which males have the external appearance of females.[31] Interference with the synthesis, release, or action of testosterone at any one of a number of different metabolic sites allows the female program, which is intrinsic in all embryos, to be phenotypically expressed in males. This interference can involve antibodies to gonadotropins, the inhibition of specific testosterone biosynthetic enzymes, the appearance of antibodies to testosterone, or blockers of testosterone receptor protein. Males who are phenotypically female can also be produced by genetic deficiencies of testosterone, biosynthetic enzymes, or androgen receptor proteins.[31]

What Proportion of Malformations Can Be Explained?

Factors have been identified that account for about one-third of congenital malformations (Table 2–1). Twenty percent to 25% appear to be due to genetic and chromosomal factors and about 10% to known environmental agents.[9] It is often asked what proportion of unexplained malformations might be due to unidentified environmental agents, particularly chemicals. This question is very difficult to answer for several reasons:

1. Most embryos are exposed to multiple environmental agents. Most women take more than one drug during pregnancy and are exposed to multiple household, industrial, and agricultural chemicals, most of which have not been tested for their teratogenicity.
2. A potentially teratogenic drug may be administered for a disorder that itself is associated with an increased frequency of malformations. For example, the in-

TABLE 2–1.

Relative Contributions of Various Causes to the Frequency of Human Malformations*

Etiology		Malformed Live Births (%)
Genetic		*20–25*
Cytogenetic abnormalities	5–10	
Mendelian inheritance	15–20	
Spontaneous mutations	<1	
Environmental (exposure of the embryo)		*10*
Maternal infections (cytomegalovirus, rubella, herpes simplex, varicella, toxoplasmosis, syphilis)	2–3	
Maternal disease states (diabetes, smoking, alcoholism, endocrinopathies, myasthenia gravis, phenylketonuria, myotonic dystrophy, systemic lupus erythematosus)	2–3	
Amnionic band syndrome	1	
Vascular disruption	1	
Drugs, chemicals, irradiation, hyperthermia	<1	
Maternal malnutrition	?	
Unknown		*65–70*
Polygenic, multifactorial	?	
Synergism	?	
Spontaneous errors of development	?	

*Adapted from Brent RL, Beckman DA: Etiology of human birth defects, with comments on the role of placental transport of human teratogens in Bellisario R, Mizejewski GJ (eds): Transplacental Disorders, Perinatal Detection, Treatment and Management. New York, Alan R Liss Inc, 1990, pp 17–36.

creased frequency of malformations in children whose mothers have a seizure disorder could be due to the teratogenicity of anticonvulsant drugs, to the disorder that is responsible for the seizures, or to the hypoxia to which the embryo may be exposed during a maternal seizure.[95]

3. Genetic differences among embryos appear to influence their susceptibilities to some drug-induced malformations.[100]

All of these possibilities must be considered in the context of the wider theories of how birth defects arise. These theories fall into several categories: (a) intrinsic biologic errors, (b) polygenic influences, (c) multifactorial influences.[9] The *intrinsic biologic error* thesis postulates that there are biologic errors inherent in the reproductive process. This would explain the origin of spontaneous mutations.[9] The *polygenic hypothesis* assumes that malformations that recur in families are due to gene abnormalities at two or more loci. If

a disorder is due to a homozygous recessive abnormality at two gene loci and the parents are heterozygous, there is a 6.25% probability that the gene will be present at all four loci in any given child of these parents and thereby manifest as a genetic disorder. This is close to the observed recurrence rate of some recessive disorders but it does not entirely explain their occurrence. For example, it does not explain why some of these disorders are occasionally discordant in monozygous twins.[9]

The *multifactorial hypothesis* postulates an interaction of modulating environmental factors with a continuum of characteristics that have multiple gene loci.[36] A large body of animal studies supports this theory but very little human data are available. Brent and Beckman[9] suggest that the following factors might be modulating influences: (1) variations in placental blood flow, (2) variations in placental transport, (3) differing sites of placental implantation, (4) maternal disorders, (5) gestational infections, (6) drug and chemical exposures during gestation. To this list can be added severe undernutrition and malnutrition because the frequencies of spina bifida, hydrocephalus, and some other central nervous system malformations doubled for children exposed as embryos to severe maternal undernutrition and malnutrition in the Dutch famine winter of 1944–1945.[101]

The Collaborative Perinatal Study (CPS) contains the data needed to explore the possible teratogenic influence of some of these factors. We have not used CPS data to explore the roles of drugs and chemicals because Heinonon et al. did not find a clear teratogenic effect for any drug used in the CPS.[40] In our explorations we defined major congenital malformations as those with the potential to shorten life span or seriously impair a child's function. In the first step of our studies χ^2 analysis was used to see if individual risk factors had a significant correlation with major malformations in the CPS (Table 2–2). Risk factors that had such a correlation were next included as independent variables in a multiple regression analysis to calculate their relative risks and attributable risks for malformations. Details of

how these analyses were conducted are found in the introduction to this book.[73]

The attributable risk analyses identified antecedents for 39% of the major malformations in the CPS (see Table 2–2). Maternal seizure disorders accounted for 12%, first-trimester maternal acetonuria for 9%, familial disorders for 4%, and maternal diabetes mellitus, placenta previa, and twins for smaller percentages of the malformations. Details of some of the risk factors are of interest. Among placental disorders placenta previa was worth exploring because it is the result of a fertilized egg implanting at an abnormal site in the uterine wall. It was associated with a 2.2-fold increase in the risk for major malformations and was the antecedent of 1% of all the major malformations in the study (see Table 2–2). Maternal hypertension was explored as a possible risk factor because it is often associated with low uteroplacental blood flow and the low flow can start early in gestation.[67,79] It was not associated with fetal malformations when all of the other risk factors were taken into consideration.

Among the *maternal disorders* during pregnancy, diabetes mellitus is a well-known teratogen if it is under poor control at the time of organogenesis (see Table

TABLE 2–2.

Risk Estimates for Possible Modulating Factors in the Genesis of Major Congenital Malformations

Risk Factors	Major Malformations per 1,000 Newborns by Specified Risk Factors*	Relative Risks (95% Confidence Intervals)	Attributable Risks (95% Confidence Intervals)
All cases	75 (4,439)		
Placenta			
Placenta previa	202 (50), $P<.001$	2.2 (1.3, 3.7)	.01 (.00, .01)
Fibrosis of terminal placental villi	163 (157), $P<.001$	1.3 (1.0, 1.7)	.01 (.00, .01)
Maternal disorders			
Gestational acetonuria	118 (468), $P<.001$	1.5 (1.3, 1.7)	.09 (.07, .11)
Diabetes mellitus	167 (149), $P<.001$	1.8 (1.3, 2.4)	.03 (.02, .04)
More than one possible mechanism			
Maternal seizure disorder	436 (348), $P<.001$	5.3 (4.7, 6.1)	.12 (.11, .14)
Twins	109 (136), $P<.001$	1.5 (1.1, 2.1)	.01 (.00, .01)
Genetic factors			
Familial disorders	107 (906), $P<.001$	1.2 (1.0, 1.4)	.04 (.03, .06)
Male infants	82 (2,320), $P<.001$	1.2 (1.1, 1.3)	.08 (.06, .11)
Population attributable risk			*.39 (.36, .42)*

Numbers of cases are in parentheses.

2–2).[77] If control is good during this period the malformation rate is reportedly close to that of the general population. In the CPS, diabetes mellitus was associated with a 1.8-fold increase in the risk of major congenital malformations and was the antecedent of 3% of the malformations in the study (see Table 2–2). Congenital malformations are part of a continuum of diabetes-related embryonic damage, with abortions being frequent if diabetes is under poor control. Experimentally it has been shown that high levels of glucose around the blastocyst cause it to degenerate. To prevent both the excess of malformations and abortions it is important to keep the average daily maternal blood glucose level less than 180 mg/dL for one or more menstrual cycles before conception. If this glycemic control is started only after pregnancy is confirmed there will be an excess of malformations because organogenesis has often begun by the fifth or sixth week after the start of the last menstrual period, the time when many pregnancies are first suspected and confirmed.

First-trimester maternal acetonuria, not associated with diabetes mellitus, was the next maternal risk factor examined. Small amounts of acetonuria are present in many normal pregnancies, but acetonuria can also be the manifestation of a mild metabolic acidosis produced by maternal fasting.[25,72] First-trimester acetonuria was associated with a 1.5-fold increase in the risk of congenital malformations and it was the antecedent of 9% of the malformations in the CPS. Other maternal risk factors analyzed were asthma, hypothyroidism, hyperthyroidism, and glomerulonephritis. None had a significant association with major malformations.

Infections were explored as possible teratogens by examining the correlations of first-trimester urinary tract infections, hepatitis, viral inclusions in the placenta, and chronic villitis with major malformations. None had a significant correlation with major malformations. A fever of 38.9° C or more in the first trimester of pregnancy was another possible risk factor for malformations that we analyzed. It was not associated with an increased frequency of malformations. The last maternal factor that we analyzed was *maternal age greater than 35 years* because waiting for 35 or more years to conceive provides many opportunities for an ovum to be damaged. In the CPS, being older than 35 years was not associated with an increased frequency of major malformations when other risk factors were taken into consideration.

Several possible teratogens fall into the category of more than one possible teratogen. A *maternal seizure disorder* is such a risk factor because any association seizures might have with malformations could have a genetic, hypoxic, or drug-related origin. A chronic maternal seizure disorder increased the risk of congenital malformations 5.3-fold and it was the antecedent of 12% of the malformations in the study (see Table 2–2). *Cigarette smoking* was also placed in the more-than-one-possible-mechanism category because it reduces uteroplacental blood flow for 5 to 20 minutes after each cigarette smoked and tobacco smoke contains hundreds of chemicals whose teratogenicity has never been tested.[60] Cigarette smoking was not associated with an increase in malformations. *Twins and triplets* were also analyzed as a risk factor for malformations because there are many published reports that malformations are more frequent in twins than in single-born children. Such malformations could be the result of the influences that produce multiple ovulation or cause a fertilized egg to divide into two eggs. Being a twin or triplet increased the risk of congenital malformations 1.5-fold and it was the antecedent of 1% of the major malformations in the study (see Table 2–2).

Possible genetic disorders were put into a single consolidated category which we termed *familial disorders*. Included were the following in parents or siblings: major congenital malformations, mental retardation, motor disorders, sensory disorders.[18] Taken together these familial disorders increased the risk for congenital malformations 1.2-fold and they were the antecedents of 4% of the major malformations in the study (see Table 2–2). Being a male increased the risk for malformations 1.2-fold and accounted for 8% of the malformations in the study (see Table 2–2).

TERATOGENS

Drugs and Chemical Compounds

Antibiotics.—*Tetracycline* and its related drug doxycycline do not appear to produce major malformations, but they should not be used during pregnancy because they deposit in fetal bones and teeth when taken after the 25th week of gestation.[76] Their use decreases linear bone growth, stains teeth, and produces enamel hypoplasia (Table 2–3).

Anticoagulants.—The use of *vitamin K antagonists* during the first trimester of pregnancy sometimes produces a syndrome termed *warfarin embryopathy*. This syndrome includes a hypoplastic nose, eye abnormalities, and stippled epiphyses.[96] The abnormalities may be directly caused by the drugs or they could be due to hemorrhages with secondary tissue atrophy and scarring. Other abnormalities found in some of the affected children include broad short hands, short distal phalanges, skull malformations, optic atrophy, and hypertelorism. In a literature review the use of warfarin (Coumarin) derivatives during the first trimester produced warfarin embryopathy, CNS abnormalities, or hemorrhage-related abnormalities in one-sixth of exposed liveborn children.[106] Warfarin exposure after the second trimester of pregnancy increases the frequencies of fetal hemorrhage and subsequent growth retardation, impaired vision, and mental retardation. Hemorrhage has also been more frequent than expected after third-trimester exposure to the drug. If anticoagulation is required during pregnancy, heparin is the drug of choice.

Anticonvulsants.—A syndrome can follow maternal treatment with a *hydantoin* anticonvulsant during early gestation.[38] Features of the syndrome include antenatal growth retardation, microcephaly, craniofacial abnormalities, developmental delays, and mental retardation. The dysmorphic craniofacial features include a short nose, mild hypertelorism, ptosis of the eyelids, strabismus, and a wide mouth. Cleft lip, cleft palate, cardiac anomalies, genitourinary anomalies, and serious limb reduction defects can also occur. At the present time the craniofacial and limb abnormalities appear to be the most constant features of the syndrome.[37] In recent

TABLE 2–3.

Drugs and Chemicals That Are Recognized or Often Claimed to Be Human Teratogens

Drugs	
Aminopterin	Methyltrexate
Androgenic hormones	Penicillamine
Busulfan	Phenytoin
Chlorobiphenyls	Polychlorinated biphenyls (PCBs)
Cocaine	Propylthiouracil
Cyclophosphamide	Tetracycline
Diethylstilbestrol	Thalidomide
Ethanol	Trimethadione
Iodine	Valproic acid
Isotretinoin (13-*cis*-retinoic acid)	Warfarin
Lithium	
Heavy Metals	
Lead	
Mercury	

years evidence has emerged that many of the features of the syndrome are genetically linked to epilepsy itself rather than to the drugs used to treat the disorder. The current view is that only hypertelorism and digital hypoplasia are clearly linked to phenytoin exposure.[29] The risk of serious developmental disturbance in phenytoin-exposed children is probably only 1% to 2%.[29] The teratogenicity of hydantoin is apparently related to oxidative metabolites that are normally eliminated by the enzyme epoxide hydrolase.[11] Low levels of epoxide hydrolase in the amniotic fluid appear to correlate with the risk of a fetus developing features of the hydantoin syndrome.[11] Cancers have been reported in a number of children who were prenatally exposed to hydantoin.[3,37]

A syndrome can also follow fetal exposure to the oxazolidine anticonvulsants *tridione, trimethadione*, and *paramethadione*. Common features include fetal growth retardation, mental retardation, speech difficulties, epicanthus, V-shaped eyebrows, irregular teeth, palatal anomalies, and low-set ears.[32] Dysmorphic facial features and cardiac defects have also been reported. The facial features include mild brachycephaly with midfacial hypoplasia, a short nose, a broadly depressed nasal bridge, low-set ears, and irregular dentition. The most frequent cardiac anomalies are septal defects and tetralogy of Fallot. Two studies have raised the possibility that antenatal damage attributed to hydantoin and tridione might be due to some intrinsic characteristic of the mothers because high rates of malformations were found in a cohort study whether or not the mothers had been treated with anticonvulsants.[95] *Valproic acid*, another anticonvulsant, reportedly can cause craniofacial malformations.[32]

Antiemetics. — No association between *antiemetics* and human birth defects has been found in multiple cohort and case-controlled studies.[44,110] Nevertheless, questions repeatedly arise about the possible teratogenic properties of an-tiemetics. None, including Bendectin (doxylamine succinate–pyridoxine hydrochloride), have been shown to cause malformations.[53]

Caffeine. — There is no good evidence that caffeine is teratogenic. Caffeine reportedly has little or no effect on birth weight, birth length, head circumference at birth, or on children's subsequent growth.[12,27] However, a dose response has been reported between the consumption of caffeinated beverages and the time it takes to become pregnant.[109] Failed ovulation was excluded as the responsible factor, so a failure of implantation and an excess of early embryo losses are mechanisms to be explored.

Cocaine. — Among the claimed effects of maternal use of cocaine during pregnancy are more frequent abortions, fetal growth retardation, congenital urogenital anomalies, neonatal necrotizing enterocolitis, and cerebral infarction.[14,15,21,75,91] The growth retardation affects body weight, body length, and head circumference.[35,113] The exposed children also have an increased frequency of neurobehavioral abnormalities in the neonatal period characterized by rapid shifts between irritability and lethargy.[13,14,75] Neurobehavioral abnormalities have been identified in some exposed fetuses.[46] These neurobehavioral abnormalities are discussed in more detail in Chapter 11.

Cocaine is metabolized very slowly in the fetus because the fetus has low plasma levels of cholinesterase.[19] Cocaine acts mainly by blocking the presynaptic re-uptake of neurotransmitters at the nerve terminals which results in increased levels of norepinephrine and dopamine. It may also alter the availability and utilization of calcium.[78] In addition, cocaine reduces blood flow from the uterus to the placenta. It has been postulated that these effects on blood flow and calcium availability may be responsible for the fetal growth retardation and urogenital malformations associated with exposure to the drug.[15] Poor maternal nutrition may also play a role in the fetal growth retardation because cocaine suppresses appetite.[19,113]

Cytotoxic Agents.—Cytotoxic agents exert their effect on rapidly dividing cells so it is not surprising that they can lead to abortion, produce a malformed embryo, stunt fetal growth, and cause systemic toxicity that persists after birth. When given in the first week after conception, these agents sometimes produce an abortion. Embryos that survive without further exposure to the agents usually develop normally. During the period of organogenesis some cytotoxic agents produce slow fetal organ growth, microcephaly, and long-term mental retardation. The cytotoxic agents that have reportedly produced malformations include the alkylating agents *busulfan* and *cyclophosphamide* and the antimetabolites *aminopterin* and *methotrexate*.[22] The risk of malformations with these agents is substantial, between 10% and 20% with both *busulfan* and *aminopterin*.[22] Synergistic teratogenic effects have been reported when two or more agents have been used in combination, when agents have been used in sequence, or when an agent has been combined with radiotherapy.[20,22,69] *Aminopterin* produces abnormalities consistent enough to have been recognized as a syndrome which includes delayed ossification of the calvarium, hypertelorism, a wide nasal bridge, micrognathia, and malformations of the external ear.[22]

Diethylstilbestrol, Norethindrone.—In 1971 Herbst et al. reported that the daughters of women who took *diethylstilbestrol (DES)* during pregnancy sometimes developed a clear cell adenocarcinoma of the vagina as teenagers or later in life.[42] The critical antenatal exposure period for this neoplasm seems to be between the 4th and 12th weeks of gestation. Since 1971, more than 400 cases of the drug-associated adenocarcinoma have been recorded in a DES tumor registry. The risk of exposed women developing this neoplasm is now estimated to be less than 1 in 1,000. This estimate will probably not change very much in the future because the prevalence of vaginal epithelial changes associated with DES exposure falls off rapidly after 26 years of age and most exposed women have passed this age.[103]

Clear cell adenocarcinomas of the vagina are rare by comparison with the nonneoplastic genital abnormalities that follow DES exposure. These nonneoplastic abnormalities include the development of glandular epithelium in the vagina (vaginal adenosis) or in the portio of the cervix (cervical extropion). Malformations have also been described in the vagina and in the uterus of the exposed women. Cysts in the epididymis, cryptorchidism, hypogonadism, and diminished spermatogenesis have been reported in some males antenatally exposed to DES.[41] Virilization of the external genitalia has been reported in female fetuses following maternal treatment with high doses of *norethindrone* during pregnancy.[93]

Dioxin Derivatives.—These agents are among the most toxic substances known and they occur as contaminants in many substances, including herbicides and the commonly used wood preservative pentachlorophenol. The herbicide *Agent Orange* is a combination of the dioxin derivatives 2,4-D and 2,4,5-T. Widespread spraying of forests during the Vietnam War resulted in reports of an increased frequency of malformations, abortions, and stillbirths.[74] Large quantities of 2,4,5-T were sprayed in parts of Oregon some years ago to increase the productivity of commercial forests. Spontaneous abortions reportedly increased in the sprayed areas in the months that followed the spraying.[23] On the other hand, a study from New Zealand found no increase in miscarriages, stillbirths, or congenital malformations after contact with the compound.[99]

Ethanol.—The *fetal alcohol syndrome* has been extensively investigated. The most common findings are fetal growth retardation, microcephaly, mental retardation, midfacial hypoplasia, and short palpebral fissures in a child born to a chronic alcoholic mother.[27,52] Ptosis, strabismus, a long flat philtrum, and a long convex upper lip are also common. Less frequent features of the syndrome include hyperactivity, speech problems, atrial and ventricular septal defects of the heart, renogenital malformations, hemangiomas, aberrant palmar creases, hypoplasia of the nails, and restrictions of joint movements.[49] An abnormally low uteroplacental blood flow may contribute to the growth retardation.[51] Clarren et al. described brain abnormalities in four infants with the syndrome which were caused by the failure of neuronal migrations.[16] Although the type of the defect was the same in all four cases, the location of the malformations varied from case to case, which may explain some of the clinical variations in psychomotor performance reported with the syndrome. Alcohol is metabolized to acetaldehyde in the liver by the cytoplasmic enzyme alcohol dehydrogenase. It has been claimed that acetaldehyde causes the fetal alcohol syndrome through its inhibiting effects on DNA synthesis, placental amino acid transport, and the development of the fetal brain.[58]

Mental retardation is the most sensitive manifestation of fetal damage due to maternal alcohol abuse. Such mental retardation, along with fetal growth retardation, the presence of minor malformations, and a history of excessive maternal alcohol intake during pregnancy are the minimal criteria for the diagnosis of the fetal alcohol syndrome. The actual amount and duration of alcohol consumption needed to produce features of the syndrome have not been determined. However, it is widely recognized that an occasional alcoholic drink during pregnancy does not produce the syndrome. Six of the 23 identified alcoholic women in the CPS had children with features of the syndrome. Unfortunately, there was no systematic attempt made to assess alcohol consumption in the CPS so many alcoholics were probably not recognized and therefore not recorded.

Laxatives. — Data from the CPS show no association between individual drugs in this category and congenital malformations.[40] However, the *anthraquinone laxatives* cross the placenta and therefore probably should not be used during pregnancy.[40]

Marijuana. — The main active ingredient in marijuana is δ-9-tetrahydrocannabinol. It is fat-soluble, crosses the placenta easily, particularly in early gestation, and may persist in the fetus for as long as 30 days.[47,55,57] Fetal growth retardation has been reported in the children of marijuana users, independent of other factors that retard fetal growth.[113] The growth retardation is reported to affect body weights and body lengths but not head circumference. Marijuana is teratogenic in some animals and there are several reports of malformed children following maternal marijuana use during pregnancy.[1,6] However, none of these reports establish marijuana as a teratogen because other potentially teratogenic drugs were likely being used by the gravidas who were smoking marijuana.

There is one report that marijuana use during pregnancy increased the risk of children exposed in utero subsequently developing nonlymphoblastic leukemia.[80] Tetrahydrocannabinol has been found to stimulate monocytes to mature partially, so this might be the biologic link between marijuana and nonlymphoblastic leukemia if such a link exists.[70,80]

Amphetamines. — Newborns of mothers who used methamphetamine during pregnancy are sometimes growth-retarded at birth and have abnormal sleep patterns, poor feeding, tremors, and hypertonia in the neonatal period.[75] Amphetamine use during pregnancy in therapeutic doses did not affect fetal growth or survival in the CPS.[71]

Methylmercury. — In 1953 a neurologic disorder that included mental confusion, convulsions, and coma developed in some residents of Minamata, a town in southern

Japan.[54] About 38% of the affected individuals died. Six percent of the children born between 1955 and 1959 in the town developed cerebral palsy with accompanying mental retardation. The mothers of these children had all eaten fish and shellfish from Minamata Bay, which contained high concentrations of mercury compounds derived from local factories. Other epidemics have occurred in Niigata, Japan, and in Iraq. Methylmercury is an inexpensive and effective fungicide which has often been used to treat seed grains. Methylmercury-treated wheat was responsible for the epidemic in Iraq. Methylmercury poisoning produces an atrophy of the granular layer of the cerebellum and a spongiose softening in the visual cortex and other cortical areas of the brain. A polyneuritis can also occur. The lesions are permanent.

Epidemics like those in Japan and Iraq are not the only threat posed by methylmercury. Certain freshwater fish in the United States, Canada, and Sweden are also contaminated by methylmercury. In these locations mercury effluent from paper mills and chloralkali plants has passed into the bottom sediments of nearby lakes, where microorganisms have converted the mercury into methylmercury which has then been picked up by resident fish. There is a continuing concern that gravidas might eat too much of such contaminated fish with resultant subtle methylmercury damage to the brains of their fetuses.[107] There are also varying levels of methylmercury in some saltwater fish, mainly swordfish and sharks.

Polychlorinated and Polybrominated Biphenyls (PCBs). — These compounds are widely used in heat exchangers and in plasticizers. They mainly reach children through breast milk, but placental transfer also occurs.[2] There have been two epidemics in which cooking oil contamination led to sizable transplacental transfers of *PCBs* to fetuses.[81] The children have had deeply pigmented skin, low birth weights, enlarged sebaceous glands in their eyelids, hypoplastic deformed nails, and abnormal pigmentation of their gums, nails, and groin.[61] There are two reports of subtle neurologic dysfunction following transplacental transfers of PCBs.[82] Not all of the long-term effects of transplacental PCB transfer may yet be known because contaminated children excrete the chemical very slowly over a period of many years.[81]

Penicillamine. — *Penicillamine*, a heavy metal chelator, was initially developed to treat Wilson's disease, a disorder that produces copper retention. In recent years the drug has been widely employed in the treatment of rheumatoid arthritis, scleroderma, other autoimmune disorders, and cystinuria. Most human pregnancy outcomes have been normal after the drug was used but there have been several cases of cutis laxa, a disorder characterized by lax skin, hyperextensible joints, and occasionally other anomalies.[85] Most of these children have died. Cutis laxa disappeared after a time in two survivors suggesting that once the drug has been cleared from the body normal collagen production can resume.[85]

Sedatives. — More information is available about *phenobarbital* than about any other sedative. The CPS found no increase in congenital malformations with the use of this drug.[38] Smaller studies have reported increased frequencies of cleft lip, cleft palate, and congenital heart disease, but these reports are difficult to evaluate because they included epileptics who took more than one anticonvulsant drug. Recently there has been a report that benodiazepine drugs, taken in large amounts, produce fetal growth retardation, cleft lip, and facial features that resemble the characteristic findings of the fetal alcohol syndrome.[59]

Thalidomide. — *Thalidomide* is the most famous of all teratogenic drugs. Phocomelia was caused by maternal ingestion of as little as 100 mg of the drug between the fourth and the sixth weeks of gestation. Other organs were also often affected, but the most obvious findings were the reduction deformities of the limbs. The association of phocomelia with nasal hemangioma, hearing loss, duodenal stenosis, and other defects has been termed the *thalidomide syndrome*.[63] Tissues from animals that are sensitive to thalidomide teratogenesis can convert the drug to a reactive arene oxide metabolite, whereas tissues from insensitive species cannot make the conversion.[33] It is postulated that this metabolite is the teratogenic factor.

Vitamin A Congeners. — Starting in 1954 more than a hundred studies have found that large quantities of vitamin A and various analogs of vitamin A are teratogenic in experimental animals.[86] Teratogenicity for humans did not become clear until 1983. Then microcephaly, various central nervous system lesions, low-set or absent ears, abnormal auditory canals, facial dysmorphia, micrognathia, cleft palate, thymus hypoplasia, and cardioaortic defects, particularly coarctation of the aorta, were reported following the use of low doses of the vitamin A congener *isotretinoin*.[84,86] Brain abnormalities have included hydrocephalus, posterior fossa cysts, cortical blindness, and facial palsy. Spontaneous abortions are also frequent.[86] Subsequently another vitamin A congener, *etretinate*, has been found to produce similar malformations.[39] It appears that the intake of vitamin A itself must exceed 25,000 units/day for teratogenesis to occur.

Other Chemicals. — *Nitrosamines* are mutagenic and are widely distributed in the food supply, including preserved meats, beer, and Scotch whiskey. No credible information on their teratogenicity has been published and it will be difficult to obtain such information because most of the general population in the industrial nations is frequently exposed. Studies undertaken in Eastern Europe have shown no higher frequency of congenital malformation in neonates from communities heavily polluted with nitrosamines than from communities with little or no such pollution.[83] The same is also true of some studies in the United States and in Great Britain.[4,64] Such studies have not been analyzed for spontaneous abortions and it is well known that most malformed embryos are spontaneously aborted early in pregnancy, often without the affected women knowing that they are pregnant.[65] There has been a claim that the wives of workers exposed to vinyl chloride have increased frequencies of fetal and neonatal losses.[48]

There have been claims that *spermicides* used in early gestation increase the frequency of Down's syndrome, but overall there is no convincing evidence that this is true.[87,90] *Spermicides* reportedly do not increase the frequency of spontaneous abortions.[45]

IONIZING RADIATION

Irradiating experimental animals in the first postconceptual week leads to small litters but to no other discernible abnormalities.[43] During subsequent weeks when organogenesis is taking place, irradiation can produce malformations, retard growth, kill embryos, and increase the frequency of neoplasms in later life.[68] There is also an increased frequency of functionally significant central nervous system abnormalities following heavy doses of radiation administered in utero at that time.[7,68] The best human data on the effects of in utero radiation exposure come from the survivors of the atomic bombings of Hiroshima and Nagasaki. No statistically significant long-term effects have been reported on the frequencies of stillbirth, neonatal death, or chromosomal abnormalities.[94] However, the in utero radiation has produced microcephaly and mental retardation. This was most frequent in those who were exposed between the 8th and 15th weeks of gestation. No visceral, limb, or other malformations have been present unless a child was growth-retarded at birth, was microcephalic, or had a readily apparent eye malformation. However, 30 years after the event survivors have begun to experience an increased frequency of malignant neoplasms. An in utero exposure dose of 156 rads (1.56 Gy) is estimated to have doubled the frequencies of cancers of many types, not just leukemias and lymphomas.[7,94,111]

Taking all of the human and experimental data into consideration, mental impairment is probably the most sensitive measure of antenatal radiation damage. The central nervous system is not more sensitive to ionizing radiation than other organs, but it is more likely to be damaged than other organs because it maintains its sensitivity to radiation throughout gestation and the neonatal period, whereas other organs can be malformed only from the second to the fourth weeks after conception.[8] Brent reasons that significant exposures between the second and fourth weeks will be rare and will usually result in abortion. He points out that almost all studies of human fetal radiation exposures of less than 5 rads (0.05 Gy) have failed to show an increase in fetal malformations and that the information from animal studies suggests that exposures of 50 rads (0.5 Gy) or less should not produce malformations.[8] It is not known if smaller doses of radiation can cause abortions before the fertilized egg has implanted.

Currently used diagnostic x-ray equipment that is used during the first trimester of pregnancy rarely exposes an embryo to more than 3 rads (0.03 Gy), a very small dose by comparison with the dose that was received by most pregnant women at Hiroshima and Nagasaki. All of the people in Hiroshima and Nagasaki who are deformed or mentally impaired as the result of in utero exposure to the atomic bombs received hundreds of rads of exposure. The radiation received by most fetuses in the United States totals less than 1 rad (0.01 Gy). About 55% of this comes from radon gas, which collects in buildings; 27% from other natural sources including cosmic rays, radiation from buildings and isotopes that are ingested; less than 1% from the nuclear power industry; and 18%

from other man-made sources.[8] In past decades embryos and fetuses sometimes received high doses of radiation during diagnostic procedures. Long-term follow-ups from the Oxford Survey of Childhood Cancer show that x-ray examinations conducted in Great Britain between 1953 and 1979 are being followed by an increasing number of malignant neoplasms. The most recent analyses calculate one cancer death for each 990 antenatal radiation exposures.[30,56] If these data are taken at face value, as many as half of fatal childhood cancers could be radiogenic in origin. This is almost certainly a large overestimate because children living in communities where there is a high level of background radiation have not had significantly increased rates of childhood cancer.[36]

VIDEO DISPLAY TERMINALS

Computers and word processors emit radiation levels that are seldom measurable above the background level with the exceptions of extremely low frequency magnetic field emissions and static electricity. To date, studies on animals using frequencies and levels of induced current density that duplicate the emissions of display terminals have failed to produce an increase in pregnancy failures or malformations.[5] Epidemiologic studies of human exposures have also failed to find a significant increase in the frequency of malformations after exposures to video display terminals.[5]

ULTRASOUND

Ultrasound and microwave emissions are very different from x-rays and gamma rays because they do not produce ionization. Studies to date have produced no evidence in humans that ultrasound or microwave emissions produce birth defects, impair psychomotor development, or cause childhood neoplasms. Ultrasound also has been found to have no effect on fetal or postnatal growth up to 6 years of age.[62,66] There is one report that repeated ultrasound exposures are followed by reduced birth weights, but the disorders that led to the ultrasound examinations may have been responsible for the low birth weights.[66]

HYPERTHERMIA

There are many reports of associations between maternal hyperthermia during pregnancy and congenital malformations, but whether or not a causal relationship exists is unsettled.[97] There is strong evidence that hyperthermia can be teratogenic in experimental animals, but this cannot be directly extrapolated to humans because experimentally induced fever is very different in its genesis from the genesis of most fever in human pregnancies. In the first place, there is no consistency in the association of malformations with hyperthermia in human studies.[105] There were 165 gravidas in the CPS who reported temperatures of 38.9° C or higher in the first trimester of pregnancy. None of the offspring of these pregnancies had phenotypic abnormalities like those that have been attributed to hyperthermia in previously published studies.[17] It might seem that studying the effects of gravidas taking sauna baths would be an appropriate way to investigate the teratogenesis of hyperthermia since infections and other nonthermal influences are presumably absent. A large proportion of Finnish women visit the sauna during early pregnancy where they are exposed to temperatures of 70 to 80° C for 10 to 20 minutes. Studies of these women have focused on the central nervous system and orofacial defects that have most often been attributed to hyperthermia. No increase in such malformations has been identified.[89] For all of these reasons it is far from established that hyperthermia is teratogenic in humans.

There does not appear to be much to fear from the emissions of microwave ovens. Such ovens produce heat, but the protections built into them and the fact that their electromagnetic emissions dissipate rapidly at short distances probably makes them harmless to embryos and fetuses.

THE FETAL PERIOD

Since organogenesis is completed before the start of the second trimester of pregnancy, injuries to organs during the second and third trimesters do not result in malformations. However, injuries during this period may produce specific lesions and fetal growth retardation, often with an accompanying deficit in the number of cells in the affected organs. *Antithyroid drugs* taken by mothers during the second and third trimesters can produce hypothyroidism or goiter in infants.[92] Chloroquine, streptomycin, and *dihydrostreptomycin* can produce deafness.[92,104] There are reports that *isoniazid*, in the absence of supplementary vitamin B_6, can damage fetal brains.[104]

Aspirin, indomethacin, and *naproxen* act by inhibiting the synthesis of prostaglandins from arachidonic acid. They readily pass the placenta and have been shown to cause severe constriction and occasionally closure of the ductus arteriosus in the fetus.[88] This increases pulmonary arterial pressure in the fetus. When used chronically, these drugs can lead to an increase in the mass of muscle in the small pulmonary arteries, resulting in persistent pulmonary arterial hypertension in the newborn, a disorder that is difficult to manage clinically. Reports that aspirin use during the first trimester of pregnancy causes cardiac malformations have been disputed.[108,111]

REFERENCES

1. Abel EL: Fetal, neonatal and adult effects of prenatal exposure to marijuana, in *Marijuana, tobacco, alcohol and reproduction.* Boca Raton, Fla, CRC Press, 1983, pp 31–33.

2. Allen JR, Barsotti DA: The effect of transplacental and mammary movement in PCB's on

infant rhesus monkeys. *Toxicology* 1976; 6:331–340.

3. Allen RW Jr: Fetal hydantoin syndrome and malignancy. *J Pediatr* 1984; 105:681.

4. Barltrop D: Chemical and physical environmental hazards for children, in Barltrop D(ed):, *Paediatrics and the Environment. Unigate Paediatric Workshops, No. 2, 1974.* London, The Fellowship of Postgraduate Medicine, 1975, pp 11–15.

5. Blackwell R, Chang A: Video display terminals and pregnancy. A review. *Br J Obstet Gynaecol* 1988; 95:446–453.

6. Bogdanoff B, Rorke LB, Yanoff M, Warren WS: Brain and eye abnormalities. *Am J Dis Child* 1972; 123:145–148.

7. Brent RL: Radiation teratogenesis. *Teratology* 1980; 21:281–298.

8. Brent RL: The effect of embryonic and fetal exposure to X-ray, microwaves, and ultrasound: Counseling the pregnant and non-pregnant patient about these risks. *Semin Oncol* 1989; 16:347–368.

9. Brent RL, Beckman DA: Etiology of human birth defects, with comments on the role of placental transport of human teratogens, in Bellisario R, Mizejewski GJ (eds): *Transplacental Disorders, Perinatal Detection, Treatment and Management.* New York, Alan R Liss, Inc, 1990, pp 17–36.

10. Britten RJ, Davidson EH: Gene regulation for higher cells: a theory. *Science* 1969; 165:349–357.

11. Buehler BA, Delimont D, Van Waes M, Finnell RH: Prenatal prediction of risk of the fetal hydantoin syndrome, *N Engl J Med* 1990; 322:1567–1572.

12. Caan BJ, Goldhaber MK: Caffeinated beverages and low birthweight: A case-control study. *Am J Public Health* 1989; 79:1299–1300.

13. Chasnoff IJ, Burns KA, Burns WJ: Cocaine use in pregnancy: Perinatal morbidity and mortality. *Neurotoxicol Teratol* 1987; 9:291–293.

14. Chasnoff IJ, Griffith DR, MacGregor S, Dirkes K, Burns KA: Temporal patterns of cocaine use in pregnancy, perinatal outcome. *JAMA* 1989; 261:1741–1744.

15. Chavez GF, Mulinare J, Cordero JF: Maternal cocaine use during early pregnancy as a risk factor for congenital urogenital anomalies. *JAMA* 1989; 262:795–798.

16. Clarren SK, Alvord EC Jr, Sumi SM, Streissuth AP, Smith DW: Brain malformations related to prenatal exposure to ethanol. *J Pediatr* 1978; 92:64–67.

17. Clarren SK, Smith DW, Harvey MAS, Ward RH, Myrianthopoulos NC: Hyperthermia, a prospective evaluation of a possible teratogenic agent in man. *J Pediatr* 1979; 95:81–83.

18. *The Collaborative Study on Cerebral Palsy, Mental Retardation and Other Neurological and Sensory Disorders of Infancy and Childhood Manual.* Bethesda, Md, US Department of Health, Education and Welfare, 1966.

19. Cregler LL, Mark H: Medical complications of cocaine abuse. *N Engl J Med* 1986; 315:1495–1500.

20. Diamond I, Anderson MM, McCreadie SR: Transplacental transmission of busulfan in a mother with leukemia. Production of fetal malformation and cytomegaly. *Pediatrics* 1960; 25:85–90.

21. Dixon SD, Bejar R: Brain lesions in cocaine and methamphetamine exposed neonates. *Pediatr Res* 1988; 23:405A.

22. Doll DC, Ringenberg S, Yarbro JW: Antineoplastic agents and pregnancy. *Semin Oncol* 1989; 16:337–346.

23. Environmental Protection Agency: 2,4,5-T and Silvex. *Fed Register* 1979; 44:15, 874.

24. Evans HJ, Fletcher J, Torrance M, Hargreave TB: Sperm abnormalities and cigarette smoking, *Lancet* 1981; 1:627–629.

25. Felig P, Lynch V: Starvation in human pregnancy: Hypoglycemia, hypoinsulinemia, and hyperketonemia. *Science* 1970; 170:990–992.

26. Fraser FC: Interactions and multiple causes, in Wilson JG, Fraser FC (eds): *Handbook of Teratology.* New York, Plenum Press, 1977, p 445.

27. Fried PA, O'Connell CM: A comparison of the effects of prenatal exposure to tobacco, alcohol, cannabis and caffeine on birth size and subsequent growth. *Neurotoxicol Teratol* 1987; 9:79–85.

28. Fuhrmann K, Reiher H, Semmler K, Glockner E: The effect of intensified conventional insulin therapy before and during pregnancy on the malformation rate in offspring of diabetic mothers. *Exp Clin Endocrinol* 1984; 83:173–177.

29. Gaily E, Granstrom ML, Hiilesmaa V, Bardy A: Minor anomalies in offspring of epileptic mothers. *J Pediatr* 1988; 112:520–529.

30. Gilman EA, Kneale GW, Knox EG, Steward AM: Pregnancy, X-rays and childhood cancers: Effects of exposure age and radiation dose. *J Soc Radiol Protection* 1987; 8:3–8.

31. Goldman AS: Critical periods of prenatal toxic insults, in *Drug and Chemical Risks to*

the Fetus and Newborn. New York, Alan R Liss Inc, 1980.

32. Goldman AS, Zackai EH, Yaffe S: Fetal trimethadione syndrome. in Sever JL, Brent RL (eds): *Teratogen Update, Environmentally Induced Birth Defect Risks.* New York, Alan R Liss Inc, 1986, pp 35–38.

33. Gordon GB, Spielberg SP, Blake DA, Balasubramanian V: Thalidomide teratogenesis: Evidence for a toxic arene oxide metabolite. *Proc Natl Acad Sci USA* 1981; 78:2545–2548.

34. Gregg NM: Congenital cataract following German measles in the mother. *Trans Ophthalmol Soc Aust* 1941; 3:35–46.

35. Hadeed AJ, Siegel SR: Maternal cocaine use during pregnancy: Effect on the newborn infant. *Pediatrics* 1989; 84:205–210.

36. Hanson GP, Komarov E: Health effects in residents of high background radiation regions, in *Biological Effects of Low Level Radiation.* Vienna, International Atomic Energy Agency, 1983.

37. Hanson JW: Fetal hydantoin effects. in Sever JL, Brent RL (eds): *Teratogen Update, Environmentally Induced Birth Defect Risks.* New York, Alan R. Liss Inc, 1986, pp 29–33.

38. Hanson JW, Smith DW: The fetal hydantoin syndrome. *J Pediatr* 1975; 87:285–290.

39. Happle R, Traupe H, Bounameaux Y, Fisch T: Teratogene Wirkung von Etretinat beim Menschen. *Deutsch Med Wochenschr* 1984; 109:1476–1480.

40. Heinonen OP, Slone D, Schapiro S: *Birth Defects and Drugs in Pregnancy.* Littleton, Mass, Publishing Sciences Group, 1977, p 516.

41. Herbst AL, Scully RE, Robboy SJ, Welch WR: Complications of prenatal therapy with diethylstilbestrol. *Pediatrics* 1978; 62 (suppl):1151–1159.

42. Herbst AL, Ulfelder H, Poskanzer DC: Adenocarcinoma of the vagina: Association of maternal stilbestrol therapy with tumor appearance in young women. *N Engl J Med* 1971; 284:878–881.

43. Hoffman DA, et al: *Effects of Ionizing Radiation on the Developing Embryo and Fetus, a Review.* Washington, DC, US Department of Health and Human Services, DHHS Publication No 81–123.

44. Holmes LB: Bendectin, in Sever JL, Brent RL (eds): *Teratogen Update, Environmentally Induced Birth Defect Risks.* New York, Alan R. Liss Inc, 1986, pp 53–59.

45. Huggins G, Vessey M, Flavel R, Yeates D, McPherson K: Vaginal spermicides and outcome of pregnancy, findings in a large cohort study. *Contraception* 1982; 25:219–230.

46. Hume RF Jr, O'Donnell KJ, Stanger CL, Killam AP, Gingras JL: In utero cocaine exposure: Observations of fetal behavioral state may predict neonatal outcome. *Am J Obstet Gynecol* 1989; 161:685–690.

47. Idanpaan-Heikkila J, Fritchie GE, Englert LF, Ho BT, McIsaac WM: Placental transfer of tritiated-1-tetrahydrocannabinol. *N Engl J Med* 1969; 281:330.

48. Infante PF, Wagoner JK, McMichael AJ, Waxweiler RJ, Falk H: Genetic risks of vinyl chloride. *Lancet* 1976; 1:734–735.

49. Iosub S, Fuchs M, Bingol N, Gromisch DS: Fetal alcohol syndrome revisited. *Pediatrics* 1981; 68:475–479.

50. Jankowski CG: Radiation and pregnancy, putting the risks in proportion. *Am J Nurs* 1986; 86:261–265.

51. Jones PJH, Leichter J, Lee M: Placental blood flow in rats fed alcohol before and during gestation. *Life Sci* 1981; 29:1153–1159.

52. Jones KL, Smith DW: The fetal alcohol syndrome. *Teratology* 1975; 12:1–10.

53. Kalter H, Warkany J: Congenital malformations. *N Engl J Med* 1983; 308:424–431.

54. Katsuma M: *Minamata Disease.* Kunamoto, Japan, Kunamoto University Press, 1969.

55. Klausner HA, Dingell JV: The metabolism and excretion of delta-9-tetrahydrocannabinol in the rat. *Life Sci* 1971; 10:49–59.

56. Knox EG, Stewart AM, Kneale GW, Gilman EA: Prenatal irradiation and childhood cancer. *J Soc Radiol Protection* 1987; 7:3–15.

57. Kreuz DS, Axelrod J: Delta-9-tetrahydrocannabinol: Localization in body fat. *Science* 1973; 179:391–393.

58. Kumar SP: Fetal alcohol syndrome, mechanisms of teratogenesis. *Ann Clin Lab Sci* 1982; 12:254–257.

59. Laegreid L, Olegard R, Walstrom J, Conradi N: Teratogenic effects of benzodiazepine use during pregnancy. *J Pediatr* 1989; 114:126–131.

60. Lehrovirta P, Forss M: The acute effect of smoking on intervillous blood flow of the placenta. *Br J Obstet Gynaecol* 1978; 85:729–731.

61. Longo LD: Environmental pollution and pregnancy; risks and uncertainties for the fetus and infant. *Am J Obstet Gynecol* 1980; 137:162–173.

62. Lyons EA, Dyke C, Toms M, Cheang M: In utero exposure to diagnostic ultrasound: A 6-year follow-up. *Radiology* 1988; 166:687–690.

63. McBride WG: Thalidomide and congenital abnormalities. *Lancet* 1961; 2:1358.

64. McNeil J, Ptasnik J: Evaluation of long-term effects of elevated blood lead concentrations in asymptomatic children, in Proceedings of International Symposium on Recent Advances in the Assessment of the Health Effects of Environmental Pollution. Paris, June 24–28, 1974.

65. Miller JF, Williamson E, Glue J, Gordon YB, Grudzinskas JG, Sykes A: Fetal loss after implantation. *Lancet* 1980; 2:554–556.

66. Moore RM Jr., Diamond EL, Cavalieri RL: The relationship of birth weight and intrauterine diagnostic ultrasound exposure. *Obstet Gynecol* 1988; 71:513–517.

67. Morris N, Osborn SB, Wright HP: Effective circulation of the uterine wall in late pregnancy. *Lancet* 1955; 1:323–325.

68. Mossman KL, Hill LT: Radiation risks in pregnancy. *Obstet Gynecol* 1982; 60:237–242.

69. Mulvihill JJ, McKeen EA, Rosner F, Zarrabi H: Pregnancy outcome in cancer patients. *Cancer* 1987; 60:1143–1150.

70. Murison G, Chubb CBH, Maeda S, Gemmell MA, Huberman E: Cannabinoids induce incomplete maturation of cultured human leukemia cells. *Proc Natl Acad Sci USA* 1987; 84:5414–5418.

71. Naeye RL: Maternal use of dextroamphetamine and growth of the fetus. *Pharmacology* 1983; 26:117–120.

72. Naeye RL: Maternal body weight and pregnancy outcome. *Am J Clin Nutr* 1990; 52:273–279.

73. Naeye RL, Peters EC, Bartholomew M, Landis JR: Origins of cerebral palsy. *Am J Dis Child* 1989; 143:1154–1161.

74. National Research Council: *The Effects of Herbicides in South Vietnam: Part A. Summary and Conclusions Prepared for Department of Defense.* Washington, DC, National Research Council, 1974.

75. Oro AS, Dixon SD: Perinatal cocaine and methamphetamine exposure: Maternal and neonatal correlates. *J Pediatr* 1987; 111:571–578.

76. Ravid R, Toaff R: On the possible teratogenicity of antibiotic drugs administered during pregnancy, a prospective study. *Adv Exp Med Biol* 1972; 27:505–510.

77. Reece EA, Hobbins JC: Diabetic embryopathy: Pathogenesis, prenatal diagnosis and prevention. *Obstet Gynecol Surv* 1986; 41:325–335.

78. Ritchie JM, Greene NM: Local anesthetics, in Gilman AG, Goodman LS, Rall TW, Murad F (eds): *The Pharmacologic Basis of Therapeutics*, ed 7. New York, Macmillan Publishing Co, 1985, pp 309–310.

79. Robertson WB, Brosens I, Dixon G: Uteroplacental vascular pathology. *Eur J Obstet Gynecol Reprod Biol* 1985; 5:47–65.

80. Robison LL, Buckley JD, Daigle AE, Wells R, Benjamin D, Arthur DC, Hammond GD: Maternal drug use and risk of childhood nonlymphoblastic leukemia among offspring. *Cancer* 1989; 63:1904–1911.

81. Rogan WJ: PCBs and cola colored babies: Japan 1968, and Taiwan, 1979, in Sever JL, Brent RL (eds): *Teratogen Update, Environmentally Induced Birth Defect Risks.* New York, Alan R Liss Inc, 1986, pp 127–130.

82. Rogan WJ, Gladen BC, McKinney JD, Carreras N, Hardy P, Thullen J, Tinglestad J, Tully M: Neonatal effects of transplacental exposure to PCBs and DDE. *J Pediatr* 1986; 109:335–341.

83. Rokicki W, Latoszkiewicz K, Krasnodebski J: Congenital malformations and the environment. *Acta Paediatr Scand [Suppl]* 1989; 360:140–145.

84. Rosa FW: Teratogenicity of isotretinoin. *Lancet* 1983; 2:513.

85. Rosa FW: Penicillamine, in Sever JL, Brent RL (eds): *Teratogen Update, Environmentally Induced Birth Defect Risks.* New York, Alan R Liss Inc, 1986, pp 71–75.

86. Rosa FW, Wild AL, Kelsey FO: Vitamin A congeners. in Sever JL, Brent RL (eds): *Teratogen Update, Environmentally Induced Birth Defect Risks.* New York, Alan R Liss Inc, 1986, pp 61–70.

87. Rothman KJ: Spermicide use and Down's syndrome. *Am J Public Health* 1982; 72:399–401.

88. Rudolph AM: The effects of nonsteroidal antiinflammatory compounds on fetal circulation and pulmonary function. *Obstet Gynecol* 1981; 58:36S–67S.

89. Saxen L, Holmberg PC, Nurminen M, Kuosma E: Sauna and congenital defects. *Teratology* 1982; 25:309–313.

90. Shapiro S, Slone D, Heinonen OP, Kaufman DW, Rosenberg L, Mitchell AA, Heimrich SP: Birth defects and vaginal spermicides. *JAMA* 1982; 247:2381–2384.

91. Telsey AM, Merrit TA, Dixon SD: Cocaine exposure in a term neonate. *Clin Pediatr* 1988; 27:547–550.

92. Schardein JL: *Drugs as Teratogens.* Cleveland, CRC Press, 1976.

93. Schardein JL: Congenital abnormalities and hormones during pregnancy: A clinical review. *Teratology* 1980; 22:251–270.

94. Schull WJ, Otake M, Neel JV: Genetic effects of the atomic bombs, a reappraisal. *Science* 1981; 213:1220–1227.

95. Shapiro S, Stone D, Hartz SC, Rosenberg L, Siskind V, Monson RR: Anticonvulsants and parental epilepsy in the development of birth defects. *Lancet* 1976; 1:272–275.

96. Shaul WL, Hall JG: Multiple congenital anomalies associated with oral anticoagulants. *Am J Obstet Gynecol* 1977; 127:191–198.

97. Shiota K: Neural tube defects and maternal hyperthermia in early pregnancy: Epidemiology in a human embryo population. *Am J Med Genet* 1982; 12:281–288.

98. Skakkebaek NE, Philip J, Rafaelsen OJ: LSD in mice: Abnormalities in meiotic chromosomes, *Science* 1968; 160:1246–1248.

99. Smith AH, Matheson DP, Fisher DO, Chapman CJ: Preliminary report of reproductive outcomes among pesticide applicators using 2,4,5-T. *N Z Med J* 1981; 93:177–179.

100. Spielberg SP: Pharmacogenetics and the fetus. *N Engl J Med* 1982; 307:115–116.

101. Stein Z, Susser M, Saenger G. et al: *Famine and Human Development.* New York, Oxford University Press, 1975.

102. Uchida IA, Holunga R, Lawler C: Maternal radiation and chromosomal aberrations. *Lancet* 1968; 2:1045–1049.

103. Ulfelder H: DES, transplacental teratogen and possible carcinogen, in Sever JL, Brent RL (eds): *Teratogen Update, Environmentally Induced Birth Defect Risks.* New York, Alan R Liss Inc, 1986, pp 19–21.

104. Warkany J: Antituberculous drugs, in Sever JL, Brent RL (eds): *Teratogen Update, Environmentally Induced Birth Defect Risks.* New York, Alan R Liss Inc, 1986, pp 45–49.

105. Warkany J: Hyperthermia, in Sever JL, Brent RL (eds): *Teratogen Update, Environmentally Induced Birth Defect Risks.* New York, Alan R Liss Inc, 1986, pp 181–187.

106. Warkany J: Warfarin embryopathy, in Sever JL, Brent RL (eds): *Teratogen Update, Environmentally Induced Birth Defect Risks.* New York, Alan R Liss Inc, 1986, pp 23–27.

107. Weiss B, Doherty RA: Methylmercury poisoning. in Sever JL, Brent RL (eds): *Teratogen Update, Environmentally Induced Birth Defect Risks.* New York, Alan R Liss Inc, 1986, pp 119–121.

108. Werler MM, Mitchell AA, Shapiro S: The relation of aspirin use during the first trimester of pregnancy to congenital cardiac defects. *N Engl J Med* 1989; 321:1639–1642.

109. Wilcox A, Weinberg C, Baird D: Caffeinated beverages and decreased fertility. *Lancet* 1988; 2:1453–1456.

110. Witter FR, King TM, Blake DA: The effects of chronic gastrointestinal medication on the fetus and neonate. *Obstet Gynecol* 1981; 58:79S–84S.

111. Yoshimoto Y, Kato H, Schull WJ: Risk of cancer among children exposed in utero to A-bomb radiations, 1950–84. *Lancet* 1988; 2:665–669.

112. Zierler S, Rothman KJ: Congenital heart disease in relation to maternal use of Bendectin and other drugs in early pregnancy. *N Engl J Med* 1985; 313:347–352.

113. Zuckerman B, Frank DA, Hingson R, *et al:* Effects of maternal marijuana and cocaine use on fetal growth. *N Engl J Med* 1989; 320:762–768.

CHAPTER 3

Maternal Nutrition and Pregnancy Outcome

FETAL GROWTH

A human newborn weighs only about 5% of its mother's weight and it has 9 months to acquire the nutrients that it needs from its mother. Thus, it might seem that maternal nutrition would not influence fetal growth. In fact, maternal nutrition *does* affect fetal growth but often in ways that have been difficult to understand. Various homeostatic mechanisms in mothers and fetuses appear to minimize variations in fetal growth over a wide range of maternal nutritional states. An example of these homeostatic mechanisms in operation was evident at the peak of the 1944–1945 Dutch famine when birth weights decreased only about 9% from prefamine levels.[46]

Pregravid Nutritional Stores

Findings from the Collaborative Perinatal Study (CPS) and other studies give clues to some of the mechanisms by which maternal nutrition affects fetal growth.[25,30] Birth weights had a strong, positive correlation with maternal pregravid body weights in the CPS (Figs 3–1 and 3–2). There is evidence that most women who weigh more than 43.5 kg before pregnancy have ample nutritional stores to meet fetal needs because in the CPS the birth weights of their children were very little affected by maternal pregnancy weight gain (see Figs 3–1 and 3–2).[12] Women usually store 3 kg or more of depot fat during the first two trimesters of pregnancy as an energy bank, part of which is normally mobilized during the third trimester when the caloric needs of the fetus are at their peak.[12] There is a

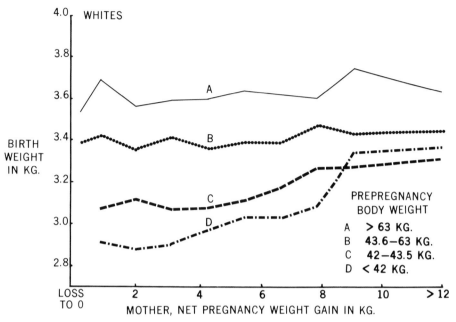

FIG 3–1.
Both maternal prepregnancy body weight and net pregnancy weight gain had a strong positive correlation with birth weights in full-term whites in the CPS. Net pregnancy weight gain is the total pregnancy weight gain at delivery minus the weight of the fetus and placenta.

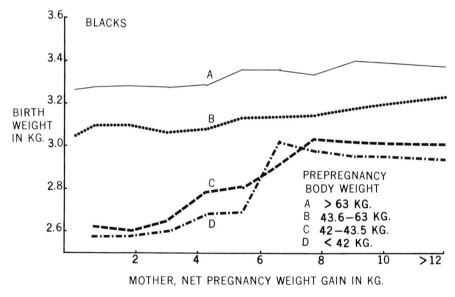

FIG 3–2.
Birth weights were about 10% less in blacks than in whites but had the same relationships with maternal prepregnancy body weight and pregnancy weight gain.

contrast between the role of this stored fat in well-nourished and poorly nourished gestations. In well-nourished gravidas caloric (energy) intake has a strong, positive correlation with the amount of fat that is stored, but there is little relationship between this fat accretion, a gravida's energy expenditures for physical activity, and infant birth weight, presumably because both fat stores and intake are adequate to meet all maternal and fetal needs.[16] In this setting of caloric sufficiency birth weights have a strong correlation with maternal lean body mass.[15]

Fat storage and release plays a large role in fetal growth when gravidas are undernourished. In a study which we conducted in Addis Ababa, Ethiopia, pregnant women were able to obtain and consume less than 60% of the calories and less than 70% of the protein recommended by the World Health Organization.[34] The newborns were 6% to 7% lighter than US newborns of the same gestational age.[34] This growth retardation correlated with maternal triceps skinfold thickness during pregnancy.[35] In normally nourished gestations triceps skinfold thickness increases in the first two trimesters of pregnancy and decreases in the third, reflecting early pregnancy storage of fat and its release in late gestation to meet the increasing energy needs of the fetus and the continuing needs of the gravida. Ethiopian women who had skinfold thickness increases and decreases as great as those in the United Kingdom and United States had neonates as heavy as those in the United Kingdom and United States. This suggests that the growth potential of Ethiopian fetuses may be as great as the growth potential of fetuses in the industrial nations. If this is true for many other Third World populations, the same fetal growth curves may be applicable for most of the world's population groups and triceps skinfold thickness could be widely used to assess the status of maternal energy reserves in studies of fetal growth.

Some other aspects of fetal growth in Addis Ababa are also of interest. Subcutaneous fat cells were smaller and testicular descent more often delayed in undernourished than in normally nourished neonates.[34] The most undernourished neonates also had a relative undergrowth of their cerebellums.[34] The cerebellum may be susceptible to the growth-limiting effects of undernutrition because it is the fastest-growing part of the brain during the last trimester of pregnancy when undernutrition has its greatest effect on fetal growth.[4] Maternal undernutrition appears to exert much of its effect on fetal growth by restricting maternal blood volume expansion and by keeping gestational blood pressure relatively low, which in turn keeps uteroplacental blood flow at a low level.[20,25–27,34,35] In general, the fetal brain is more protected from the effects of undernutrition than other organs because undernutrition does not restrict blood flow to the brain as much as it does to other body organs.[3]

Maternal Pregnancy Weight Gain

Maternal weight gain at the end of pregnancy minus the weight of the neonate and placenta is termed "net pregnancy weight gain" in many of our studies. It is mainly a measure of nutrients incorporated into maternal tissues, breast growth, the weight of the amniotic fluid, maternal blood volume increase, and the weight of other extracellular fluids accumulated during pregnancy. In the CPS net pregnancy weight gain had a strong positive correlation with birth weights when mothers were underweight before pregnancy (see Figs 3–1 and 3–2).[34] This correlation decreased and finally disappeared as mothers' pregravid body weights increased. This suggests that the fetuses of overweight mothers were amply supplied with the nutrients required for their growth, even when these mothers had a low pregnancy weight gain, whereas the fetuses of thin mothers were more dependent for energy and perhaps other nutrients on maternal food intake during pregnancy. Maternal pregravid body weight and net pregnancy weight gain had a strong positive correlation with placental weights.[34] The correlation with neonates' head circumferences and body lengths were weaker, suggesting that brains and bones have a high priority on available nutrients.[34] Maternal pregravid weight had no correlation with body length or head circumference at birth when net pregnancy weight gain exceeded

8 kg (Figs. 3–3 and 3–4). Maternal height had a strong correlation with birth weights, lengths, and head circumferences, independent of maternal pregravid body weight and pregnancy weight gain.[34] This goes along with the previously mentioned finding that maternal lean body mass strongly affects fetal growth.[15] Both are likely reflections of maternal genetic influences on fetal growth.

Maternal pregnancy weight gain has been found to have a greater effect on birth weights, birth lengths, and head circumferences when gravidas are adolescents

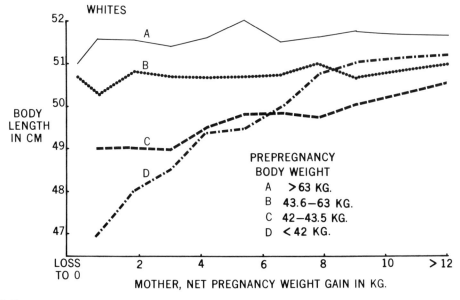

FIG 3–3.
On a percentage basis maternal pregravid body weight and pregnancy weight gain had less effect on children's body length at birth than on body weight. Pregravid body weight had no effect on birth length when maternal net pregnancy weight gains exceeded 8 kg.

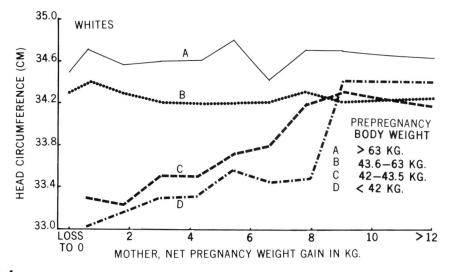

FIG 3–4.
On a percentage basis maternal pregravid body weight and pregnancy weight gain had less effect on head circumference at birth than on body weight. Maternal pregravid body weight had no effect on head circumference when maternal net pregnancy weight gains exceeded 8 kg.

than when they are adults (Figs 3–5 and 3–6).[9,47] This is presumably because the fetuses of adolescents have to compete for nutrients with the growth needs of their mothers.[27] Scholl et al. have shown that as early as 12 weeks' gestation there is a significant association between the amount of weight gain adolescents have accumulated and the birth weights of their infants.[43] This correlation increases in strength as pregnancy progresses. The weight gains of pregnant adolescents should be recorded when they enter the prenatal health care system and closely monitored until delivery.

Caloric Requirements of Pregnancy

Prentice et al. have provided details on the number of calories required by gravidas to avoid fetal growth retardation.[39] In their study, the threshold at which maternal calories affected fetal growth varied with the level of energy expended by their Gambian subjects. During the periods of the year when agricultural endeavors required little physical work, Gambian

gravidas gained 1.3 kg/month, which included a substantial deposition of subcutaneous fat on an intake of only 1,500 kcal/day. The mean birth weight of their infants, adjusted for gestational age, was 2.95 ± 0.4 kg. On the same caloric intake during the months when agricultural work required a high energy expenditure, the women gained only 0.3 kg/month and mean birth weights adjusted for gestational age fell to 2.74 ± 0.5 kg. A dietary supplement averaging 431 kcal/day during the season of hard physical work increased birth weights by 8% to the level present during the months when energy expenditures were low. The same level of supplementation during the months when energy expenditures were low did not increase birth weights. These findings suggest that the intake threshold in Gambian gravidas for a positive energy balance was only 1,500 kcal/day when energy expenditures were low.

A study which we conducted in Ethiopia produced similar findings.[34] Women consuming 1,500 to 1,600 kcal and 45 to 50 g of protein per day had full-term

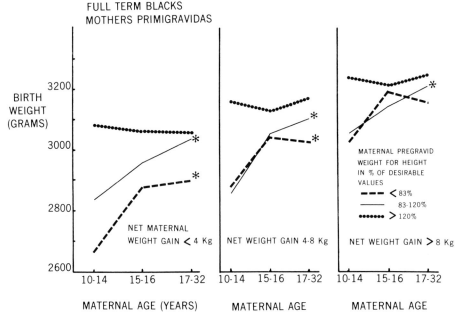

FIG 3–5.
Pregnancy weight gains had a much larger effect on birth weights when mothers were very young (just beyond menarache) than when they were older. *P < .05 for increase in birth weight with increasing maternal age.

neonates who weighed approximately 3.3 kg when gravidas engaged in light physical work vs. 3.1 kg when the work required heavy physical exertion.[34] Just prior to the hunger winter of 1944–1945, Dutch gravidas had a ration of 1,500 kcal/day. These women lost weight during pregnancy but their neonates were normally grown.[46] When caloric intakes decreased to as low as 400 kcal/day during the hunger winter, birth weights decreased markedly while body lengths and head circumferences were less affected.[46] Neonates who were in utero

during the second and third trimesters were much more growth-retarded than those exposed to the severe maternal undernutrition only during the first trimester of pregnancy.

The effects of maternal nutritional supplements on fetal growth can be influenced by the bulk of the food that is eaten. In a study which we conducted, Zulu women not engaged in agricultural work were given daily supplements starting at midgestation.[42] Prior to receiving the supplements the women had a daily intake of approximately 1,500 kcal and 50 g of

TABLE 3–1.

Relationship of Maternal Acetonuria to Perinatal Mortality Rates*

	Maternal Pregnancy Weight Gain (% of Optimal Values)†				
Maternal Status	<25%	25%–54%	55%–79%	80%–120%	>120%
Acetonuria absent	65 (2,372)	37 (2,372)	34 (3,791)	23 (5,402)	31 (2,261)
Acetonuria present	117 (162)	46 (344)	36 (557)	23 (768)	70 (301)
	$P < .05$	$P > .1$	$P > .1$	$P > .1$	$P < .005$

*Perinatal mortality rates are shown as fetal plus neonatal deaths per 1,000 births. Numbers of cases are in parentheses.
†Optimal weight gain = 12 kg at full term. Values are prorated at early gestational ages.

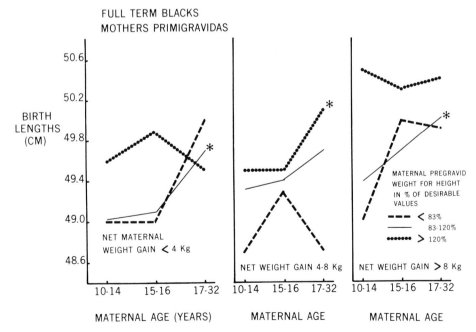

FIG 3–6.
Pregnancy weight gains had a much larger effect on birth lengths when mothers were very young (just beyond menarche) than when they were older. *Asterisk* indicates $P < .05$ for increase in birth length with increasing maternal age.

protein. One group of the women received a high bulk daily supplement of 773 kcal consisting of maize and beans, which were the main constituents of their usual daily food.[34] A second group received a supplement of much lower bulk containing 697 kcal, consisting of 100 g of dry skimmed milk added to maize. A third group received pills that contained no calories or protein. Women in this last group gained 8.0 kg between midgestation and term, those on the high bulk supplement gained 8.3 kg, and those on the low bulk supplement gained 8.1 kg. Adjusting for gestational ages at delivery, mean birth weights were 10% greater with the low bulk supplement than with either the high bulk supplement or the pills (Fig. 3–7). Women who received the high bulk supplement claimed that the supplements left them so satiated that they could eat very little at their evening meal. Those on the lower bulk supplement claimed the supplement did not reduce their food consumption at the evening meal. This raises the possibility that high bulk diets can restrict fetal growth by limiting maternal caloric intake.

Protein Requirements

Changes that appear to conserve protein for fetal use take place in maternal metabolism during pregnancy. According to Naismith, women and their fetuses must synthesize about 920 g of new protein during pregnancy.[37] Not all investigators have observed an appreciable increase in protein intake by healthy women during pregnancy, so what are the mechanisms by which this new protein is provided? Munro has shown that adults require about 40 g of dietary protein per day to maintain a positive nitrogen balance.[21] A reduction of less than 10% in maternal amino acid catabolism would enable these 40 g to meet the requirements of both mothers and their fetuses. In rats, levels of enzymes that control protein catabolism decrease during pregnancy, with a resultant decrease in protein catabolism and reduced levels of plasma urea.[37] The same decrease in maternal plasma levels of urea takes place in human pregnancies.[12]

There may be still other means by which protein is made available to the fetus without requiring an increase in

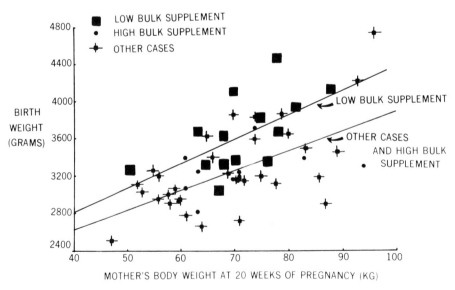

FIG 3–7.
Birth weights of full-term Zulu infants were greater when their mothers received low bulk than when they received high bulk dietary supplements during pregnancy.

maternal dietary protein intake. In rats, maternal protein is released in late pregnancy when fetal demands are high.[36,37] There is evidence that the same protein release takes place in humans. Naismith has shown that the maternal excretion of 3-methylhistidine rises during the last trimester of pregnancy.[37] This amino acid is liberated by the normal catabolism of muscle protein and is not reutilized, so its increased urinary excretion is likely the result of an accelerated catabolism of maternal muscle protein.

Zinc

Mothers with growth-retarded fetuses have been reported to have a lower zinc intake than mothers whose babies are growing normally.[45] Simmer and Thompson have suggested that zinc depletion might be a marker of poor general nutrition because they observed a correlation between low zinc intake, low maternal gestational fat reserves, and fetal growth retardation.[45] Strict vegetarians and those who diet to lose weight can have a very low zinc intake. Zinc deficiency can also result from heavy sweating. There are claims that severe maternal zinc deficiency can be teratogenic in both animals and in humans.[10,19] Normally zinc moves from the maternal plasma into maternal leukocytes, the placenta, and the fetus during pregnancy, which lowers blood plasma levels of zinc in the gravida.[1] This movement of zinc is reduced in pregnancies in which fetal growth is slow, which leaves maternal plasma levels higher and leukocyte levels lower than is the case with normal fetal growth.[1,45]

Other Nutritional Requirements

There are a number of other settings in which nutritional deficiencies have been speculated to affect pregnancy outcome. Oral contraceptives can depress the body of several micronutrients, and it has been argued that women who are taking oral contraceptives should switch to a barrier method of contraception and eat a balanced diet for several months before they plan to conceive. The value of this advice is unproven but might be most important for strict vegetarians and for women taking phenytoin (Dilantin), both of which can deplete the body of folic acid.

MECHANISMS THAT REGULATE NUTRIENT DELIVERY TO THE FETUS

Some of the homeostatic mechanisms that enable undernourished and malnourished women to produce only mildly growth-retarded neonates are now known. Some of these mechanisms appear to be mediated through the influence of maternal blood pressure on uteroplacental blood flow. In the CPS peak diastolic blood pressures increased with increases in both maternal pregravid body weight and net pregnancy weight gain (Figs 3–8 and 3–9). In the CPS, underweight mothers who had low pregnancy weight gains had growth-retarded neonates when their peak third-trimester diastolic blood pressures were less than 61 mm Hg (Fig. 3–10).[26] This growth retardation largely disappeared when peak diastolic blood pressures were between 61 and 99 mm Hg. Birth weights became independent of blood pressure levels as mothers' pregravid body weights and net pregnancy weight gains increased (see Fig. 3–10).

Findings from other studies provide additional evidence that maternal nutrition exerts some of its effects on fetal growth by affecting maternal blood pressure, which in turn influences the delivery of nutrients to the fetus through its effects on uteroplacental blood flow. Diastolic blood pressure normally decreases at the end of the first trimester of pregnancy, remains low during the second trimester, and then slowly rises to near prepregnancy levels during the third trimester. Diastolic blood pressure did not increase

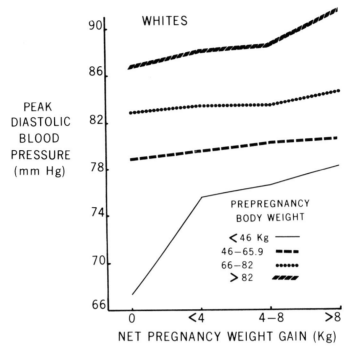

FIG 3–8.
Peak diastolic blood pressures increased in whites with both maternal pregravid body weight and pregnancy weight gain in the CPS.

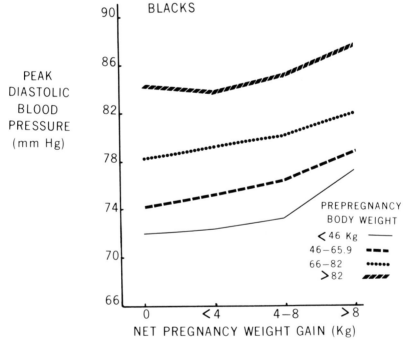

FIG 3–9.
Peak diastolic blood pressures also increased in blacks with pregravid body weight and pregnancy weight gain. However, these blood pressures were lower in blacks than in whites in every category of maternal pregravid body weight and pregnancy weight gain (see Fig 3–8).

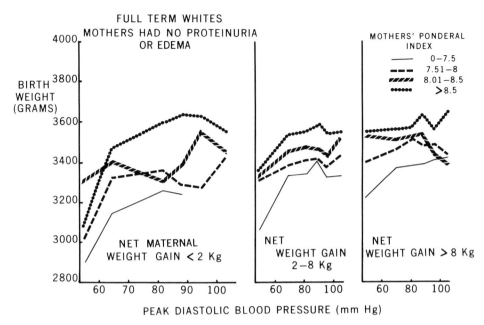

FIG 3–10.
Birth weights in the CPS increased with maternal blood pressure up to a peak maternal diastolic pressure of about 99 mm Hg. This effect was greatest in thin women who had a low pregnancy weight gain. Women with low ponderal index values were thin pregravid, while those with high values were overweight.

during the third trimester in most members of the group of severely undernourished gravidas that we studied in Addis Ababa. When diastolic pressures remained low, birth weights averaged 3.0 kg at term. A few of the undernourished women had a normal rise in diastolic blood pressure during the third trimester. The newborns of these women had an average birth weight of 3.3 kg, suggesting that the higher pressures resulted in a high nutrient delivery to their fetuses. Grunberger et al. also found that third-trimester blood pressure levels affect fetal growth.[7] They reported that uteroplacental blood flow and birth weights were much lower when maternal gestational blood pressures were consistently below 111/66 mm Hg than when pressures were higher. In some experimental animals there is a direct correlation between the size of uteroplacental blood flow and the transplacental transfer of materials across the placenta to the fetus.[49]

PERINATAL MORTALITY

Pregnancy Weight Gain

It has long been known that fetal and neonatal death rates are higher when women are underweight before pregnancy and have low pregnancy weight gains than when they have a normal or high pregravid weight for height and a normal weight gain (Fig 3–11).[22] In the Dutch hunger winter of 1944–1945 the frequency of stillbirths markedly increased, even when maternal malnutrition was relieved after the first trimester.[46] Death rates were also very high from birth until 3 months of age in infants exposed to severe maternal undernutrition during the second and third trimesters. In the CPS, underweight women who had low pregnancy weight gains had increased frequencies of acute chorioamnionitis and disorders that produce chronic low blood flow from the uterus to the placenta.[34] Far more striking were the increases in the

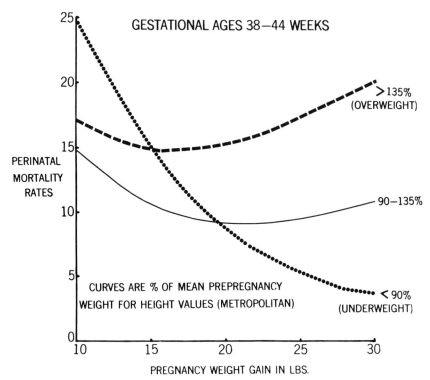

FIG 3–11.
Women in the CPS who were underweight for height before pregnancy had high perinatal mortality rates with low pregnancy weight gains and very low perinatal mortality rates with high pregnancy weight gains. Pregnancy weight gain had very little effect on perinatal mortality when women were overweight for height before pregnancy.

case fatality rates for these and other disorders, which suggests that stress from a variety of different causes was more often fatal when thin women had low pregnancy weight gains.[34] Case fatality rates are the death rate from a disorder once it is in progress. Further analyses disclosed that about one-third of the high perinatal mortality associated with low maternal pregnancy weight gain was in women who had acetonuria during pregnancy that was not due to diabetes mellitus (see Table 3–1, p. 27).[34]

Mild acetonuria has no untoward consequences with a normal pregnancy weight gain, so why was it a marker for high mortality with a low pregnancy gain? Fasting is one possible explanation. When gravidas fast in the third trimester, hypoglycemia, hyperketonemia, acetonuria, and other evidences of metabolic acidosis develop after about 20 hours, whereas it takes 2 to 4 days of fasting for the nonpregnant to become acidotic.[5,20,22] Hepatic glyconeogenesis is reduced under these circumstances, and the placenta responds by an increased release of chorionic somatomammotropic hormone. This enhances hypoaminoacidemia and hyperketonemia through the hormone's anabolic and lipolytic actions. As a result, the levels of free fatty acids increase in the blood. Under these circumstances ketone bodies, free fatty acids, and perhaps lactate and pyruvate provide a proportion of fetal energy needs that is larger than normal. The fetus can apparently use ketone bodies to form structural lipids and provide cellular energy. The fetal heart and other organs can also utilize free fatty acids for energy. However, it is not certain that all of the fetal organs can use these substitute fuels as effectively as glucose, which is their normal fuel. This may be one reason why fetal and neonatal mortality increased when CPS gravidas had acetone in their urine.

Acetonuria had some interesting seasonal variations in the CPS that support the thesis that it is sometimes the consequence of fasting. Acetonuria was most frequent at those times in the year when maternal weight gain was low and least frequent when maternal weight gains were high.[34] Specifically, it was least frequent between Thanksgiving and Christmas and then sharply increased in frequency after New Year's Day. It is tempting to attribute these changes to feasting during the holiday season and fasting after New Year's Day to compensate for high weight gains during the holiday season.

Maternal Blood Volume Increase

In the CPS only about a third of the excessive fetal and neonatal mortality associated with low pregnancy weight gain was associated with acetonuria, so there must be additional causes of the perinatal deaths associated with the low weight gains. There is evidence that low maternal blood volume expansion is one of these causes. Maternal blood volume normally increases by more than 1 L during pregnancy.[11] This expansion is characteristically less in low- than in high-weight-gain gestations.[11,12] It has been shown that a subnormal blood volume expansion leads to low uteroplacental blood flow, and low uteroplacental blood flow is a well-known cause of both stillbirth and neonatal death.[7,33] When pregnancy weight gains were low in the CPS, perinatal mortality rates were much lower when laboratory evidences of high blood volume expansion were present than when they were absent.[34] In our analyses the principal markers of a low blood volume expansion were a high maternal hemoglobin value and the absence of ankle edema in late gestation. When gestational blood volume expansion is normal, hemoglobin and hematocrit values fall because plasma volume increase makes a larger contribution to the blood volume expansion than does an increase in red cell number. Ankle edema in the absence of hypertension is a marker for a high maternal blood volume expansion.[12] Women whose hemoglobin levels were still high in the third trimester and women who had no ankle edema had perinatal mortality rates that were higher than expected (Figs 3–12 and 3–13).

Maternal Weight for Height

Overweight women have long been known to have more stillbirths and children who die as neonates than the nonoverweight. The usual explanations are that overweight gravidas more often have diabetes mellitus, hypertension, twins, and trauma-prone macrosomic infants than the nonoverweight.[6,8,13,14] We recently discovered that this problem was not limited to the overweight. In the CPS, perinatal mortality rates progressively increased with pregravid maternal weight for height so that very thin gravidas had the lowest rate of antenatal and neonatal losses. Perinatal mortality rates progressively increased with maternal weight for height from a value of 37/1,000 for offspring of thin gravidas, to 48/1,000 for children of normal-weight women, to 56/1,000 for offspring of the slightly overweight and to 121/1,000 for children of very overweight gravidas (Tables 3–2 and 3–3).[29] These findings are for infants of all gestational ages. The offspring of very thin mothers had a particularly low perinatal mortality rate when their mothers had a pregnancy weight gain of 12 kg or more (see Fig 3–11).[22] A recent British study had a similar finding for infants born preterm.[18]

Preterm births were by far the most important reason why perinatal mortality rates increased with maternal pregravid body weight for height (see Table 3–2). This increase of preterm births was mainly the result of deliveries between 24 and 30 weeks' gestation caused by acute chorioamnionitis and by twin fetuses. Both of

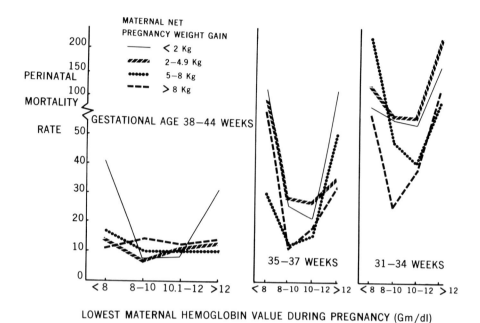

FIG 3–12.
Perinatal mortality rates were high when gravidas had high hemoglobin values in late gestation.

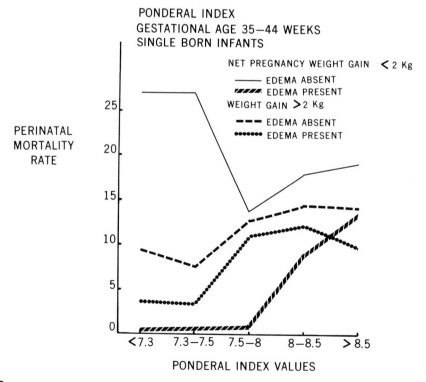

FIG 3–13.
Perinatal mortality rates were highest in normotensive gestations when ankle edema was absent late in gestation.

TABLE 3–2.

Estimated (Corrected) Perinatal Mortality Rates for Various Risk Factors With Increasing Relative Maternal Pregravid Body Weight

Pregnancy Risk Factors	Maternal Weight			
	Thin	Normal	Mildly Overweight	Overweight
Maternal				
Age 35–50 yr	1.1	2.4	4.5	10.9
Diabetes mellitus	0	0.5	0.6	12.4
Low pregnancy weight gain	1.1	1.0	0.6	0
Hypertension	0.4	0	0	0
Race: black	1.0	0	0	0
Low socioeconomic status	0	0	0	0
Fetal				
Preterm birth	19.8	25.6	27.4	58.0
Malformations	2.2	5.3	3.9	7.3
Twins, triplets	0	0.5	0.6	1.2
Neonatal				
Respiratory distress syndrome	2.2	2.4	1.7	1.2
Other disorders	9.5	10.6	16.6	29.9
Total	37.3	48.3	55.9	120.9

TABLE 3–3.

Maternal Pregravid Weight for Height and Perinatal Mortality*

Pregravid Weight for Height	Born Preterm	Born Full Term
Whites		
Thin	177 (106)	9 (41)
Normal	218 (345)	12 (174)
Slightly over-weight	234 (60)	16 (40)
Very over-weight	255 (30)	19 (24)
	$P < .02$	$P < .01$
Blacks		
Thin	124 (119)	10 (33)
Normal	122 (348)	14 (159)
Slightly over-weight	164 (100)	14 (41)
Very over-weight	177 (65)	34 (61)
	$P < .001$	$P < .001$

*Fetal plus neonatal deaths per 1,000 births. Numbers of deaths are in parentheses.

these risk factors are well-known causes of preterm birth.[34] The increase of twins was entirely in pairs with dichorionic placentas (Table 3–4). Over 90% of the twins who have dichorionic placentas are dizygotic, so the positive correlation of such twinning with maternal pregravid weight for height was due either to more frequent multiple ovulation or to an increase in the survival rate of two embryos with increasing maternal pregravid weight for height.

Other factors that contributed to the mortality increase with increasing maternal pregravid body weight were more frequent older gravidas (35–50 years of age), gravidas with diabetes mellitus, and children with major congenital malformations (see Table 3–2). Obesity has a well-

TABLE 3–4.

Twins and Maternal Weight for Height*

Pregravid Weight for Height	Monochorionic Twins per 1,000 Births	Dichorionic Twins per 1,000 Births
Thin	7 (67)	9 (93) $P<.05$
Normal	5 (156)	14 (441) $P<.001$
Slightly over-weight	6 (52)	21 (196) $P<.001$
Very overweight	6 (24)	25 (102) $P<.001$
	$P>.1$	$P<.001$

*Numbers of twin pairs are in parentheses.

TABLE 3–5.

Maternal Pregravid Weight for Height: Its Association With Gestational Acetonuria, Perinatal Death, and Major Congenital Malformations in the Newborn*

Pregravid Weight for Height	Congenital Malformations per 1000 Births†	
	No Acetonuria	2+–4+ Acetonuria
Thin	41 (145)	53 (16) $P<.1$
Normal	45 (409)	65 (52) $P<.005$
Slightly over-weight	54 (168)	95 (28) $P<.002$
Very overweight	59 (88)	93 (21) $P<.05$

*Mothers with diabetes mellitus were excluded from these analyses.
†Numbers of children with malformations are in parentheses.

known role in some of these risk factors, a speculative or unknown role in others. It is not surprising that women 35 to 50 years of age had higher pregravid body weights than younger women, because fatness increases with age in well-nourished populations and it has long been recognized that being over 34 years of age increases the risks of stillbirth and neonatal death.[34] The association between being overweight and having diabetes mellitus is also well known. Both the need for insulin and refractoriness to its action increase with fatness.[38] In our analyses the correlation between a mother being overweight and congenital malformations in her offspring was independent of maternal age, diabetes mellitus, cigarette smoking, and being a twin. Most of the increase in malformations was in children whose mothers had acetone in their urine during the first trimester of pregnancy (Table 3–5). Why acetonuria is a marker for teratogenesis remains to be determined.

The correlation of low socioeconomic status with high perinatal mortality disappeared when maternal pregravid weight for height and other nonsocioeconomic risk factors for perinatal death were taken into consideration (see Table 3–2).[29] The correlation of being black with high perinatal mortality also nearly disappeared when maternal pregravid weight for height was taken into consideration (see Table 3–2).[29] This suggests that being black and having a low socioeconomic status are often secondary to maternal weight for height as risk factors for high perinatal mortality. This, of course, does not exclude the possibility that pregravid weight for height is a surrogate for other, as yet unidentified, risk factors.

Maternal Gestational Anemia

There are many causes of maternal anemia during pregnancy, some congenital but most acquired. One or more hemoglobin values below 8 g/dL was associated with a high perinatal mortality rate in the CPS (see Fig 3–12).[31] Deficiencies of iron and folic acid are the most frequent causes of maternal gestational anemia in the absence of hemorrhage and parasites, so they can be added to the list of nutritional factors that affect pregnancy outcome.

The dietary requirement for folic acid doubles during pregnancy. A severe megaloblastic anemia sometimes develops in folate-deficient women that can threaten the life of both mother and fetus. Such deficiencies are most frequent in tropical areas where the food supply is folate-deficient during certain times of the year. There are old reports that folate deficiency predisposes to spontaneous abortions and fetal malformations, but recent studies have failed to confirm these claims.

The dietary requirements for iron increase markedly during pregnancy. Iron-supplemented gravidas have hemoglobin levels about 1 g/dL higher than do unsupplemented gravidas. As a result, most US women receive iron supplements during pregnancy. Controlled studies have never been undertaken to determine whether this supplementation and the resulting higher hemoglobin values improve pregnancy outcome.

Zinc Deficiency

A maternal dietary deficiency of zinc can increase perinatal mortality in addition to its possible influence on fetal growth. In Ethiopia a deficiency of dietary zinc often leads to levels of zinc in the amniotic fluid that are too low to make the amniotic fluid antimicrobial.[34,48] This lack of antimicrobial activity in turn is associated with a high frequency of amniotic fluid bacterial infections. Such a zinc-linked deficiency of antimicrobial activity appears to be rare in the United States.[2]

Vitamin D Deficiency

Vitamin D deficiency with resultant rickets is common in some African children as the result of mothers keeping them indoors, out of sight of the "evil eye," during early childhood. Rickets in early childhood often produces a small pelvic outlet which in turn results in many obstructed labors when the affected girls reach reproductive age.[31] This was the second most frequent cause of fetal and neonatal death in a 1975 study which we conducted in Addis Ababa.[31,34] It is also a major cause of maternal death during labor in affected populations.

Iodine Deficiency

Iodine deficiency leads to endemic goiter in areas of the world where the iodine content of the soil, water, and plants is low and food from outside areas is not consumed. Goitrogens are also present in some of these diets. The affected mothers sometimes produce cretins.

PREMATURITY

There is evidence that maternal undernutrition may predispose to preterm birth. The disorders that are responsible for most preterm labors, namely acute chorioamnionitis, abruptio placentae, and the disorders of low uteroplacental blood flow, are all more frequent when maternal pregnancy weight gains are low.[22,28]

CIGARETTE SMOKING AND NUTRITION

As a group cigarette smokers have lower pregnancy weight gains than non-

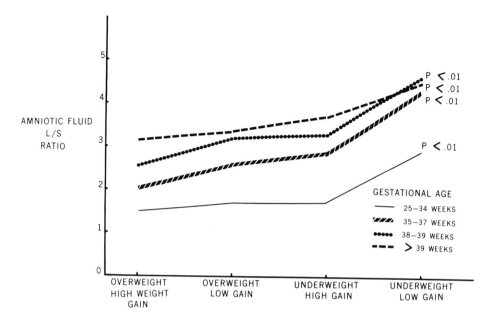

FIG 3–14.
Fetal lungs matured most rapidly when women were thin pregravid and had a low pregnancy weight gain. *L/S ratio* = lecithin-to-sphingomyelin ratio.

smokers, so it has been suggested that the unfavorable effects of maternal cigarette smoking on pregnancy outcome might be ameliorated by increasing maternal food intake during pregnancy. This possibility has never been fully tested, but in the CPS a high maternal pregnancy weight gain did not protect against the increased frequency of placental abruptions in cigarette smokers.[24,34]

CAFFEINE CONSUMPTION AND PREGNANCY OUTCOME

Two large studies have reported no relationship between the consumption of caffeine-containing beverages during early pregnancy and congenital malformations.[17,40] In one of these studies, low birth weights and short gestations were more frequent when women were heavy coffee drinkers, but these effects disappeared when the analyses were controlled for other personal habits and women's demographic characteristics.[17]

FETAL LUNG MATURATION

Several studies have shown that at any given gestational age fetal lung maturation is accelerated when gravidas are underweight before pregnancy and have a low pregnancy weight gain (Fig 3–14).[32,34,41] Women who are in these two categories have smaller pregnancy blood volume increases and smaller uteroplacental blood flows than women who are not in these risk categories.[7,12] Several studies have shown that low uteroplacental blood flow accelerates fetal lung maturation.[41,44]

REFERENCES

1. Adeniyi FAA, The implications of hypozincemia in pregnancy. *Acta Obstet Gynecol Scand* 1987; 66:579–582.

2. Appelbaum PC, Shulman G, Chambers NL, et al: Studies on the growth-inhibiting property of amniotic fluids from two United States population groups. *Am J Obstet Gynecol* 1980; 137:579–582.

3. Creasy R, DeSweet M, Kahanpar KV, et al: Pathophysiological changes in the fetal lamb with growth retardation, in Comline KS, Cross KW, Dawes GS, et al: *Fetal and Neonatal Physiology.* Cambridge, England, Cambridge University Press, 1973, p 398.

4. Dobbing J, Sands J: Quantitative growth and development of human brain. *Arch Dis Child* 1973; 48:757–767.

5. Felig P, Lynch V: Starvation in human pregnancy, hypoglycemia, hypoinsulinemia and hyperketonemia. *Science* 1970; 170:990–992.

6. Garbaciak JA Jr, Richter M, Miller S, Barton JJ: Maternal weight and pregnancy complications. *Am J Obstet Gynecol* 1985; 152:238–245.

7. Grunberger W, Leodolter S, Paraschalk O: Maternal hypotension, fetal outcome in treated and untreated cases. *Gynecol Obstet Invest* 1979; 10:32–38.

8. Harrison GG, Udall JN, Morrow G: Maternal obesity, weight gain in pregnancy and infant birth weight. *Am J Obstet Gynecol* 1980; 136:411–412.

9. Horon IL, Strobino DM, MacDonald HM: Birth weights among infants born to adolescent and young adult women. *Am J Obstet Gynecol* 1983; 146:444–449.

10. Hurley LS, Swenerton H: Congenital malformations resulting from zinc deficiency in rats. *Proc Soc Exp Biol Med* 1966; 123:692–696.

11. Hytten FE, Chamberlain GVP: *Clinical Physiology of Obstetrics.* Oxford, England, Blackwell Scientific Publications, 1980.

12. Hytten FE, Leitch IL: *The Physiology of Human Pregnancy.* Oxford, England, Blackwell Scientific Publications, 1964.

13. Johnson SR, Kolberg BH, Varner MW, Railsback LD: Maternal obesity and pregnancy. *Surg Gynecol Obstet* 1987; 164:431–437.

14. Kleigman RM, Gross T: Perinatal problems of the obese mother and her infant. *Obstet Gynecol* 1985; 66:299–306.

15. Langhoff-Roos J, Lindmark G, Gebre-Medhin M: Maternal fat stores and fat accretion during pregnancy in relation to infant birthweight. *Br J Obstet Gynaecol* 1987; 94:1170–1177.

16. Langhoff-Roos J, Lindmark G, Kylberg E, Gebre-Medhin M: Energy intake and physical activity during pregnancy in relation to maternal fat accretion and infant birthweight. *Br J Obstet Gynaecol* 1987; 94:1178–1185.

17. Linn S, Schoenbaum SC, Monson RR, et al: No association between coffee consumption and adverse outcomes of pregnancy. *N Engl J Med* 1982; 306:141–145.

18. Lucas A, Morley R, Cole TJ, Bamford MF, Boon A, Crowle P, Dossetor JFB, Pearse R: Maternal fatness and viability of preterm infants. *Br Med J* 1988; 296:1496–1497.

19. Marsal K, Furgyik S: Zinc concentrations in maternal blood during pregnancy and post partum, in cord blood and amniotic fluid. *Acta Obstet Gynecol Scand* 1987; 66:653–656.

20. Metzger BE, Ravnikar V, Vileisis RA, et al: Accelerated starvation and the skipped breakfast in late normal pregnancy. *Lancet* 1982; 1:588–592.

21. Munro HN: in Wilkinson AW (ed): *Parenteral Nutrition.* London, Churchill Livingstone, 1972, p 34.

22. Naeye RL: Weight gain and the outcome of pregnancy. *Am J Obstet Gynecol* 1979; 135:3–9.

23. Naeye RL: The duration of maternal cigarette smoking, fetal and placental disorders. *Early Hum Dev* 1979; 3:229–237.

24. Naeye RL: Cigarette smoking and pregnancy weight gain. *Lancet* 1980; 1:765–766.

25. Naeye RL: Nutritional/nonnutritional interactions that affect the outcome of pregnancy. *Am J Clin Nutr* 1981; 34:727–737.

26. Naeye RL: Maternal blood pressure and fetal growth. *Am J Obstet Gynecol* 1981; 141:780–787.

27. Naeye RL: Teenaged and pre-teenaged pregnancies: Consequences of the fetal-maternal competition for nutrients. *Pediatrics* 1981; 67:146–150.

28. Naeye RL: Pregnancy hypertension, placental evidences of low uteroplacental blood flow and spontaneous preterm delivery. *Hum Pathol* 1989; 20:441–444.

29. Naeye RL: Maternal body weight and pregnancy outcome. *Am J Clin Nutr* 1990; 52:273–279.

30. Naeye RL, Blanc WA, Paul C: Effects of maternal nutrition on the human fetus. *Pediatrics* 1973; 52:494–503.

31. Naeye RL, Dozor A, Tafari N, et al: Epidemiologic features of perinatal death due to obstructed labor in Addis Ababa. *Br J Obstet Gynaecol* 1977; 84:747–750.

32. Naeye RL, Freeman RK, Blanc WA: Nutrition, sex and fetal lung maturation. *Pediatr Res* 1974; 2:200–204.

33. Naeye RL, Friedman EA: Causes of perinatal death associated with gestational hypertension and proteinuria. *Am J Obstet Gynecol* 1979; 133:8–10.

34. Naeye RL, Tafari N: *Risk Factors in Pregnancy and Diseases of the Fetus and Newborn.* Baltimore, Williams & Wilkins Co, 1983, pp 29–42.

35. Naeye RL, Tafari N: Biologic bases for international fetal growth curves. *Acta Paediatr Scand* [Suppl] 1985; 319: 164–169.

36. Naismith DJ: The foetus as a parasite. *Proc Nutr Soc* 1969; 28:35–41.

37. Naismith DJ: Diet during pregnancy, a rationale for prescription, in Dobbing J (ed): *Eating for Two.* London, Academic Press, 1981, p 21.

38. Olefsky JM: Insulin resistance and insulin action, an in-vitro and an in-vivo perspective, *Diabetes* 1981; 30:148–169.

39. Prentice AM, Watkinson M, Whitehead RG, et al: Prenatal dietary supplementation of African women and birthweight. *Lancet* 1983; 1:489–492.

40. Rosenberg L, Mitcheell AA, Shapoiro S, et al: Selected birth defects in relation to caffeine containing beverages. *JAMA* 1982; 247:1429–1432.

41. Ross S, Naeye RL: Racial and environmental influences on fetal lung maturation. *Pediatrics* 1981; 687:790–795.

42. Ross SM, Nel E, Naeye RL: Differing effects of low and high bulk maternal dietary supplements during pregnancy. *Early Hum Dev* 1985; 10:295–302.

43. Scholl TO, Hediger ML, Ances IG, Belsky DH, Salmon RW: Weight gain during pregnancy in adolescence: Predictive ability of early weight gain. *Obstet Gynecol* 1990; 75:948–953.

44. Sher G, Statland BE, Knutzen VK: Identifying the small for gestational age fetus on the basis of enhanced surfactant production. *Obstet Gynecol* 1983; 61:13–14.

45. Simmer JM, Thompson RPH: Maternal zinc and intrauterine growth retardation. *Clin Sci* 1985; 68:395–399.

46. Stein Z, Susser M, Saenger G, et al: *Famine and Human Development.* New York, Oxford University Press, 1975.

47. Stevens-Simon C, McAnarney ER: Adolescent maternal weight gain and low birth weight: A multiifactorial mode. *Am J Clin Nutr* 1988; 47:948–953.

48. Tafari N, Ross SM, Naeye RL, et al: Failure of bacterial growth inhibition of amniotic fluid. *Am J Obstet Gynecol* 1977; 128:187–189.

49. Wilkening RB, Anderson S, Martensson L, et al: Placental transfer as a function of uterine blood flow. *Am J Physiol* 1982; 242:H429–436.

CHAPTER 4

Fetal Growth

Abnormal fetal growth is common and has many causes. Some are associated with a high perinatal morbidity and mortality and are followed by impaired growth and psychomotor development in childhood while others have no untoward clinical consequences. The bad outcomes are widely known, so fetal growth retardation is often assumed to be an intrinsic indicator of high risk without reference to its genesis.[54] This assumption can be misleading. Many years ago van den Berg and Yerushalmy analyzed liveborn infants in New York City and found that fetal growth retardation had a positive correlation with congenital anomalies but a negative association with neonatal death.[108] This chapter explores the causes of fetal growth retardation, and analyzes growth retardation by its individual causes for perinatal death and for long-term growth retardation and neurologic abnormalities.

THE CELLULAR BASIS OF ANTENATAL GROWTH RETARDATION

Antenatal growth is accomplished through complex interactions between cell multiplication, tissue induction, cell migration, and differentiation. All of these processes are affected by the extracellular environment, including cell-to-cell recognition systems and the release of hormonal messengers, such as peptide growth factors.[28] The last-named include potentiators and inhibitors of growth and differentiation that appear and disappear in a programmatic manner at predetermined times and places. Organogenesis is regulated by a matrix of molecules that influence the pace of cell multiplication, the onset of differentiation, and the direction in which cells migrate. Cell-to-cell adhesion molecules, some classified as cadherins, assemble dispersed embryonic cells to form organs.[9,28,32] Cadherins also determine the manner in which cells of different types become placed next to one another.

Peptide growth factors are protein and glycoprotein hormones which influence cell replication and initiate tissue differentiation.[28] Some of the better known of these factors are insulin-like growth factors (IGF-I, IGF-II), epidermal growth factor (EGF), transforming growth factor-alpha, fibroblast growth factor, and platelet-derived growth factor. Each has a spectrum of cell types whose growth it stimulates. These effects are less specific for cell multiplication than for differentiation. However, each plays a precise role in the cycle of cell replication. Each prepares a cell to enter the next stage of the replication cycle, so for a cell to replicate it must be exposed to a specific sequence of these peptide growth factors. Growth-inhibiting factors also have a role in this process, but their biologic actions are less well defined than are the roles of the growth potentiating factors. The peptide growth factors also augment and antagonize the onset of cellular differentiation. These various growth potentiators and inhibitors appear and disappear in tissue structures coincident with major events of morphogenesis and differentiation.[28] In human fetuses these growth factors are identified in almost every tissue in combination with specific binding proteins which are within or on cells.[29]

The environment in which the embryo or fetus lives appears to have a major effect on tissue levels of the peptide growth factors. In this regard fetal growth is somewhat different from postnatal growth, which is governed mainly by genetic factors. Placental insufficiency,

disorders that reduce uteroplacental blood flow, and protracted maternal undernutrition all slow fetal growth and are accompanied by reduced tissue levels of some growth factors.[48] For example, adequate levels of fetal insulin and IGF-II are required to maintain normal fetal growth.[22] Maternal blood levels of somatostatin are reportedly inversely related to birth weights in full-term born infants.[117] This had led to the suggestion that low maternal somatostatin levels are related to an efficient storage of the nutrients in the fetus which facilitates fetal growth. However, for the most part fetal growth is not directly affected by maternal hormone levels. Insulin, thyroxine, and the pituitary hormones do not cross the placenta in physiologically significant amounts. Levels of these hormones in the fetus are, of course, important. Insulin promotes anabolism, thyroid hormones stimulate neuronal maturation, and pituitary hormones are necessary for gonadal and enzymic development. Pituitary growth hormone promotes both beta cell replication in the pancreatic islets and their release of insulin.[94] There is a possibility that underproduction of growth hormone by the fetus retards fetal growth. Rochiccioli et al. recently reported that 16 of 24 children who were growth-retarded at birth and still growth-retarded at several years of age had a growth hormone deficiency at the older age.[92] The administration of growth hormone rapidly accelerated the growth of 9 of these children.

FETAL GROWTH FACTORS

Genetic vs. Environmental Influences

Studies have shown marked differences in birth weights between population groups around the world (Table 4–1).[31,47] Whether these differences are genetic or environmental in origin has been long debated. Genetic influences are unquestionably present. Women who were growth-retarded at birth are at increased risk of giving birth to small-for-gestational age infants.[36] The fact that male fetuses

TABLE 4–1.

Mean Birth Weights From Various Nations and Their Population Groups*

Place	Group	Year(s)	Mean Birthweight (kg)
New Guinea	Lumi	1962–1967	2.40
	Coastal	1979	2.70
	Highland	1979	3.10
India	Bombay		2.58
	Lower class	1963	
	Lower middle class	1963	2.80
	Upper middle class		2.95
	Upper class		3.25
Congo	Pygmies	1959	2.64
Gambia	Before new crops harvested	1979	2.78
	After new crops harvested	1979	2.94
USSR	Uzbek	1960–1961	3.22
	Kazaks	1960–1961	3.27
	Russian	1960–1961	3.32
Tahiti	Papeete	1950–1954	3.29
United Kingdom		1946–1964	3.35
Norway	Bergen	1955	3.45

*Data taken mainly from Meredith HV: Hum Biol 1970; 42:217.

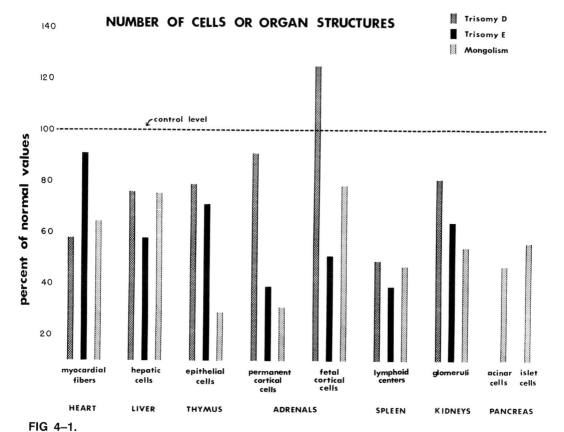

FIG 4–1.
The pattern of growth retardation associated with chromosomal abnormalities varies greatly from one autosomal disorder to another.

grow more rapidly than female fetuses has also been cited as evidence for a mainly genetic control of antenatal growth. Genes could explain this difference between the sexes without resolving the underlying questions of gene vs. environment because genetically programmed higher levels of testosterone in male fetuses could be responsible for their more rapid growth.[114] Most chromosomal disorders, with the exception of the multiple X and Y syndromes, result in some degree of fetal growth retardation which usually persists after birth. This is evidence that the genetic control of fetal growth involves gene loci that are widely distributed through the autosomes. Additional evidence for many genes affecting fetal growth is the strikingly different patterns of fetal growth retardation associated with trisomies 13, 18, and 21 (Fig 4–1).[65,96,97]

The genetic influences that affect fetal growth appear to originate mainly in the maternal genome. This was dramatically shown many years ago by Walton and Hammond, who crossed large Shire horses with small Shetland ponies and demonstrated that newborn foals were similar in size to foals of the pure breeds to which the mothers belonged.[112] Recently, modern genetic technology has confirmed that maternal genes play the major role in controlling fetal growth in experimental animals.[91] Postnatal growth is, of course, strongly influenced by genes from both parents.

All of this evidence that genes strongly influence fetal growth is not proof that the major differences in fetal growth between human populations are mainly genetic in origin. For example, it is not easy to explain by genetic mechanisms why most of the differences in fetal growth between populations first appear in late gestation (Fig 4–2).[25] Late gestation is the time when fetal needs for nutrients are at their peak and nutritional deprivation is most apt to slow fetal growth at that time. A relative deficiency of nutrients is the presumed reason why fetal growth normally decelerates in late gestation and then accelerates after birth (Fig 4–3). The pla-

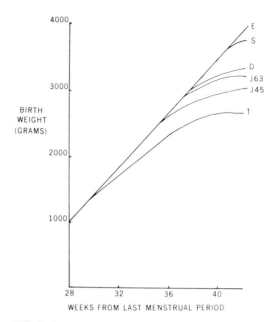

FIG 4–2.
Smoothed birth-weight curves for several populations show that differences in birth weights originate almost entirely in differing rates of growth during late gestation. *E* = extrapolated curve; *S* = Sweden; *D* = Denver; J63 = Japan 1963; J45 = Japan 1945; T = twins. (From Gruenwald P: *The Placenta and Its Maternal Supply Line.* Baltimore, University Park Press, 1975, p 10. Used by permission.)

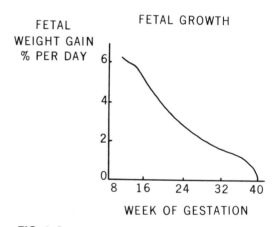

FIG 4–3.
Growth of the embryo and fetus between 8 and 40 weeks' gestation.

centa reaches its maximum capacity to deliver nutrients to the fetus before term, and if maternal blood flow to the placenta is low or the placenta is growth-retarded, nutrients delivered to the fetus are less than normal and fetal growth retardation

TABLE 4–2.

Risk Estimates for Low Birth Weights (<3 kg) for Full-Term Born Infants

Risk Factors	No. of Newborns With Birth Weights <3 kg per 1,000 Newborns With Specified Risk Factors*	Relative Risks (95% Confidence Intervals)†	Attributable Risks (95% Confidence Intervals)†
All cases	319 (12,523)		
Maternal factors			
Thin before pregnancy	426 (2,766), $P<.001$	**2.1** (2.0, 2.3)	**.09** (.08, .10)
Short height (<152 cm)	403 (2,183), $P<.001$	**1.8** (1.7, 1.9)	**.08** (.07, .09)
Smoked >10 cigarettes/day	406 (3,107), $P<.001$	**1.9** (1.8, 2.1)	**.06** (.04, .07)
Low socioeconomic status	375 (5,385), $P<.001$	**1.2** (1.1, 1.3)	**.04** (.03, .06)
Age 10–16 yr	456 (867), $P<.001$	**1.9** (1.7, 2.2)	**.03** (.02, .03)
Blue collar worker	344 (6,970), $P<.001$	**1.2** (1.1, 1.3)	**.03** (.01, .05)
Net pregnancy weight gain < 2 kg	323 (997), $P>.001$	**1.2** (1.1, 1.3)	**.01** (.01, .02)
Unevenly accelerated placental maturation	374 (425), $P<.1$	**1.5** (1.3, 1.8)	**.01** (.00, .01)
Peak diastolic blood pressure <60 mm Hg	470 (146), $P<.001$	**1.3** (1.0, 1.8)	**.01** (.00, .01)
Parental mental retardation	427 (161), $P<.001$	**1.4** (1.0, 2.0)	**.01** (.00, .01)
Fetal factors			
Race: black	407 (6,751), $P<.001$	**1.9** (1.7, 2.1)	**.23** (.22, .24)
Sex: female	378 (7,262), $P<.001$	**1.7** (1.6, 1.8)	**.19** (.18, .21)
Twin or triplet	812 (389), $P<.001$	**9.6** (8.9, 10.5)	**.02** (.02, .03)
Major congenital malformations	461 (119), $P<.001$	**1.4** (1.0, 2.0)	**.01** (.00, .01)
Population attributable risk			**.79** *(.75, .82)*

*Numbers of cases are in parentheses.
†Significant values are in boldface.

results.[68,80] In other instances the mother's nutritional reserves may be depleted before late gestation so that homeostatic mechanisms come into play that further restrict the transfer of her nutrients to the fetus. These homeostatic mechanisms are discussed in Chapter 1.

If both genetic and environmental factors strongly influence fetal growth, it is important to identify their relative roles in individual populations because environmental causes of low birth weight often increase fetal and neonatal mortality, whereas most genetic influences do not have this effect. To try to obtain some new information on this issue we undertook a number of studies using both data from the Collaborative Perinatal Study (CPS) and data from African populations. The nature of the CPS data base and the methods we employed to analyze it are described in the introduction to this book. Very briefly, χ^2 and multiple logistic regression analyses were used to identify factors that were significantly associated with abnormal fetal growth. A method described by Bruzzi et al. for estimating attributable risks from logistic regression models was utilized to estimate the relative contribution of each potential growth factor when adjusted for all of the other growth factors in the model.[5] We first analyzed for factors that may affect birth weight, birth length, and head circumference (Tables 4–2 through 4–4). The risk factors that were found to have a significant association with these birth measurements were then reanalyzed to see if they had an association with perinatal death, with long-term neurologic abnormalities, or with growth retardation at 7 years of age (Tables 4–5 through 4–10).

Based on attributable risk estimates, explanations were found for 79% of birth weights less than 3 kg in full-term born infants in the CPS (see Table 4–2). Forty-five percent of the identified risk was related to maternal factors and 55% to

TABLE 4–3.

Risk Estimates for a Short Body Length (< 48 cm) at Birth in Full-Term Born Infants

Risk Factors	No. of Newborns With Birth Lengths <48 cm per 1,000 Newborns With Specified Risk Factors*	Relative Risks (95% Confidence Intervals)†	Attributable Risks (95% Confidence Intervals)†
All cases	215 (8,798)		
Maternal factors			
Smoked >10 cigarettes/day	265 (2,147), P<.001	**1.7** (1.5, 1.8)	**.08** (.07, .09)
Thin before pregnancy	265 (1,847), P<.001	**1.4** (1.4, 1.5)	**.07** (.06, .08)
Low socioeconomic status	253 (3,772), P<.001	**1.2** (1.2, 1.3)	**.07** (.05, .09)
Short height (<152 cm)	291 (1,578), P<.001	**1.6** (1.5, 1.7)	**.06** (.05, .07)
Net pregnancy weight gain < 2 kg	230 (749), P<.001	**1.1** (1.0, 1.2)	**.01** (.00, .01)
Unevenly accelerated placental maturation	240 (289), P<.005	**1.4** (1.2, 1.7)	**.01** (.00, .01)
Age 10–16 yr	281 (563), P<.001	**1.2** (1.0, 1.4)	**.01** (.00, .01)
Fetal factors			
Race: black	271 (4,842), P<.001	**1.7** (1.7, 1.8)	**.24** (.22, .25)
Sex: female	258 (5,279), P<.001	**1.7** (1.6, 1.8)	**.19** (.18, .21)
Twin or triplet	627 (318), P<.001	**3.9** (2.1, 7.0)	**.04** (.03, .04)
Major congenital malformations	335 (83), P<.001	**2.0** (1.5, 2.6)	**.01** (.00, .01)
Population attributable risk			**.76** (.74, .79)

Numbers of cases are in parentheses.
†Significant values are in boldface.

TABLE 4–4.

Risk Estimates for Small Head Circumference (< 34.1 cm) at Birth in Full-Term Born Infants

Risk Factors	No. of Newborns With Head Circumferences <34.1 cm per 1,000 Newborns With Specified Risk Factors*	Relative Risks (95% Confidence Intervals)†	Attributable Risks (95% Confidence Intervals)†
All cases	136 (5,987)		
Maternal factors			
Thin before pregnancy	182 (1,329), P<.001	**1.6** (1.5, 1.6)	**.08** (.07, .09)
Low socioeconomic status	167 (2,619), P<.001	**1.2** (1.1, 1.3)	**.05** (.04, .07)
Short height (<152 cm)	189 (1,023), P<.001	**1.5** (1.4, 1.6)	**.04** (.03, .05)
Smoked >10 cigarettes/day	169 (1,436), P<.001	**1.7** (1.6, 1.8)	**.03** (.02, .04)
Parental mental retardation	243 (101), P<.001	**2.1** (1.3, 3.3)	**.01** (.00, .01)
Fetal factors			
Sex: female	178 (3,823), P<.001	**2.1** (2.0, 2.1)	**.29** (.28, .31)
Race: black	180 (3,357), P<.001	**1.9** (1.8, 2.0)	**.24** (.23, .26)
Twin or triplet	412 (221), P<.001	**4.5** (4.1, 5.0)	**.02** (.01, .02)
Major congenital malformations	252 (73), P<.001	**2.0** (1.6, 2.8)	**.01** (.00, .01)
Population attributable risk			**.74** (.66, .82)

Numbers of cases are in parentheses.
†Significant values are in boldface.

fetal factors (see Table 4–2). The major maternal factors were being thin pregravid, being short in height, smoking cigarettes during pregnancy, and having a low socioeconomic status. All but maternal cigarette smoking during pregnancy still influenced children's body weight at 7 years (see Tables 4–5 and 4–6). The two major fetal factors that affected antenatal growth were being black and female. The only major factor that lost its correlation before 7 years was maternal cigarette smoking during pregnancy. The only fetal factor that still had a large effect at 7 years

TABLE 4–5.

Risk Estimates for Low Body Weights (<20 kg) at 7 Years of Age for Full-Term Born Infants

Risk Factors	No. of 7-Year-Old Children <20 kg in Body Weight per 1,000 Children With Specified Antenatal Risk Factors*	Relative Risks (95% Confidence Intervals)†	Attributable Risks (95% Confidence Intervals)†
All cases	108 (4,698)		
Maternal factors			
Thin before pregnancy	163 (1,176), P<.001	**1.8** (1.7, 1.9)	**.12** (.11, .13)
Short height (<152 cm)	177 (958), P<.001	**2.0** (1.9, 2.2)	**.09** (.08, .10)
Low socioeconomic status	120 (1,879), P<.001	**1.2** (1.1, 1.2)	**.05** (.04, .06)
Parental mental retardation	144 (60), P<.01	**1.6** (1.0, 2.5)	**.01** (.00, .01)
Fetal factors			
Sex: female	132 (2,845), P<.001	**1.7** (1.6, 1.7)	**.23** (.21, .24)
Race: black	113 (2,110), P<.001	**1.2** (1.0, 1.4)	**.02** (.01, .02)
Major congenital malformations	135 (39), P>.1	**1.4** (1.0, 1.9)	**.01** (.00, .01)
Population attributable risk			**.53** (.49, .58)

Numbers of cases are in parentheses.
†Significant values are in boldface.

TABLE 4–6.

Risk Estimates for Small Head Circumference (<50 cm) at 7 Years of Age in Full-Term Born Infants

Risk Factors	No. of 7-Year-Old Children With Head Circumferences <50 cm per 1,000 With Specified Antenatal Risk Factors	Relative Risks (95% Confidence Intervals)†	Attributable Risks (95% Confidence Intervals)†
All cases	218 (9,458)		
Maternal factors			
Low socioeconomic status	258 (4,055), P<.001	**1.3** (1.2, 1.4)	**.10** (.08, .11)
Blue collar worker	238 (5,360), P<.001	**1.2** (1.1, 1.3)	**.06** (.04, .09)
Short height (<152 cm)	281 (1,520), P<.001	**1.4** (1.4, 1.5)	**.05** (.04, .05)
Smoked >10 cigarettes/day	230 (1,961), P<.001	**1.4** (1.3, 1.6)	**.04** (.03, .05)
Thin before pregnancy	249 (1,780), P<.001	**1.2** (1.1, 1.4)	**.04** (.03, .05)
Parental mental retardation	394 (164), P<.001	**1.7** (1.1, 2.7)	**.01** (.00, .01)
Fetal factors			
Sex: female	282 (6,047), P<.001	**1.3** (1.1, 1.4)	**.34** (.32, .34)
Race: white	250 (4,655), P<.001	**1.6** (1.5, 1.7)	**.10** (.08, .12)
Major congenital malformations	214 (62), P>.1	**1.9** (1.4, 2.6)	**.01** (.00, .01)
Population attributable risk			**.73** (.70, .77)

Numbers of cases are in parentheses.
†Significant values are in boldface.

of age was being female. Being black was now a very minor factor, so its influence on fetal growth might be environmental. Most of the maternal factors associated with slow fetal growth did not increase the risk of perinatal death or of long-term neurologic abnormalities when other risk factors were taken into consideration (see tables 4–7 through 4–10). This raises the possibility that these maternal factors are genetic, surrogates for genetic factors, or if they are environmental, that their influence on growth and development is not detrimental.

Four risk factors for fetal growth retardation also were risks for increased perinatal mortality or for long-term neurologic abnormalities. These were low maternal weight gain during pregnancy, gestational hypertension with proteinuria, being a twin or triplet, and congenital malformations. When children with one

TABLE 4–7.

Risk Estimates for Fetal or Neonatal Death by Birth Weight Category in Full-Term Born Infants

| Risk Factors | Birth Weight Percentiles* | | | |
	1–10	11–100	1–10	11–100
	Perinatal Deaths in Risk Categories (%)†		Relative Risks (95% Confidence Intervals)	
All cases	**1.1** (46)	0.3 (122), $P < .001$		
Maternal Factors				
Thin before pregnancy	0	0.2 (4)	**0.3** (0.1, 0.7)	**0.1** (0.0, 0.6)
Short height (102–153 cm)	0.9 (9)	0.5 (35), $P > .1$	0.9 (0.6, 1.3)	**1.8** (1.2, 2.7)
Net pregnancy weight gain < 2 kg	**1.6** (18)	0.4 (32), $P < .001$	**1.9** (1.0, 4.1)	1.0 (0.6, 1.9)
Unevenly accelerated placental maturation	2.9 (2)	0	**2.0** (1.0, 4.0)	0.4 (0.1, 9.2)
Smoked > 10 cigarettes/day	**1.0** (13)	0.4 (25), $P < .001$	1.0 (1.7, 1.3)	1.3 (0.8, 2.0)
Age 10–16 yr	**1.3** (3)	0.2 (4) $P < .01$	1.1 (0.4, 2.0)	0.6 (0.2, 1.6)
Low socioeconomic status	**1.3** (21)	0.3 (46), $P < .001$	1.4 (0.8, 2.1)	0.9 (0.6, 1.3)
Blue collar worker	**1.1** (26)	0.3 (66), $P < .001$	0.9 (0.4, 1.7)	0.9 (0.6, 1.3)
Parental mental retardation	0	0.6 (2)	**0.5** (0.3, 0.8)	1.8 (0.4, 7.2)
Fetal factors				
Sex: female	**1.2** (24)	0.3 (51), $P < .001$	1.9 (0.6, 1.8)	0.8 (0.6, 1.1)
Race: black	**1.2** (22)	0.4 (62), $P < .001$	1.0 (0.5, 2.1)	1.3 (0.9, 1.9)
Twin or triplet	**5.3** (16)	2.2 (7), $P < .05$	**7.2** (4.0, 13.2)	**5.1** (2.7, 13.5)
Major congenital malformations	**4.8** (21)	1.8 (56), $P < .001$	**30.3** (14.8, 63.4)	**9.9** (7.0, 14.3)

Significant values are in boldface.
†Numbers of cases are in parentheses.

TABLE 4–8.

Risk Estimates for Neurologic Abnormalities at 7 Years of Age by Birth Weight Category in Full-Term Born Infants

| Risk Factors | Birth Weight Percentiles* | | | |
	1–10	11–100	1–10	11–100
	Neurologic Abnormalities in Risk Category (%)†		Relative Risks (95% Confidence Intervals)	
All cases	**7.4** (193)	4.0 (1,065), $P < .001$		
Maternal Factors				
Thin before pregnancy	**10.3** (24)	4.4 (75), $P < .001$	1.4 (0.9, 2.4)	1.1 (0.9, 1.4)
Short height (102–153 cm)	**7.8** (50)	3.9 (198), $P < .001$	1.0 (0.9, 1.1)	0.9 (0.6, 1.3)
Net pregnancy weight gain < 2 kg	**6.6** (47)	4.2 (257), $P < .01$	0.7 (0.4, 1.3)	**1.4** (1.2, 1.7)
Unevenly accelerated placental maturation	**12.2** (5)	3.4 (7), $P < .01$	**1.4** (1.0, 2.0)	**0.9** (0.5, 1.8)
Smoked > 10 cigarettes/day	**8.3** (71)	4.8 (235), $P < .001$	**1.4** (1.0, 2.0)	**1.7** (1.3, 2.3)
Age 10–16 yr	**7.1** (11)	3.2 (45), $P < .01$	0.9 (0.5, 1.9)	0.8 (0.6, 1.1)
Low socioeconomic status	**7.4** (74)	4.5 (420), $P < .001$	0.9 (0.5, 1.9)	0.8 (0.6, 1.3)
Blue collar worker	**7.6** (110)	4.1 (571), $P < .001$	1.0 (0.7, 1.4)	1.0 (0.9, 1.2)
Parental mental retardation	6.9 (2)	7.7 (19), $P > .1$	0.9 (0.2, 4.0)	**2.0** (1.3, 3.1)
Fetal factors				
Sex: female	**7.2** (99)	3.3 (440), $P < .001$	1.0 (0.7, 1.3)	**0.7** (0.6, 0.8)
Race: black	**8.0** (95)	3.7 (463), $P < .001$	**1.4** (1.0, 1.9)	**0.8** (0.7, 0.9)
Twin or triplet	**8.2** (16)	4.3 (20), $P < .05$	**1.2** (1.0, 1.6)	1.0 (0.6, 1.9)
Major congenital malformations	**20.1** (52)	7.6 (154), $P < .001$	**3.9** (2.7, 5.6)	**2.1** (1.8, 2.5)

Significant values are in boldface.
†Numbers of cases are in parentheses.

TABLE 4–9.

Risk Estimates for Perinatal Death by Birth Head Circumference in Full-Term Born Infants

	Head Circumference Percentiles*			
	1–10	11–100	1–10	11–100
	Perinatal Deaths in Risk Category (%)†		Relative Risks (95% Confidence Intervals)	
Risk Factors				
All cases	**1.2** (33)	0.3 (135), $P < .001$		
Maternal factors				
Thin before pregnancy	0	0.1 (4)	**0.2** (0.0, 0.6)	**0.3** (0.2, 0.9)
Height	**1.0** (7)	0.5 (37), $P < .05$	1.1 (0.4, 2.6)	**1.6** (1.1, 2.5)
Net pregnancy weight gain < 2 kg	**1.5** (10)	0.4 (40), $P < .001$	0.7 (0.2, 3.3)	1.3 (0.8, 2.3)
Unevenly accelerated placental maturation	4.8 (7)	0	**3.7** (1.0, 10.7)	0.4 (0.1, 1.2)
Smoked > 10 cigarettes/day	**1.3** (12)	0.4 (28), $P < .001$	1.1 (0.5, 2.5)	1.3 (0.8, 2.0)
Age 10–16 yr	**1.8** (3)	0.2 (4), $P < .001$	2.3 (0.6, 9.5)	0.5 (0.2, 1.3)
Low socioeconomic status	**0.9** (10)	0.4 (57), $P < .02$	0.7 (0.3, 1.7)	1.1 (0.8, 1.6)
Blue collar worker	**1.3** (19)	0.3 (73), $P < .001$	1.4 (0.7, 3.2)	0.8 (0.6, 1.1)
Parental mental retardation	0	0.5 (2)	0.6 (0.1, 17.9)	1.5 (0.4, 2.7)
Fetal factors				
Sex: female	**1.0** (14)	0.3 (61), $P < .001$	0.6 (0.3, 1.2)	0.9 (0.6, 1.3)
Race: black	**0.9** (11)	0.4 (73), $P < .02$	**0.5** (0.3, 1.0)	**1.5** (1.0, 2.2)
Twin or triplet	**6.6** (10)	2.8 (13), $P < .02$	**7.2** (3.3, 16.1)	**8.1** (4.4, 14.7)
Major congenital malformations	**4.5** (14)	1.9 (63), $P < .005$	**5.3** (2.5, 10.9)	**10.1** (7.2, 14.2)

*Significant values are in boldface.
†Numbers of cases are in parentheses.

TABLE 4–10.

Risks for Neurologic Abnormalities at 7 Years of Age by Head Size at Birth in Full Term Born Infants

	Head Circumference Percentiles*			
	1–10	11–100	1–10	11–100
	Neurologic Abnormalities in Risk Category (%)†		Relative Risks (95% Confidence Intervals)	
Risk Factors				
All cases	**7.8** (134)	4.1 (1,124), $P < .001$		
Maternal factors				
Thin before pregnancy	**11.8** (18)	4.6 (81), $P < .001$	1.6 (.09, 2.9)	1.1 (0.9, 1.4)
Height	**8.4** (35)	4.0 (213), $P < .001$	1.0 (0.7, 1.6)	0.9 (0.8, 1.1)
Net pregnancy weight gain < 2 kg	**10.5** (11)	4.1 (263), $P < .005$	1.4 (0.8, 2.6)	**1.3** (1.1, 1.6)
Unevenly accelerated placental maturation	8.7 (2)	4.4 (10), $P > .1$	1.1 (0.3, 3.4)	1.2 (0.6, 2.1)
Smoked > 10 cigarettes/day	**9.0** (44)	5.0 (262), $P < .001$	**1.3** (1.0, 1.7)	**1.3** (1.1, 1.5)
Age 10–16 yr	6.6 (7)	3.4 (49), $P < .1$	0.7 (0.3, 1.6)	0.8 (0.6, 1.1)
Low socioeconomic status	**8.6** (61)	4.5 (433), $P < .001$	1.4 (0.9, 2.1)	**1.2** (1.1, 1.4)
Blue collar worker	**7.3** (69)	4.3 (612), $P < .001$	0.7 (0.5, 1.1)	1.1 (0.9, 1.2)
Parental mental retardation	14.3 (4)	6.9 (17), $P > .1$	2.2 (0.7, 6.8)	**1.8** (1.1, 2.9)
Fetal factors				
Sex: female	**7.5** (71)	3.4 (468), $P < .001$	0.9 (0.6, 1.3)	**0.7** (0.6, 0.8)
Race: black	**7.4** (61)	3.9 (497), $P < .001$	0.9 (0.6, 1.3)	**0.9** (0.8, 1.0)
Twin or triplet	**17.8** (16)	3.0 (10), $P < .001$	**3.3** (1.8, 6.1)	0.7 (0.4, 1.3)
Major congenital malformations	**24.2** (38)	7.9 (168), $P < .001$	**5.2** (3.5, 7.7)	**2.2** (1.8, 2.6)

*Significant values are in boldface.
†Numbers of cases are in parentheses.

or more of these risk factors were growth-retarded at birth they were at increased risk for fetal or neonatal death and for neurologic abnormalities at 7 years of age (see Tables 4–7 and 4–8). It is important to note that in the CPS only 5% of the full-term birth weights less than 3 kg were attributable to one or more of these four risk factors. Thus, only 1 in 20 cases of fetal growth retardation with an identified cause was due to a disorder that increased the risk for fetal or neonatal death or for long-term neurologic abnormalities.

Based on attributable risk estimates, explanations were found for 76% of the full-term birth lengths less than 48 cm in the CPS (see Table 4–3). Forty percent of the identified risk was associated with maternal factors and 60% with fetal factors. The major risk factors were almost identical with those associated with low birth weights (see Table 4–2).

Explanations were found for 74% of the small head circumferences at birth in the CPS (see Table 4–4). The fetal risk factors were the same as those associated with low body weight and short body length at birth (see Tables 4–2 through 4–4). Maternal factors had less influence on head circumferences at birth than on birth weights and lengths (see Tables 4–2 through 4–4). To be specific, maternal cigarette smoking during pregnancy had less effect on head circumferences than on the other body measurements of newborns. Mother being a teenager and having blue collar–type work outside of the home was mainly a risk for low birth weight (see Tables 4–2 through 4–4). With one exception, the factors that were risks for a small head circumference at birth were still a risk at 7 years of age. The exception was race. Being black was a risk for small head circumference at birth, being white a risk for small head circumference at 7 years (see Tables 4–4 and 4–6).

All of these findings show that it is a mistake to consider fetal growth retardation, including a small head circumference at birth, a risk for perinatal death or for long-term neurologic abnormalities in full-term born infants unless specific maternal or neonatal co-risk factors are also present. This generalization does not apply to preterm born infants for two reasons. First, preterm fetal growth standards are generally inaccurate because many of the disorders that lead to preterm birth also retard fetal growth.[42,80] As a result, many preterm born infants who are considered to be normally grown are instead growth-retarded.[76] Second, many very low-birth-weight preterm born infants sustain brain damage in the neonatal period. This damage is so frequent that it overshadows the influence of growth-retarding disorders.

Congenital Malformations

Many but not all infants with major congenital malformations are growth-retarded at birth. In the industrial nations congenital malformations are a leading cause of death in growth-retarded neonates.[80,105] The growth retardation is usually due to a subnormal number of cells in body organs.[60] Not all organs are uniformly affected and the pattern often varies from one disorder to another. At various stages of embryonic development, events that temporarily slow cellular division will malform organs that are in critical stages of being formed, while already formed organs will only be retarded in their growth. Events that slow cell multiplication and limit individual cell growth during fetal life also produce growth-retarded neonates.

Congenital malformations sometimes exert secondary effects on fetal growth. Congenital abnormalities in the pituitary sometimes lead to secondary underdevelopment of the pituitary-dependent end organs. For example, absence of the pituitary leads to adrenal and thyroid hypoplasia, a subnormal number of nephrons, and hypoplastic renal tubules.[77] Congenital cardiac malformations sometimes lead to complex abnormalities in other organs. In the normal fetus, inferior vena caval blood, which is rich in oxygen and nutrients from the placenta, is selectively shunted to the left atrium and thence to the brain and heart, where many of its nutrients and much of its oxygen are extracted. Blood returning from these sites is in turn selectively shunted to the right ventricle and then to the abnormal viscera and placenta by means of the ductus arteriosus. Transposition of the great vessels and other cardiac malformations that mix blood in the atria from the superior and inferior venae cavae produce cellular hypertrophy in many fetal organs.[62] This is presumably because abdominal viscera are perfused by blood that has higher-than-normal levels of nutrients, including glucose. The pancreas responds by increasing insulin output.[79] Glucose in conjunction with insulin increases cell size in many organs. As a result, cellular hypertrophy is striking in the abdominal organs of neonates with transposition of the great vessels and other cardiovascular malformations that are in the category of cyanotic congenital heart disease.[62]

In the CPS congenital malformations that were serious enough to shorten life span or affect a child's health and function were associated with an increased frequency of fetal growth retardation. The greatest risk was for a small head circumference; the least risk was for a low birth weight (see Tables 4–2, 4–3, 4–4). These findings are somewhat deceptive because the near-normal birth weight of many children with cyanotic types of congenital heart disease is due to the hypertrophied cells in many of their organs. These same organs often have a marked deficiency in cell number. This is presumably one reason why CPS children with major malformations were growth-retarded at 7 years of age (see Tables 4–5, 4–6). There are reports that rather severe placental insufficiency is associated with some trisomic disorders.[116] This raises the possibility that placental insufficiency might account for part of the fetal growth retardation that is characteristic of these chromosomal disorders.

Congenital Infections

Growth retardation is common in neonates who have antenatally acquired viral or bacterial infections.[76,80] Several viruses, by their actions on fetal organs, retard fetal growth. It is less clear why some neonates with antenatal bacterial infections are growth-retarded.

The viral infections that retard fetal growth are usually persistent in character. The best known are the infections due to rubella, cytomegalovirus, and herpesvirus. The rubella virus disseminates through the embryo when mothers are infected during the first 8 to 10 weeks of pregnancy. The infections often persist through fetal life and sometimes for a year or longer after birth. Growth retardation is frequent but not inevitable, and the degree to which individual organs are growth-retarded varies greatly from one fetus to another (Fig 4–4).[73] Cellular necrosis is one explanation for the growth retardation, but an even more important mechanism is the mitotic inhibitor that is released from infected cells.[88] Most of the organ malformations that are associated with congenital rubella are the apparent consequence of this virus-induced mitotic inhibition.

Cytomegalovirus infections have an even more unpredictable effect on antenatal growth. Early gestational infections are most apt to retard growth.[50,100] Infected infants often excrete the virus for long periods after birth. Organs of the affected neonates often have a subnormal number of cells, presumably as the result of cellular destruction.[63] Fetal growth retardation is not as frequent with cytomegalovirus infections as it is with rubella infections. Most neonates with cytomegalovirus infections are normally grown.[63]

Herpes simplex virus infection is occasionally acquired during early or midgestation, but it is most often contracted during passage through the birth canal.[4,51,99] The infections acquired during early gestation sometimes lead to fetal growth retardation, including microcephaly.

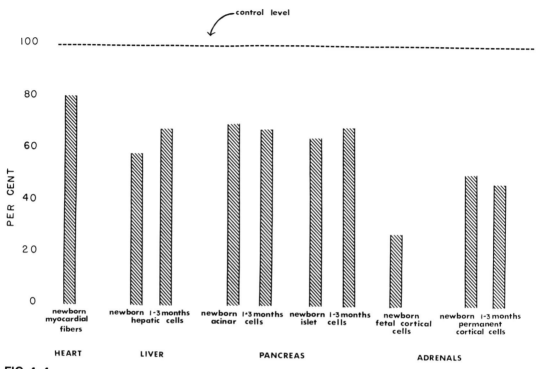

NUMBER OF CELLS IN ORGANS
CONGENITAL RUBELLA

FIG 4–4.

The growth retardation of most organs in newborns with congenital rubella is due to a subnormal number of cells in many organs.

Bacterial-induced acute chorioamnion-itis has been found to be the most frequent cause of preterm delivery in every population where it has been systematically studied.[80] The disorder is more frequent in growth-retarded than in normally grown fetuses.[76] Since these infections usually last only a few days before initiating labor, it is difficult to see how they could cause significant growth retardation. Therefore, the possibility arises that the growth retardation in some way predisposes to acute chorioamnionitis or is the marker for some other condition that predisposes to the infection. It might be speculated that fetal undernutrition, which is a common cause of fetal growth retardation, is responsible for the undergrowth and chorioamnionitis by impairing maternal and fetal defense mechanisms against infection. Under close scrutiny this hypothesis is not credible. First, undernutrition does not usually impair fetal growth until late in gestation, and acute chorioamnionitis often develops weeks or months before undernutrition significantly retards fetal growth.[76,80] Also against the hypothesis is the fact that acute bacterial chrioioamnionitis is more frequent in the gestations of overweight than of underweight women, and overweight women rarely produce growth-retarded neonates.[71] An abnormal bacterial flora in the vagina and cervix appears to predispose to acute chorioamnionitis, so it has been suggested that some agent in this abnormal flora might predispose to fetal growth retardation. For example, a causal relationship between genital infections with *Chlamydia trachomatis, Candida al-*

bicans, and *Mycoplasma hominis* and fetal growth retardation has been postulated from the association of these infections with growth retardation.[89] Assuming such a causal relationship is risky because no linking mechanism has yet been demonstrated between bacterial or fungal flora and growth retardation.

Fetal undergrowth has also been reported with antenatal viral, bacterial, and parasitic infections in tropical settings. Included in the list of infecting agents are the human immunoviruses, leprosy, and malaria.[14,45] Many of the mothers of the affected infants have been seriously undernourished and malnourished. At present not enough is known to differentiate with confidence between the effects of this poor nutrition and the effects of the infections on fetal growth. Chronic parasitic infections reportedly can retard fetal growth. In a study conducted in Guatemala, up to 10% of fetal growth retardation was attributed to parasitic infections in malnourished women.[109] The frequency of fetal growth retardation increased with the number of parasites present, perhaps because the parasites competed with the gravidas for available nutrients.

Fetal Anemia

Fetal anemia has often been assumed to be a cause of fetal growth retardation because when it is severe it deprives the fetal organs of oxygen. It is not easy to determine if such deprivation retards fetal growth because most of the disorders that cause anemia also restrict the delivery of nutrients to the fetus. We undertook two lines of investigation to try to determine if anemia by itself retards fetal growth. Severe Rh erythroblastosis fetalis is a disorder that deprives fetal organs of oxygen but not of nutrients. It does not appear to retard fetal growth (Fig 4–5).[64] Next we looked at severe fetal anemia of other origins. No independent association was found between these other types of fetal anemia and fetal growth retardation.

Placental Disorders

The placenta is fetal tissue, so many growth disorders that involve the fetus also affect the placenta. However, there is a strong possibility that different genes regulate placental and fetal growth, so their growth may not always be genetically linked. Specifically, paternal genes strongly influence placental growth while maternal genes have the dominant role in fetal growth.[91] Normally the placenta grows much more rapidly than the fetus in early gestation and much more slowly than the fetus in late gestation. Fetal growth progressively decelerates during the last 2 months of gestation owing to limitations in the placental transport of nutrients needed by the fetus (see Fig 4–3).[107] Although fetal growth slows, it rarely stops or reverses. Among the postterm children in the CPS who died just before or just after birth without malformations, those who had a normal body weight had a normal number of cells in their organs. Those who were growth-retarded had the greatest cell deficit in their spleen, thymus, and adrenals, a pattern that is typical for late gestational stress (Fig 4–6).

Acquired placental disorders explained no more than 1% of the growth retardation in the CPS. Most such disorders are in the category labeled "unevenly accelerated placental maturation" (see Tables 4–2 and 4–3). The disorders that most often produce this uneven villous maturation are preeclampsia and eclampsia.[80] The placenta often fails to grow to a normal size when preeclampsia exerts its effect early in gestation. Low uteroplacental blood flow is the factor that damages and reduces the growth of the placenta in preeclampsia.[66,68,80] Disorders in this category explained approximately 1% of low birth weights and birth lengths in the CPS (see Tables 4–2 and 4–3). There were no effects of these disorders on head circumference at birth or on body dimensions at 7 years of age (see Tables 4–4 through 4–6).

Is small placental size in itself an

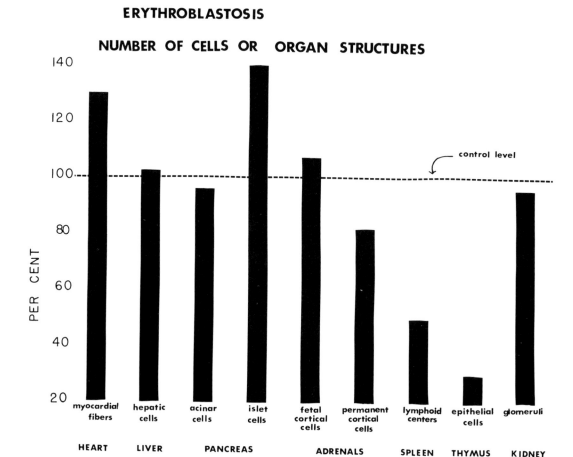

FIG 4–5.
Only the lymphoid organs have a significant deficiency of cells in neonates with severe Rh erythroblastosis fetalis.

important restrictor of fetal growth? The answer is probably yes because fetal growth normally slows in late gestation and then accelerates after birth, an indication that nutrient delivery to the fetus restricts fetal growth in late gestation (Fig 4–3). Small placental size is also associated with fetal growth retardation in a number of congenital disorders in which a primary growth disturbance is presumably present. These disorders are discussed in Chapters 6 and 7 and include single umbilical artery, velamentous insertion of the umbilical cord, marginal insertion of the umbilical cord, an abnormally short umbilical cord, membranous placenta, and circumvallate placenta.

Preterm Birth

There are many reports in recent years of a high frequency of growth retardation among infants spontaneously born preterm.[42,80] This was also true in the CPS, particularly among those born preterm as the result of acute chorioamnionitis and major congenital malformations being present.[76] It has been reported that tocolysis more often fails when fetuses are growth-retarded.[42] This could be due to the high frequency of acute chorioamnionitis among the preterm born. Labors initiated by acute chorioamnionitis cannot be stopped and acute chorioamnionitis was the most frequent cause of spontaneous preterm birth in the CPS.[80,93] Mothers

PROLONGED GESTATION
NUMBER OF CELLS
OR ORGAN STRUCTURES

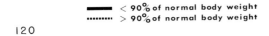

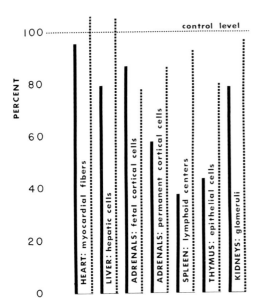

FIG 4–6.
The organs of most postterm neonates had a normal number of cells. Those who were growth-retarded had the greatest deficiency in cell number in their lymphoid organs and adrenal glands.

who themselves were born preterm reportedly deliver an increased frequency of growth-retarded but not preterm children.[36]

MATERNAL FACTORS

Maternal Fatness and Pregnancy Weight Gain

Most aspects of nutrition are covered in Chapter 3. The analyses in this chapter are therefore limited to a brief consideration of the effects of nutrition on fetal growth in the context of other factors that also influence fetal growth.

The factor that has the greatest impact on fetal growth is maternal pregravid body weight (see Table 4–2).[3,80] Maternal pregravid body weights were obtained by interview at the first clinic visit for antenatal medical care. Maternal pregravid body weight appears to exert its influence through its positive correlations with maternal pregnancy plasma volume expansion and uteroplacental blood flow.[18,19,26,31,80] The clinical features of this plasma volume expansion have been well described and include the presence of ankle edema and a drop in maternal hemoglobin and hematocrit values before midgestation as the result of hemodilution.[24]

In the CPS a mother being very thin pregravid had a larger influence on birth weight than any other maternal factor (see Table 4–2). It explained 9% of the 1st to 10th percentile birth weights in the study. Its influence on head circumference and body length was nearly as great (see Tables 4–3 and 4–4). By contrast, net maternal pregnancy weight gain had only a very small influence on birth weight and no influence on either birth length or head circumference. It also had no influence on body measurements at 7 years of age (see Tables 4–3 through 4–6). Maternal net pregnancy weight gain had an effect on fetal growth only when women were thin or had a normal pregravid weight for height.[67,71]

Maternal Gestational Blood Pressure

There was a strong, positive correlation in the CPS between maternal pregravid fatness and peak diastolic blood pressures during pregnancy (see Chapter 3).[68,80] CPS women who had a low pregravid body weight and a low net pregnancy weight gain very often had lower-than-normal blood pressures during pregnancy. When the pressure remained low through the third trimester, neonates were as growth-retarded as neonates in severely undernourished Third World populations (Fig 4–7). When proteinuria was absent,

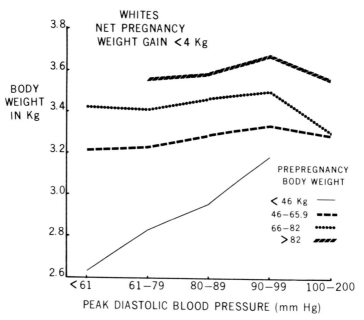

FIG 4–7.
Full-term birth weights increased with maternal blood pressure when white women were thin before pregnancy and had low pregnancy weight gains.

birth weights markedly increased in whites as third-trimester blood pressure increased up to a diastolic level of 99 mm Hg (see Fig 4–7). Increasing blood pressures did not have this effect on fetal growth when maternal pregravid body weights exceeded 66 kg. Increasing blood pressures did not accelerate fetal growth in blacks, even when gravidas were underweight pregravid and had a low net pregnancy weight gain (Fig 4–8).

The significance of maternal hypertension for fetal growth was very different when proteinuria was present. When proteinuria was present, birth weights started to decline at a peak diastolic pressure of only 85 mm Hg (Fig 4–9). Fetal growth was most retarded when hypertension and proteinuria developed before late pregnancy.[17] The slow fetal growth in these circumstances is presumably caused by lower-than-normal blood flow from the uterus to the placenta. The usual reason for this blood flow being low is that trophoblastic cells fail to remodel uterine spiral arteries completely early in pregnancy, leaving segments of these arteries in a narrow, constricted state.[34] The fail- ure to remodel these arteries is the first identified event in the genesis of pre- eclampsia and eclampsia. Increased vaso- constriction of the uterine arteries and decreases in maternal blood volume later in gestation also contribute to the reduc- tion in uteroplacental blood flow when proteinuria accompanies hypertension.[12] The proteinuria is mainly the result of renal damage caused by vasoconstriction. This enhanced vasoconstriction some- times also produces proliferative and ne- crotic lesions in the uterine arteries.[11] These lesions likely further restrict blood flow to the placenta. Low maternal car- diac output, consequent to a low plasma volume, also contributes to the low utero- placental blood flow.[83]

The fetal growth retardation that ac- companies hypertension and low utero- placental blood flow has well-defined fea- tures. The growth of the fetal brain and bone are less impaired than the growth of the adrenals, liver, and lymphoid or- gans.[61] Cells in the most growth-retarded organs have a subnormal volume of cyto- plasm and in some instances are also subnormal in number.[61]

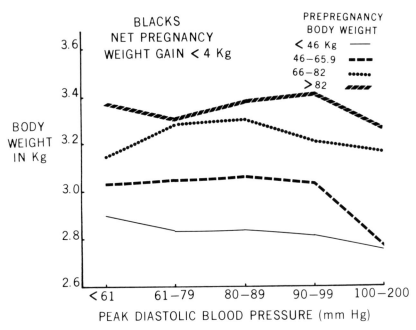

FIG 4–8.
Unlike in whites, birth weights did not significantly increase in blacks with increases in maternal blood pressure.

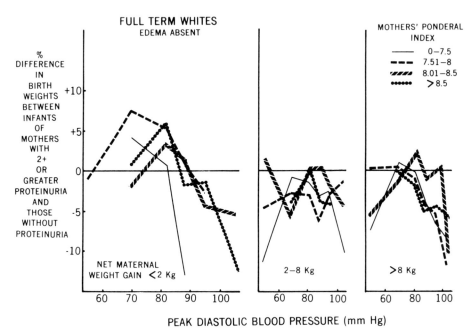

FIG 4–9.
When pregnant women developed proteinuria during pregnancy, birth weights declined at peak diastolic blood pressures greater than 84 mm Hg. When proteinuria was absent this birth weight decline did not start until a diastolic blood pressure level of 99 mm Hg was reached.

When severe, fetal growth retardation in this setting can be accompanied by a high resistance in the placental circulation, hypertension in the fetal circulation, low fetal-to-placental blood flow, fetal renal failure, oligohydramnios, fetal metabolic acidosis, and stillbirth or neonatal death.[6,7,80,116] Nicholaides et al. have reported that the metabolic acidosis and resulting deterioration of the fetal circulation can sometimes be reversed by the administration of 55% oxygen to the gravida.[82] Fetal growth retardation due to chronic low uteroplacental blood flow accelerates pulmonary and liver maturation but its other effects are unfavorable. It is associated with increased frequencies of mild mental retardation, learning disorders, poor coordination, short attention span, and hyperactivity syndromes.[111] Details of the association between chronic low uteroplacental blood flow and the subsequent brain dysfunctions produced by these pregnancies can be found in Chapter 11.

Maternal Gestational Anemia

Another factor that we analyzed for its effect on fetal growth was severe maternal anemia during pregnancy. Some cases of gestational anemia have a congenital origin or are due to blood loss, while others are due to iron or folic acid deficiency and thus fall in the nutritional category. We defined maternal anemia as one or more hemoglobin values of 8 g/dL or less after midgestation. Such anemia had no effect on fetal growth when other growth factors were taken into consideration.

Nausea, Vomiting, Anorexia Nervosa, Bulimia

It has long been known that nausea during early pregnancy is a good prognostic sign for fetal growth and full-term delivery. The frequency of both preterm birth and fetal growth retardation increase when nausea is absent.[106] The effects of vomiting after the first trimester appear to depend on what happens to maternal body weight. If body weight decreases, the frequency of fetal growth retardation increases. Anorexia nervosa and bulimia have no effect on pregnancy outcome if they are in remission.[101] If either is active at the time of conception the disorder usually continues or worsens during pregnancy and there is a high risk of both fetal growth retardation and problems with postpartum breast feeding.[101] Women who are anorectic or bulimic should be advised to delay pregnancy until their disorder is in full remission.

Maternal Age

In the Third World most women have their first pregnancy as teenagers, usually within 1 to 2 years of menarche. Teenage pregnancies are also frequent in the United States and other industrial nations. Teenagers do not complete their own body growth until 1 to 2 years after the onset of menarche and there is evidence in the CPS that the growth needs of such mothers sometimes compete for available nutrients with the growth needs of their fetuses.[69] In the CPS 10- to 16-year-old mothers had growth-retarded neonates by comparison with older mothers (see Tables 4–2 through 4–4). The only exception was the head circumference of neonates, which was not affected by maternal age. Overweight 10- to 16-year-old mothers had normally grown neonates, suggesting that they had enough nutritional reserves to support their own as well as fetal growth needs (Figs 4–10 and 4–11). The growth retardation in children of 10- to 16-year-old mothers disappeared by 7 years of age (see Table 4–5).[69] All of these findings support the possibility that the growth retardation of many neonates of 10- to 16-year-old mothers is nutritional in origin. For example, maternal undernutrition affects birth weight more than head circumference and the growth-inhibiting effects of maternal undernutrition characteristically disappear after birth if the growth retardation at birth is not too severe.[80] The fact that overweight teenage gravidas did not produce growth-retarded

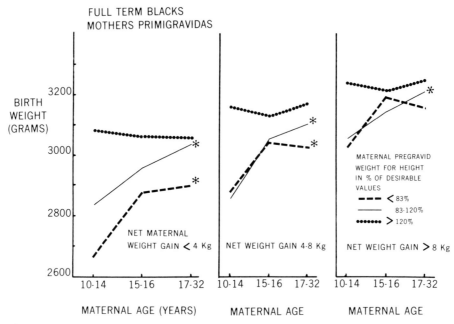

FIG 4–10.

Very young mothers, just beyond their menarache, had lighter newborns than older mothers when the data were stratified by maternal pregravid weight for height and pregnancy weight gain. *P < .05 for increase in birth weight with increasing maternal age.

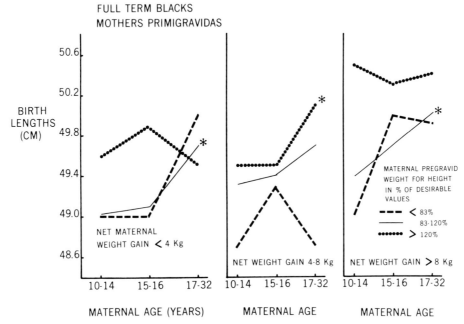

FIG 4–11.

Birth lengths were less affected than birth weights by very young maternal age.

neonates is further evidence that maternal age was not the primary factor that limited fetal growth.

Maternal Parity

It has long been known that mothers' first-born children are smaller at birth than their subsequently born children. In some instances this could be due to the very young age of some primigravidas whose own growth needs compete with their fetuses for available nutrients.[69] Some of the smaller size of first-born infants could also be due to preeclampsia, which is mainly a disorder of first pregnancies. Data collected in the CPS were analyzed to see if there are additional explanations for the increase in birth weights with increasing parity.

Most women in the CPS weighed more at the start of their second than at the start of their first pregnancies. This greater pregravid weight in second pregnancies explained almost all of the higher birth weights of the second-born infants (Fig 4–12). Part of the weight a woman gains during pregnancy is adipose tissue. When some of this fat is retained between pregnancies, it likely provides a source of calories that can be mobilized to support maternal needs and fetal growth in the next pregnancy. How is this caloric reserve mobilized? Pregravid body weight has a positive correlation with maternal pregnancy blood volume expansion, and a large blood volume expansion correlates with a large uteroplacental blood flow.[26,31] There is indirect evidence that blood volume expansion increases with parity. Two of every three women in the CPS had lower third-trimester hemoglobin values in their second pregnancy than in their first pregnancy, suggesting a larger expansion of plasma volume (hemodilution) and, hence, a larger blood volume expansion in the second pregnancy. Lower hemoglobin values in second pregnancies correlated with higher birth weights (Fig 4–13). Second-born

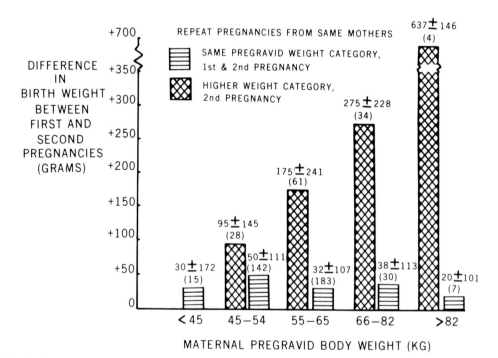

FIG 4–12.
The larger birth weights of second-born than of first-born infants were related to mothers' greater pregravid body weights in their second pregnancies.

infants who were larger at birth than their first-born siblings lost their growth advantage by 7 years of age.

Frequent Childbearing

There has long been a suspicion that frequent childbearing can deplete maternal nutrients and thereby slow fetal growth in subsequent pregnancies. In a Brazilian study interpregnancy intervals of 6 months or less increased the risk of fetal growth retardation by 38%.[15] Growth retardation was most frequent in the offspring of women who had a low pregravid body weight. In a study which we conducted in New York City, successive pregnancies in underweight women produced progressively more undergrown neonates when pregnancy weight gains were low (Fig 4–14).[75] This supports the thesis that undernourished women sometimes undergo progressive nutritional depletion during the course of successive pregnancies, and this depletion can retard fetal

growth. A recent study from Boston found that an interpregnancy interval of 18 months or less increased the risk of fetal growth retardation.[40] This analysis took maternal pregravid weight, pregnancy weight gain, gestational blood pressure, maternal age, parity, and many other risk factors into consideration, so nutritional depletion may not explain all of the increased risk of fetal growth retardation when women have short intervals between pregnancies.

Maternal Blood Volume

It has been known for many years that maternal blood plasma volume increases during pregnancy, starting as early as the fourth week after conception.[31] It appears that a fairly constant level of blood volume expansion is normally maintained until term.[19] In both normotensive and hypertensive gestations there is a strong positive correlation between the size of this blood volume expansion and fetal growth. In a

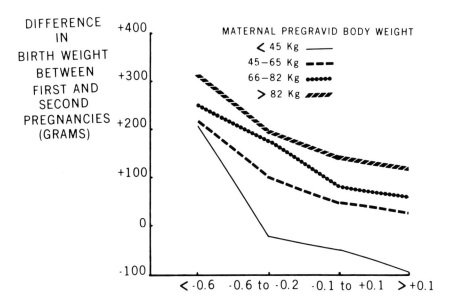

CHANGES IN LOWEST MATERNAL HEMOGLOBIN VALUE
BETWEEN FIRST AND SECOND PREGNANCIES (gm/dl)

FIG 4–13.
Maternal hemoglobin values were lower and birth weights higher in second than in first pregnancies, presumably because hemodilution associated with blood volume expansion and consequent uteroplacental blood flow were greater in second pregnancies.

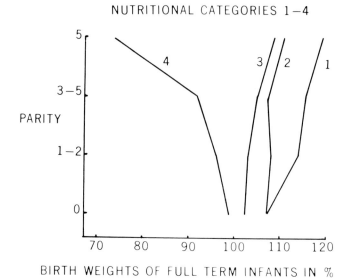

FIG 4–14.
Successive pregnancies in underweight women produced progressively more undergrown neonates at term when pregnancy weight gains were low. Nutritional categories: *(1)* Women who were overweight pregravid and had a large pregnancy weight gain. *(2)* Women who were overweight pregravid and had a low weight gain. *(3)* Women who were underweight pregravid and had a large weight gain. *(4)* Underweight women who had a low pregnancy weight gain.

prospective study Gallery et al. found that gravidas who developed preeclampsia had a normal early gestational plasma volume expansion followed by a plasma volume contraction in the third trimester.[19] The plasma volume contraction always preceded the onset of hypertension. This raises the possibility that plasma volume contraction plays an important role in the fetal growth retardation that often accompanies preeclampsia and eclampsia. This possibility is supported by two other findings. Gestational hypertension has on occasion been reduced by the administration of oncotic plasma volume expanders and gravidas with the largest plasma volume expansions have had the largest neonates, independent of their blood pressure levels.[1,18]

In the CPS there was a strong inverse correlation between the lowest maternal hemoglobin value recorded during the third trimester of pregnancy and birth weight (Fig 4–15). The simplest explanation is that low hemoglobin values usually reflected hemodilution due to a large plasma volume expansion, which in turn insured a large uteroplacental blood flow and an ample supply of nutrients to the fetus.

Gestational Edema

Hytten and Leitch reported many years ago that normotensive gravidas who developed edema in their hands and faces had heavier newborns than nonedematous women.[31] Data from the CPS provide some additional information about this finding. The frequency of such edema had positive correlations with maternal pregravid body weight, maternal gestational blood pressure, and maternal net pregnancy weight gain (Fig 4–16). The edema was also associated with an accelerated fetal growth as long as blood pressures were below the hypertensive range (Fig 4–17). According to Hytten and Leitch, women who develop such edema mobilize their fat stores more rapidly in late gestation than do women who are not edematous.[31] Gallery et al. found that edema is more frequent in those who have the largest blood volume expansion, while the

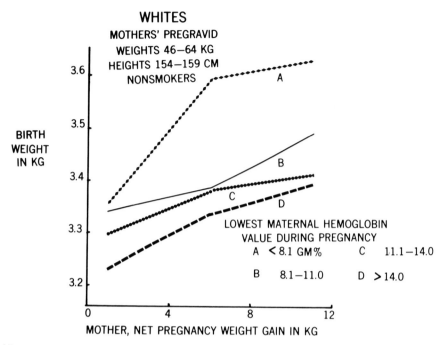

FIG 4–15.
Women with the lowest third-trimester hemoglobin values had the heaviest newborns in full-term gestations.

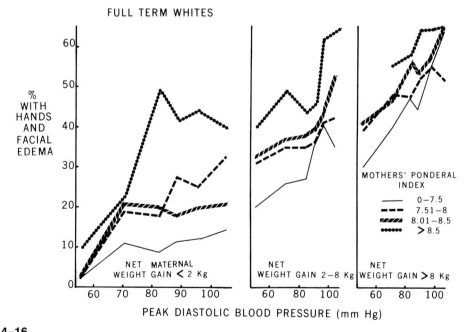

FIG 4–16.
The frequency of hands and facial edema increased with increases in maternal pregravid body weight, pregnancy blood pressure, and pregnancy weight gain.

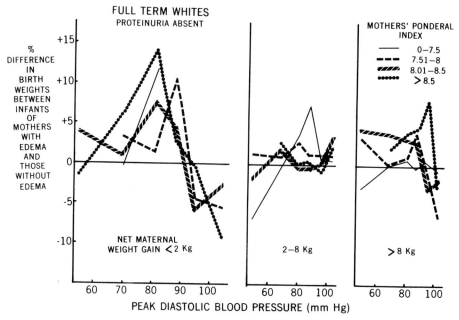

FIG 4–17.
Hands and facial edema were associated with accelerated fetal growth except in women who were hypertensive during pregnancy.

reverse is true in hypertensive gravidas.[19] As previously mentioned, late gestational blood volume has a strong, positive correlation with uteroplacental blood flow, which in turn has a positive correlation with fetal growth.[26]

Diuretics were given to some normotensive gravidas in the CPS solely because they had ankle and facial edema. Such use reduces both maternal blood volume and uteroplacental blood flow, and it reduced birth weights in low but not in high-maternal-weight-gain gestations in the CPS (Fig 4–18).[68] There would seem to be a simple explanation for these findings. Prior to starting the diuretics pregnancy blood volume expansion was presumably less in the low-weight-gain than in the high-weight-gain gestations. A moderate decrease in the large blood volumes of the high-weight-gain gestations presumably did not reduce uteroplacental blood flow below fetal needs, whereas a similar reduction in the initially lower blood volume of the low-weight-gain gravidas may have reduced their uteroplacental blood flow to a level that deprived

fetuses of needed nutrients which thereby restricted their growth.[68]

Diabetes Mellitus

The introduction of insulin into clinical practice in 1922 made pregnancy possible for many women with diabetes mellitus. Fetal macrosomia was soon recognized as a complication of their gestations. There are many standards for fetal macrosomia. Some consider macrosomia to be present when birth weights exceed 4.2 kg. Such weights are reportedly frequent when diabetic gravidas have average daily blood glucose levels greater than 130 mg/dL in the third trimester of pregnancy.

Macrosomic neonates of diabetic mothers have abnormally large deposits of adipose tissue and an accelerated growth of their long bones, so they are both obese and unusually long at birth.[57] All organs except the brain are large for gestational age, while the heart, liver, and adrenals are also large for body weight. These organ enlargements are mainly due to a greater-than-normal mass of cytoplasm in

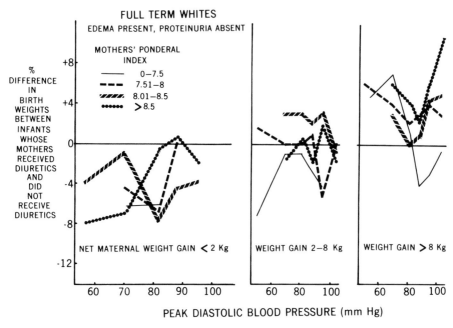

FULL TERM WHITES
EDEMA PRESENT, PROTEINURIA ABSENT

FIG 4–18.
Birth weights were lower when women with low pregnancy weight gains took diuretics in the third trimester of pregnancy than when they did not take diuretics.

organ enlargements are mainly due to a greater-than-normal mass of cytoplasm in individual parenchymal cells rather than to an increase in cell number.[57,79] Newborns of latent diabetic and prediabetic mothers sometimes also have macrosomia and organomegaly.[79] Pedersen was the first to propose a credible explanation for the fetal macrosomia associated with maternal diabetes mellitus.[85] Maternal hyperglycemia produces fetal hyperglycemia, which in turn stimulates hypersecretion of insulin by the fetal pancreas.[86] Insulin is strongly lipogenic and the protein anabolic actions of insulin and glucose explain most of the macrosomia of the affected neonates. There is a direct correlation between the degree to which these neonates are overgrown and the volume of insulin-producing islet tissue in their pancreases.[57] It is not completely known how insulin exerts its effects. Some evidence suggests that it enhances IGF-I secretion.[21] Another possibility is that high levels of insulin are anabolic by binding to IGF-I receptors.[21]

Five percent to 10% of infants of diabetic mothers are growth-retarded at birth. Organs in these infants are subnormal in size owing to both a subnormal number of cells and a low volume of cytoplasm in individual parenchymal cells.[57] These abnormalities are characteristic evidences of fetal undernutrition.[58] Fetal growth retardation is most frequent when diabetic mothers have advanced arterial and arteriolar disease, so this vascular disease is a widely accepted explanation for the associated fetal growth retardation.

In some cases fetal growth retardation starts very early in diabetic gestations and is accompanied by a retardation in placental growth.[87] Pedersen et al. have suggested that the delay in placental growth may be the factor that slows fetal growth.[87] At the present time fetal growth retardation in diabetic gestations is sometimes related to the improper management of blood glucose levels. Fetal growth retardation occurs when average maternal daily blood glucose levels are maintained at less than 110 mg/dL.

In the CPS, diabetes mellitus was not a risk for fetal growth retardation. Part of the explanation may be that we included maternal fatness as an independent variable in our analyses and the birth weights of infants of diabetic mothers reportedly correlate more with maternal fatness than with maternal age or the severity of the diabetes.[44]

Working During Pregnancy

We have conducted three studies of the effects on fetal growth of women working during pregnancy. Two of these studies used data from the CPS and the third analyzed the effects of work on fetal growth in Addis Ababa, Ethiopia.[78,104] All of these studies found that mothers' work, under some circumstances, slowed fetal growth. That was also the conclusion of a Guatemalan study which found that manual work and work that required continuous standing increased the risk of fetal growth retardation.[38] A study from Zaire found that work in late gestation most often retarded fetal growth.[43]

In the CPS, birth weights of full-term infants were lower when women continued to work outside of their homes after the 28th week of gestation than when they quit work earlier in gestation. The only exceptions were infants whose mothers had sit-down work and no children at home to care for when they returned home from work (Fig 4–19). Birth weights were most affected by maternal work when women were underweight pregravid, had a low pregnancy weight gain, or were hypertensive during pregnancy (Fig 4–20). The apparent effects of work on birth weights were not due to shorter gestations or to lower maternal pregnancy weight gains.[78] Unlike birth weights, birth lengths and head circumferences were not reduced when women worked outside of their homes during pregnancy.[78] Such work did not affect children's body weights, heights, or head circumferences at 7 years of age.

The fact that work had its greatest effect when women had a low pregravid body weight, a low pregnancy weight gain, or were hypertensive during pregnancy supports the possibility that work produced its growth-retarding effect by restricting uteroplacental blood flow. The sparing by

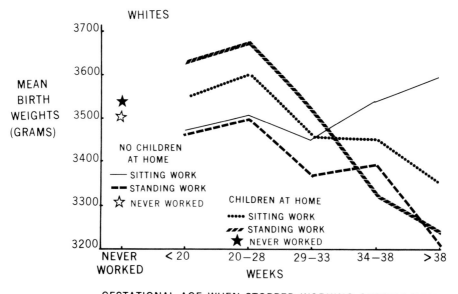

FIG 4–19.
Birth weights of full-term infants were progressively lower when women continued to work outside of their homes after the 28th week of gestation. The only exception was infants whose mother had sit-down work and no children at home.

maternal work of neonates' body length and head circumference is also characteristic of the growth retardation caused by low uteroplacental blood flow during late gestation.[25,34]

Fetal growth retardation was much greater with stand-up than with sit-down work. There are reports that maternal plasma volume and cardiac output are lower in the upright than in the recumbent position, so the continuous upright position required by stand-up work may potentiate fetal growth retardation by further reducing uteroplacental blood flow.[102] In the CPS, women who continued stand-up work after the 37th week of gestation had a fivefold greater frequency of large placental infarcts than women who remained at home or whose employment outside the home required only sit-down work during late gestation.[78] This further strengthens the possibility that stand-up work reduces uteroplacental blood flow because such low flow is an important antecedent of placental infarcts.[66] Finally, hemoglobin values in full-term CPS neonates were

higher when gravidas worked after 37 weeks of gestation than when they quit work outside of their homes before midgestation (Fig 4–21). These differences were greatest in thin gravidas who had a low pregnancy weight gain. These findings are evidence that maternal work, under some circumstances, reduces late gestational uteroplacental blood flow enough to produce mild fetal hypoxemia. This conclusion is deduced from the fact that CPS neonates who were exposed to chronic low uteroplacental blood flow disorders had higher hemoglobin values than neonates not exposed to these disorders.

Exercise During Pregnancy

It cannot be assumed from the studies just described on the effects of maternal work on fetal growth that regular maternal exercise during pregnancy retards fetal growth. With rare exceptions gravidas exercise for only short periods of time, so that the fetus is likely exposed to only

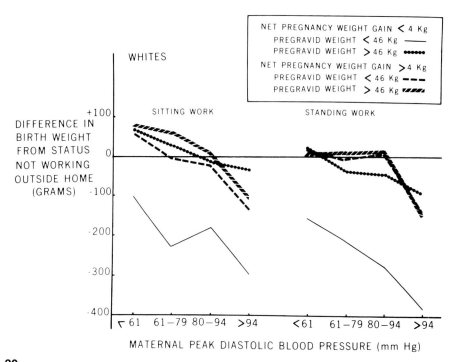

FIG 4–20.
The fetal growth retardation associated with women working during pregnancy was greatest when women were hypertensive, were underweight pregravid, and had a low pregnancy weight gain.

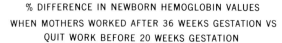

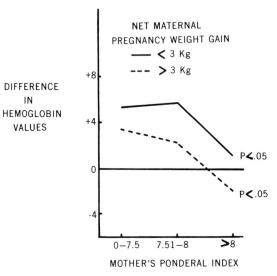

FIG 4–21.
Hemoglobin values in full-term neonates were higher when their mothers continued to work outside of their homes after 36 weeks' gestation.

short periods of reduced uteroplacental blood flow. To date, studies have shown no detrimental effects of regular exercise during pregnancy on fetal growth or on fetal well-being as long as gravidas were in good general health and had no pregnancy-initiated disorders.[30] Questions have been raised about protracted exercise during very early gestation that markedly raises core body temperature because high temperatures in experimental animals have occasionally been teratogenic.[35]

Fetal Macrosomia

Maternal diabetes mellitus is not the only disorder that predisposes to fetal macrosomia. The following nondiabetic factors also accelerate fetal growth: high maternal pregravid weight for height, high pregnancy weight gain, and maternal gestational hypertension without proteinuria.[68,80] There are literature reports that high parity and advanced maternal age also predispose to fetal macrosomia, but as explained earlier in this chapter, these associations are likely due to more pregravid body fat in older women and in multigravidas.[39,80] The major clinical complications of macrosomia are cephalopelvic disproportion and shoulder dystocia, both of which lead to fetal trauma, the need for oxytocin augmentation of labor, tears in the birth canal, postpartum hemorrhage, and cesarean sections.[39] In the CPS the more frequent need for oxytocin in overweight gravidas was in part due to the higher frequency of acute chorioamnionitis in these women.[71]

Cigarette Smoking

The effects of maternal cigarette smoking on fetal growth are covered in Chapter 5.

ANCIENT HOMEOSTATIC MECHANISMS

Many of the findings discussed earlier in this chapter raise the possibility that some of the hypertension that arises during pregnancy is the overshoot of normal homeostatic mechanisms that developed during the course of human evolution. For several million years human nutrition was dependent on hunting and gathering and was therefore subject to the fluctuations imposed by animal migrations, drought, and other weather conditions. From our studies, it appears that a woman's pregravid nutritional stores and food intake during pregnancy have a positive correlation with gestational blood volume expansion, blood pressure, uteroplacental blood flow, and hence, the rate at which maternal nutrients are transferred to the fetus. Some of the gestational hypertension seen in modern women may therefore be the hemodynamic response to these ancient mechanisms, a reflection of ample pregravid nutritional stores and a continuous high nutritional intake throughout pregnancy. This is a likely reason why a low maternal blood pressure level combined with a low weight gain is more apt to slow fetal growth when women are thin than when they are not thin. Such a slowing of nutrient delivery to the fetus would likely increase the possibility that a seriously undernourished gravida could survive pregnancy to become pregnant again at a time when food was more plentiful.

The fetus appears to adapt to the volume of maternal blood flow to the placenta.[7] The placenta often reacts to low uteroplacental blood flow by increasing its vascular resistance, which increases fetal blood pressure and reduces the blood flow from the fetus into the placenta.[6] When the fetus experiences acidosis as a result of a decrease in its supply of oxygen and glucose, the velocity of blood flow in the fetal aorta slows.[98] In this setting the fetus attempts to maintain blood flow to the placenta, heart, and brain by reducing blood flow to its other organs.[2] If this pattern is maintained over a period of time, growth retardation ensues that spares the heart and brain more than other organs.

Endocrine-metabolic mechanisms may be responsible for the relative homeostasis displayed by women and their fetuses during large swings in the available food supply. It has long been known that heat production decreases during fasting and increases during overfeeding.[37] This is mediated through the peripheral conversion of thyroxine to metabolically active triiodothyronine and through changes in sympathoadrenal activity.[37] Such changes in thermogenesis may help pregnant women to maintain their body mass while continuing the flow of nutrients to their fetuses when food is in short supply.

DRUGS

As noted in Chapter 2, there are many drugs that are teratogenic and a large proportion of malformed children are growth-retarded at birth. In addition, Chapter 2 reports on drugs that cause fetal growth retardation without producing malformations. The fetus is usually exposed to these last-mentioned growth-retarding drugs after embryogenesis has been completed. The most widely recognized of these drugs are tetracycline, the antithyroid drugs, and several drugs used by oncologists to treat malignant neoplasms.[8,95]

Fetal growth retardation has also been associated with the use of a number of psychotropic drugs including alcohol, heroin, cocaine, marijuana, methamphetamine, and pentazocine. The fetal alcohol syndrome has been extensively studied and its associated fetal growth retardation widely recognized.[16] Heroin-exposed neonates that we have studied have had growth retardation that affected all of their organs to about the same degree.[74] The brain and bones were not spared as is often the case with the growth retardation caused by undernutrition. The growth-retarded organs of heroin-exposed neonates have a subnormal number of cells, whereas the growth retardation in undernourished neonates is mainly due to the subnormal size of individual parenchymal cells unless gravidas were severely undernourished at the time they became pregnant.[74] Opiates are capable of causing significant fetal growth retardation in experimental animals, methadone having less of a growth-inhibiting effect than heroin.[33,90,103]

The fetal growth retardation associated with maternal cocaine use during pregnancy reportedly affects body weight, body length, and head circumference.[119] The fetal growth retardation associated with the use of marijuana reportedly affects birth weight and length but not head circumference.[119] Illicit methamphetamine use during pregnancy is reported to retard fetal growth but dextroamphetamine in therapeutic doses does not have this effect.[70,84] A high frequency of fetal growth retardation has been reported with maternal abuse of pentazocine during pregnancy.[113] This growth retardation starts early in gestation and affects head circumference as well as other body measurements.

A number of drugs that are teratogenic also often retard fetal growth. These drugs include busulfan, aminopterin, hydantoin, tridione, trimethadione, paramethadione, and the vitamin K antagonists.[23,115]

CHEMICALS AND RADIATION

Polychlorinated and polybrominated biphenyls ingested during pregnancy have reportedly caused fetal growth retardation in addition to other abnormalities.[41] A large proportion of African fetuses are exposed to aflatoxins during some parts of the year and there is evidence that this exposure may retard fetal growth.[10] Embryos that receive high doses of ionizing radiation are subsequently growth-retarded as fetuses and neonates.[53] Doses greater than 10 rem were required to produce fetal growth retardation after the atomic bomb blast at Hiroshima. It is rare for antenatal exposures to exceed 1 rem in North America and exposures at this level are usually cumulative over the entire pregnancy, not limited to a single exposure during embryogenesis as happened at Hiroshima. There is a report that repeated ultrasound exposures are followed by reduced birth weights, but the disorders that led to the ultrasound examinations were likely responsible for the low birth weights, not the exposure to ultrasound.[52]

TWINS

McKeown and Record reported in 1952 that twins grow as rapidly as single-born infants until about the 30th week of gestation, after which the growth of twins slows more than the growth of single fetuses (see Fig 4–2).[46] Monozygous twins grow somewhat more slowly in late gestation than dizygous twins.[72] This is mainly because mothers of dizygous twins are more often obese and the fetuses of obese gravidas usually grow to a larger size than the fetuses of thin gravidas.[71] This growth pattern was recently confirmed by analyses of data from the CPS. Twins were more often growth-retarded in birth weight, birth length, and head circumference than single-born infants, but this growth retardation of twins disappeared by 7 years of age (see Tables 4–2 through 4–6). Most twins go through a period of catch-up growth after birth and reach the size of single-born infants by 12 months of age.[56] This pattern of fetal growth retardation, followed by accelerated postnatal growth, is characteristic of fetal undernutrition. Tissue analyses show that most of the antenatal growth retardation in twins is due to a subnormal amount of cytoplasm in individual cells rather than a subnormal number of cells in organs.[59] Such a deficit of cytoplasm is characteristic of the reversible growth retardation caused by late gestational undernutrition.[58,61]

One member of a newborn twin pair is often more growth-retarded than the other. Sometimes the two partners do not share equally the placental tissue that is present. This might be expected in dizygous twins where the two members have a different genetic origin, but studies show that single egg (monozygous) twins are more often discordant in size at birth than dizygous twins.[72] This discordance is sometimes due to major congenital mal-formations, which are more frequent in one member of monozygous than of dizy-gous twin pairs. More often the discor-dance is due to an unequal exchange of blood between the monozygous partners through transplacental blood vessel anas-tomoses.[55,59] In about 85% of such un-equal parabiotic exchanges the recipient member of the pair has a larger blood volume and larger body size at birth than its donor partner.[55] In the remaining cases the recipient twin is smaller than its donor partner, so there must sometimes be nonparabiotic explanations for the dis-cordant growth.

The smaller members of discordant monozygous twin pairs sometimes have more than a deficiency of cytoplasm in their cells to explain their smaller size. When the birth weight of such a twin is less than 75% of the expected value for single-born infants of the same gestational age, the affected twin's organs commonly have a subnormal number of cells.[59] This may explain why postnatal catch-up growth sometimes fails to bring the body size of such a twin to the body size of its twin.

RACE

It has long been known that blacks have higher perinatal mortality rates and grow more slowly than whites before birth.[80] Blacks as a group are about 100 g lighter than whites at term. It should not be assumed that this slower rate of growth in some way explains the higher perinatal mortality of blacks. Analyses of the CPS data reveal that the two findings are unrelated.

The first issue to be considered is the slower growth of blacks before birth. This slower growth starts only at 32 to 34 weeks' gestation. Such a late slowing of fetal growth is most often due to an inadequate delivery of nutrients to the fetus. In the case of blacks this late slowing of growth is not due to the usual maternal factors that limit nutrient delivery to the fetus. These maternal factors include preeclampsia and eclampsia, being very thin pregravid, having a low pregnancy weight gain, working hard outside of the home during pregnancy, being very young, smoking cigarettes, having a low socioeconomic status, and having a shorter length of gestation (see Tables 4–2 through 4–4). Blacks grow more rapidly than whites after birth so blacks are clearly not genetically programmed to be undersized.[20]

Recently we found evidence that the slower growth of blacks in late gestation might be due to genetically determined lower uteroplacental blood flow. Through the microscopic examination of placentas we discovered that blacks had more ma-ture placentas than whites at every gesta-tional age in late gestation (see Chapter 7). Accelerated placental maturation is a characteristic consequence of low utero-placental blood flow, but in the case of blacks the acceleration was unusual in that it was relatively uniform, not uneven as is the case with preeclampsia and eclampsia. Second, the relationships be-tween maternal gestational blood pres-sures and fetal growth were different in blacks. When maternal proteinuria was absent, birth weights increased with in-creasing maternal blood pressure in whites but not in blacks (see Figs 4–7 and 4–8). This raises the possibility that blacks may be less able than whites to increase uteroplacental blood flow during preg-nancy by increasing their blood pressures, and the resulting lower uteroplacental blood flows in blacks accelerates their placental maturation. A clue to these find-ings may be the greater activity of the renin-angiotensin system in whites.[110] This renin-angiotensin difference may be the reason why maternal peak gestational diastolic blood pressures were about 4 mm Hg higher in whites than in blacks at every maternal pregravid body weight and pregnancy weight gain level in the CPS.[80]

Wilcox and Russell recently explained why at any given birth weight, black neonates have a higher survival rate than their white counterparts.[118] It is simply due to blacks being older than whites at any given birth weight. If comparisons take the different fetal growth rates of the two races into consideration, blacks have a higher death rate than whites.[118] This finding of Wilcox and Russell is supported by data from the CPS. Blacks had a substantially higher perinatal mortality rate than whites at every gestational age, in large part because acute chorioamnionitis and gravidas being overweight were more frequent in blacks than in whites.[71,80] These latter findings are covered in Chapters 3 and 7.

OTHER FACTORS

Analyses of the CPS data identified two other factors that correlated with fetal growth retardation. These were low socioeconomic status and mild mental retardation in one or both parents (see Tables 4–2 through 4–4). Both were still associated with growth retardation at 7 years of age, so they likely had a genetic origin or were surrogates for genetic factors that affect growth (see Tables 4–5 and 4–6). Factors that were included in the index values for socioeconomic status were family income, maternal education, and the type of employment of the head of the household. Low socioeconomic status posed as large a risk for small head circumference as it did for low body weight at birth and at 7 years of age, so it may be a surrogate for genetic factors in its association with growth retardation. If it was a surrogate for one of the disorders that limits the delivery of nutrients to the fetus, birth weight would be more affected than head circumference.

REFERENCES

1. Arias F: Expansion of intravascular volumes and fetal outcome in patients with hypertension and pregnancy. *Am J Obstet Gynecol* 1975; 123:610–616.
2. Battaglia FC, Meschia G: *An Introduction to Fetal Physiology.* Orlando, Fla, Academic Press, 1986, pp 49–99.
3. Brown J, McKay C, Abrams BF, Lederman SA, Naeye RL, Rees JM, Taffel S, Worthington-Roberts BS, Tharp TM: Report of a special panel on desired weight gains for underweight and normal weight women. *Public Health Rep* 1990; 105:24–28.
4. Brown ZA, Vontver LA, Benedetti J, Critchlow CW, Sells CJ, Berry S, Corey L: Effects on infants of a first episode of genital herpes during pregnancy. *N Engl J Med* 1987; 317:1246–1251.
5. Bruzzi P, Green SB, Byar DP, Brinton LA, Schairer C: Estimating the population attributable risk for multiple risk factors using case-control data. *Am J Epidemiol* 1985; 122:904–914.
6. Clavero JA, Negueruela J, Ortiz L, DeLos Heros JA, Modrego SP: Blood flow in the intervillous space and fetal blood flow. I. Normal values in human pregnancies at term. *Am J Obstet Gynecol* 1973; 116:340–346.
7. Clavero JA, Ortiz L, DeLos Heros JA, Negueruela J: Blood flow in the intervillous space and fetal blood flow. II. Relation to placental histology and histometry in cases with and without high fetal risk. *Am J Obstet Gynecol* 1973; 116:1157–1162.
8. Cohlan SQ, Bevelander G, Tiamsic T: Growth inhibition of prematures receiving tetracycline: A clinical and laboratory investigation of tetracycline-induced bone fluorescence. *Am J Dis Child* 1963; 105:453–461.
9. Dan-Sohkawa M, Yamanaka H, Watanabe K: Reconstruction of bipinnaria larvae from dissociated embryonic cells of the starfish, *Asterina pectinifera. J Embryol Exp Morphol* 1986; 94:47–60.
10. DeVries HR, Maxwell SM, Hendrickse RG: Foetal and neonatal exposure to aflatoxins. *Acta Paediatr Scand* 1989; 78:373–378.
11. De Wolf F, Robertson WB, Brosens I: The ultrastructure of acute atherosis in hypertensive pregnancy. *Am J Obstet Gynecol* 1975; 123:164–174.
12. Dixon HG, Browne JCM, Davey DA: Choriodecidual and myometrial blood-flow. *Lancet* 1963; 2:369–373.
13. Doll DC, Ringenberg QS, Yarabro JW: Antineoplastic agents and pregnancy. *Semin Oncol* 1989; 16:337–346.
14. Duncan ME, Fox H, Harkness RA, Rees RJW: The placenta in leprosy. *Placenta* 1984; 5:189–198.
15. Ferraz EM, Gray RH, Fleming PL, Maia TM: Interpregnancy interval and low birth weight: Findings from a case-control study. *Am J Epidemiol* 1988; 128:1111–1116.

16. Fried PA, O'Connell CM: A comparison of the effects of prenatal exposure to tobacco, alcohol, cannabis and caffeine on birth size and subsequent growth. *Neurotoxicol Teratol* 1987; 9:79–85.

17. Friedman EA, Neff RK: *Pregnancy Hypertension: A Systematic Evaluation of Clinical Diagnostic Criteria.* Littleton, Mass, PSG Publishing Co, 1977.

18. Gallery EDM, Delprado W, Gyory AZ: Plasma volume expanders in the management of pregnancy-associated hypertension. *Aust NZ J Med* 1980; 10:475.

19. Gallery EDM, Hunyor SN, Gyory AZ: Plasma volume contraction: A significant factor in both pregnancy-associated hypertension (preeclampsia) and chronic hypertension in pregnancy. *Q J Med* 1979; 48: 593–602.

20. Garn SM, Clark DC, Trowbridge FL: Tendency toward greater stature in American black children. *Am J Dis Child* 1973; 126:164–166.

21. Gluckman PD: Hormones and fetal growth. *Oxford Rev Reprod Biol* 1986; 8:1–60.

22. Gluckman PD, Butler JH, Comline R, Fowden A: The effects of pancreatectomy on the plasma-concentration of insulin-like growth factor I and factor II in the sheep fetus. *J Dev Physiol* 1987; 9:79–88.

23. Goldman AS, Zackai EH, Yaffe S: Fetal trimethadione syndrome, in Sever JL, Brent RL (eds): *Teratogen Update, Environmentally Induced Birth Defect Risks.* New York, Alan R Liss Inc, 1986, pp 35–38.

24. Goodlin RC, Dobry CA, Anderson JC, Woods RE, Quaife M: Clinical signs of normal plasma volume expansion during pregnancy. *Am J Obstet Gynecol* 1983; 145:1001–1009.

25. Gruenwald P: *The Placenta and Its Maternal Supply Line.* Baltimore, University Park Press, 1975, p 10.

26. Grunberger W, Leodolter S, Parschalk O: Maternal hypotension: Fetal outcome in treated and untreated cases. *Gynecol Obstet Invest* 1979; 10:32–38,.

27. Hanson JW, Smith DW: The fetal hydantoin syndrome. *J Pediatr* 1975; 87:285–290.

28. Hill DJ: Cell multiplication and differentiation. *Acta Paediatr Scand* [Suppl] 1989; 349:13–20.

29. Hill DJ, Clemmons DR, Wilson S, Han VKM, Strain AJ, Milner RDG: Immunological distribution of one form of insulin-like growth factor (IGF) binding protein and IGF peptides in human fetal tissues. *J Mol Endocrinol* 1989; 2:31–38.

30. Huch R, Erkkola R: Pregnancy and exercise, exercise and pregnancy. A short review. *Br J Obstet Gynaecol* 1990; 97:208–214.

31. Hytten FE, Leitch I: *The Physiology of Human Pregnancy.* Oxford, England, Blackwell Scientific Publications, 1964.

32. Johnson MH, Maro B, Takeichi M: The role of cell adhesion in the synchronization and orientation of polarization in 8-cell mouse blastomeres. *J Embryol Exp Morphol* 1986; 93:239–255.

33. Kandall SR, Albin S, Lowinson J, Berle B, Eidelman AI, Gartner LM: Differential effects of maternal heroin and methadone use on birthweight. *Pediatrics* 1976; 58:681–685.

34. Khong TY, DeWolf F, Robertson WB, Brosens I: Inadequate maternal vascular response to placentation in pregnancies complicated by pre-eclampsia and by small-for-gestational age infants. *Br J Obstet Gynaecol* 1986; 93:1049–1059.

35. Kilham L, Ferm VH: Exencephaly in fetal hamsters following exposure to hyperthermia. *Teratology* 1976; 14:323–326.

36. Klebanoff MA, Meirik O, Berendes HW: Second-generation consequences of small-for-dates birth. *Pediatrics* 1989; 84:343–347.

37. Landsberg L, Young JB: Fasting, feeding and regulation of the sympathetic nervous system. *N Engl J Med* 1978; 298:1295–1301.

38. Launer LJ, Villar J, Kestler E, De Onis M: The effect of maternal work on fetal growth and duration of pregnancy: a prospective study. *Br J Obstet Gynaecol* 1990; 97:62–70.

39. Lazer S, Biale Y, Mazor M, Lewenthal H, Insler V: Complications associated with the macrosomic fetus. *J Reprod Med* 1986; 31:501–505.

40. Lieberman E, Lang JM, Ryan KJ, Monson RR, Schoenbaum SC: The association of inter-pregnancy interval with small for gestational age births. *Obstet Gynecol* 1989; 74:1–5.

41. Longo LD: Environmental pollution and pregnancy: Risks and uncertainties for the fetus and infant. *Am J Obstet Gynecol* 1980; 137:162–173.

42. MacGregor SN, Sabbagha RE, Tamura RK, Pielet BW, Feigenbaum SL: Differing fetal growth patterns in pregnancies complicated by preterm labor. *Obstet Gynecol* 1988; 72:834–837.

43. Manshande JP, Eeckels R, Manshande-Desmet V, Vlietinck R: Rest versus heavy work during the last weeks of pregnancy: Influence on fetal growth. *Br J Obstet Gynaecol* 1987; 94:1059–1067.

44. Maresh M, Beard RW, Bray CS, Elkeles RS, Wadsworth J: Factors predisposing to and outcome of gestational diabetes. *Obstet Gynecol* 1989;; 74:342–346.

45. McGregor IA. Epidemiology, malaria and pregnancy. *Am J Trop Med Hyg* 1984; 33:517–525.

46. McKeown T, Record RG: Observations on foetal growth in multiple pregnancy in man. *J Endocrinol* 1952; 8:386–401.

47. Meredith HV: Body weight at birth of viable human infants: A worldwide comparative treatise. *Hum Biol* 1970; 42:217–264.

48. Milner RDG, Hill DJ: Interaction between endocrine and paracrine peptides in prenatal growth control. *Eur J Pediatr* 1987; 146:113–122.

49. Milner RDG, Hill DJ: Fetal growth signals. *Arch Dis Child* 1989; 64:53–57.

50. Monif GRG, Egan EA, Held B, Eitzman DV: The correlation of maternal cytomegalovirus infection during varying stages in gestation with neonatal involvement. *J Pediatr* 1972; 80:17–20.

51. Montgomery JR, Flanders RW, Yow MD: Congenital anomalies and herpesvirus infection. *Am J Dis Child* 1973; 126:364–366.

52. Moore RM Jr, Diamond EL, Cavalieri RL: The relationship of birth weight and intrauterine diagnostic ultrasound exposure. *Obstet Gynecol* 1988; 71:513–517.

53. Mossman KL, Hill LT: Radiation risks in pregnancy. *Obstet Gynecol* 1982; 60:237–242.

54. Myers SA, Ferguson R: A population study of the relationship between fetal death and altered fetal growth. *Obstet Gynecol* 1989; 74:325–331.

55. Naeye RL: Human intra-uterine parabiotic syndrome and its complications. *N Engl J Med* 1963; 268:804–809.

56. Naeye RL: The fetal and neonatal development of twins. *Pediatrics* 1964; 33:546–553.

57. Naeye RL:Infants of diabetic mothers: A quantitative, morphologic study. *Pediatrics* 1965; 35:980–988.

58. Naeye RL: Malnutrition: A probable cause of fetal growth retardation. *Arch Pathol* 1965; 79:284–291.

59. Naeye RL: Organ abnormalities in a human parabiotic syndrome. *Am J Pathol* 1965; 46:829–842.

60. Naeye RL: Unsuspected organ abnormalities associated with congenital heart disease. *Am J Pathol* 1965; 47:905–915.

61. Naeye RL: Abnormalities in infants with mothers having toxemia of pregnancy. *Am J Obstet Gynecol* 1966; 95:276–283.

62. Naeye RL: Transposition of the great arteries and prenatal growth. *Arch Pathol* 1966; 82:412–418.

63. Naeye RL: Cytomegalovirus disease, the fetal disorder. *Am J Clin Pathol* 1967; 47:738–744.

64. Naeye RL: New observations in erythroblastosis fetalis. *JAMA* 1967; 200:281–286.

65. Naeye RL: Prenatal abnormal organ and cellular growth with various chromosomal disorders. *Biol Neonate* 1967; 11:248–255.

66. Naeye RL: Placental infarction leading to fetal or neonatal death. A prospective study. *Obstet Gynecol* 1977; 50:583–588.

67. Naeye RL: Weight gain and the outcome of pregnancy. *Am J Obstet Gynecol* 1979; 135:3–9.

68. Naeye RL: Maternal blood pressure and fetal growth. *Am J Obstet Gynecol* 1981; 141:780–787.

69. Naeye RL: Teenaged and pre-teenaged pregnancies: Consequences of the fetal-maternal competition for nutrients. *Pediatrics* 1981; 67:146–150.

70. Naeye RL: Maternal use of dextroamphetamine and growth of the fetus. *Pharmacology* 1983; 26:117–120.

71. Naeye RL: Maternal body weight and pregnancy outcome. *Am J Clin Nutri* 1990; 52:273–279.

72. Naeye RL, Benirschke K, Hagstrom JWC, Marcus CC: Intrauterine growth in twins as estimated from liveborn birth-weight data. *Pediatrics* 1966; 76:409–416.

73. Naeye RL, Blanc WA: Pathogenesis of congenital rubella. *JAMA* 1965; 194:1277–1283.

74. Naeye RL, Blanc W, Leblanc W, et al: Fetal complications of maternal heroin addiction: Abnormal growth, infections and episodes of stress. *J Pediatr* 1973; 83:1055–1061.

75. Naeye RL, Blanc WA, Paul C: Effects of maternal nutrition on the human fetus. *Pediatrics* 1973; 52:494–503.

76. Naeye RL, Dixon JB: Distortions in fetal growth standards. *Pediatr Res* 1978; 12:987–991.

77. Naeye RL, Milic AMB, Blanc W: Fetal endocrine and renal disorders: Clues to the origin of hydramnios. *Am J Obstet Gynecol* 1970; 108:1251–1256.

78. Naeye RL, Peters EC: Working during pregnancy, effects on the fetus. *Pediatrics* 1982; 69:724–727.

79. Naeye RL, Sims EAH, Welsh GW, Gray MJ: Newborn organ abnormalities as a guide to abnormal maternal glucose metabolism. *Arch Pathol* 1966; 81:552–557.

80. Naeye RL, Tafari N: *Risk Factors in Pregnancy and Diseases of the Fetus and Newborn.* Baltimore, Williams & Wilkins Co, 1983.

81. Nazir MA, Pankuch GA, Botti JJ, Appelbaum PC: Antibacterial activity of amniotic fluid in the early third trimester. *Am J Perinatol* 1987; 4:59–62.

82. Nicholaides KH, Campbell S, Bradley RJ, Bilardo CM, Soothill PW, Gibb D: Maternal oxygen therapy for intrauterine growth retardation. *Lancet* 1987; 1:942–945.

83. Nisell H, Lunell NO, Linde B: Maternal hemodynamics and impaired fetal growth in pregnancy-induced hypertension. *Obstet Gynecol* 1988; 71:163–166.

84. Oro AS, Dixon SD: Perinatal cocaine and methamphetamine exposure: Maternal and neonatal correlates. *J Pediatr* 1987; 111:571–578.

85. Pedersen J: Weight and length at birth of infants of diabetic mothers. *Acta Endocrinol* 1954; 16:330–342.

86. Pedersen J: *The Pregnant Diabetic and Her Newborn,*ed 2. Baltimore, Williams & Wilkins Co, 1977.

87. Pedersen JF, Molsted-Pedersen L, Lebech PE: Is the early growth delay in the diabetic pregnancy accompanied by a delay in placental development? *Acta Obstet Gynecol Scand* 1986; 65:665–667.

88. Plotkin SA, Vaheri A: Human fibroblasts infected with rubella virus produce a growth inhibitor. *Science* 1967; 156:659–661.

89. Polk BF, Berlin L, Kanchanaraksa S, et al: Association of *Chlamydia trachomatis* and *Mycoplasma hominis* with intrauterine growth retardation and preterm delivery. *Am J Epidemiol* 1989; 129:1247–1257.

90. Raye JR, Dubin JW, Blechner JN: Fetal growth restriction following maternal narcotic administration: Nutritional or drug effect? *Pediatr Res* 1975; 9:279.

91. Reik W, Collick A, Norris ML, Barton SC, Surani MA: Genomic imprinting determines methylation of parental alleles in transgenic mice, *Nature* 1987; 328:248–251.

92. Rochiccioli P, Tauber M, Moisan V, Pienkowski C: Investigation of growth hormone secretion in patients with intrauterine growth retardation. *Acta Paediatr Scand* [Suppl] 1989; 349:42–46.

93. Romero R, Sirtori M, Oyarzun E, Avila C, Mazor M, Callahan R, Sabo V, Athanassiadis AP, Hobbins JC: Prevalence, microbiology, and clinical significance of intraamniotic infection in women with preterm labor and intact membranes. *Am Obstet Gynecol* 1989; 161:817–824.

94. Sandler S, Andersson A, Korsgren O, Tollemar J, Petersson B, Groth CG, Hellerstrom C: Tissue culture of human fetal pancreas: Growth hormone stimulates the formation and insulin production of islet-like cell clusters. *J Clin Endocrinol Metab* 1987; 65:1154–1158.

95. Schardein JL: *Drugs as Teratogens.* Cleveland, CRC Press, 1976.

96. Schneider EL, Epstein CJ: Replication rate and lifespan of cultured fibroblasts in Down's syndrome. *Proc Soc Exp Biol Med* 1972; 141:1092–1094.

97. Segal DJ, McCoy EE: Studies on Down's syndrome in tissue culture. *J Cell Physiol* 1974; 83:85–90.

98. Soothill PW, Nicolaides KH, Bilardo CM, Campbell S: Relation of fetal hypoxia in growth retardation to mean blood velocity in the fetal aorta. *Lancet* 1986; 2:1118–1120.

99. South MA, Tompkins WAF, Morris CR, Rawls WE: Congenital malformation of the central nervous system associated with genital type (type 2) herpesvirus. *J Pediatr* 1969; 75:13–18.

100. Stagno S, Pass RF, Cloud G, Britt WJ, Henderson RE, Walton PD, Veren DA, Page F, Alford CA: Primary cytomegalovirus infection in pregnancy. *JAMA* 1986; 256:1904–1908.

101. Stewart DE, Raskin J, Garfinkel PE, MacDonald OL, Robinson GE: Anorexia nervosa, bulimia and pregnancy. *Am J Obstet Gynecol* 1987; 157:1194–1198.

102. Suonio S, Simpanen AL, Olkkonen H, Harring P: Effect of the left lateral recumbent position compared with the supine and upright positions on placental blood flow in normal, late pregnancy. *Ann Clin Res* 1976; 8:22–26.

103. Taeusch HW Jr, Carson SH, Wang NS, Avery ME: Heroin induction of lung maturation and growth retardation in fetal rabbits. *J Pediatr* 1973; 82:869–875.

104. Tafari N, Naeye RL, Gobezie A: Effects of maternal undernutrition and heavy physical work during pregnancy on birth weight. *Br J Obstet Gynaecol* 1980; 87:222–226.

105. Tenovuo A, Kero P, Piekkala P, Korvenranta H, Erkkola R: Fetal and neonatal mortality of small-for-gestational age infants. *Eur J Pediatr* 1988; 147:613–615.

106. Tierson FD, Olsen CL, Hook EB: Nausea and vomiting of pregnancy and association with pregnancy outcome. *Am J Obstet Gynecol* 1986; 155:1017–1022.

107. Usher RH, McLean FH: Normal fetal growth and the significance of fetal growth retarda-

tion, in Davis J, Dobbin J: *Scientific Foundation of Paediatrics.* London, Wm Heinemann Medical Books Ltd, 1974, p 71.

108. van den Berg BJ, Yerushalmy J: The relationship of the rate of intrauterine growth of infants of low birth weight to mortality, morbidity, and congenital anomalies. *J Pediatr* 1966; 69:531–545.

109. Villar J, Klebanoff M, Kestler E: The effect on fetal growth of protozoan and helminthic infection during pregnancy. *Obstet Gynecol* 1989; 74:915–920.

110. Voors AW, Berenson GS, Shuler SE: Racial differences in blood pressure control. *Science* 1979; 204:1091–1094.

111. Walther FJ: Growth and development of term disproportionate small-for-gestational age infants at the age of seven years. *Early Hum Dev* 1988; 18:1–11.

112. Walton A, Hammond J: The maternal effects on growth and conformation in Shire horse–Shetland pony crosses. *Proc R Soc* 1938; 125B:311–335.

113. Wapner RJ, Fitzsimmons J, Ross RD et al: A quantitative evaluation of fetal growth failure in a drug-abusing population. *Natl Inst Drug Abuse Res Monogr Ser* 1980; 34:131–139.

114. Ward IL, Weisz J: Maternal stress alters plasma testosterone in fetal males. *Science* 1980; 207:328–329.

115. Warkany J: Warfarin embryopathy, in Sever JL, Brent RL (eds): *Teratogen Update, Environmentally Induced Birth Defect Risks.* New York, Alan R Liss Inc, 1986, pp 23–27.

116. Weiner CP, Williamson RA: Evaluation of severe growth retardation using cordocentesis, hematologic and metabolic alterations by etiology. *Obstet Gynecol* 1989; 73:225–229.

117. Widstrom AM, Matthiesen AS, Winberg J, Uvnas-Moberg K: Maternal somatostatin levels and their correlation with infant birth weight. *Early Hum Dev* 1989; 20:165–174.

118. Wilcox A, Russell I: Why small black infants have a lower mortality rate than small white infants: The case for population-specific standards for birth weight. *J Pediatr* 1990; 116:7–10.

119. Zuckerman B, Frank DA, Hingson R, et al: Effects of maternal marijuana and cocaine use on fetal growth. *N Engl J Med* 1989; 320:762–768.

CHAPTER 5

Effects of Maternal Cigarette Smoking on the Fetus and Neonate

Over 300 years ago King James I of England described the smoking of tobacco as "a custome lothsome to the eye, hateful to the nose, harmful to the braine, dangerous to the lungs."[24] The possible effect of smoking on pregnancy outcome first came to public notice in 1957 when Simpson reported that the frequency of low birth weights doubled when women smoked during pregnancy.[54] Since that time, many abnormalities have been reported in the pregnancies of cigarette smokers and their offspring. Reviews of the literature from the US Surgeon General have reported that maternal smoking retards fetal growth and may be a cause of abruptio placentae, placenta previa, premature rupture of the fetal membranes, preterm birth, spontaneous abortion, impaired fertility, and the sudden infant death syndrome.[49]

The poor pregnancy outcomes reported for cigarette smokers are partially counterbalanced by reports that smokers have normal pregnancy outcomes.[61] One reason for these differing reports is that most of the studies have taken no more than a few potentially confounding risk factors into consideration. Many potentially confounding risk factors need to be considered because the pregnancy outcomes being analyzed have complex origins, and cigarette smokers as a group often differ from nonsmokers in prepregnancy body weight, pregnancy weight gain, prenatal medical care, age, race, cultural origin, marital status, income, type of daily work, personal temperament, and contact with agents other than tobacco that may injure unborn children.[53,61] Most studies of smoking during pregnancy have been retrospective and have not considered most of these potentially confounding factors. Most of the published studies have also not included many major biologic risk factors for the outcomes being analyzed. For example, studies of the influence of smoking on preterm birth, stillbirth, neonatal death, and the sudden infant death syndrome (SIDS) have not taken into account the most frequent disorders that predispose to these outcomes, namely acute chorioamnionitis and the various disorders that produce low uteroplacental blood flow. The data collected by the Collaborative Perinatal Study (CPS) have the information needed to take many of these potentially confounding risk factors into consideration.[11,44] Data in the CPS were collected prospectively and include a large volume of demographic, socioeconomic, work, and lifestyle information as well as medical, laboratory, placental, and developmental data on pregnancy and its outcome. Several thousand women had more than one pregnancy in the CPS and over a thousand smoked in one pregnancy but not in another. Analyses of these paired pregnancies are potentially useful in distinguishing between the effects of smoking and other influences on pregnancy outcomes because comparing the two pregnancies of the same mother controls for many nonsmoking risk factors.

We analyzed the CPS data in a stepwise fashion to try to determine if maternal smoking affects the time it takes to become pregnant, various pregnancy disorders, and pregnancy outcomes. First, correlation coefficients were calculated to see if significant associations existed between cigarette smoking and each of 55 risk factors for pregnancy disorders and outcomes that were included in our analyses (Table 5–1). Those risk factors that had a significant correlation with cigarette smoking were then included as independent variables, along with smoking, in relative risk and attributable risk analyses for various pregnancy outcomes (see Tables 5–2 through 5–12). The analytic methods which we used are explained in the introduction to this book.[8,19,45] These methods took into consideration all of the aforementioned potentially interacting risk factors. To keep the outcome tables short and easy to understand we did not

include factors that lost their risk for an abnormal outcome when other risk factors were included in the analysis.

IMPAIRED FERTILITY

Infertility has repeatedly been reported to be more frequent among smokers than among nonsmokers.[3,15,23,34,48] Investigators have postulated that oocyte depletion or abnormalities in the mechanisms that control ovulation might be responsible for this infertility.[34] There has even been a suggestion that impaired defense mechanisms in cigarette smokers might lead to infertility by predisposing to pelvic inflammatory disease and scarring of the fallopian tubes.[9] In the CPS it took longer for smokers than for nonsmokers to conceive (Table 5–2). However, this association completely disappeared when confounding risk factors were taken into consideration (see Table 5–2). The two confounding risk factors that were responsible for the delay that smokers experienced in becoming pregnant were being over 34 years in age and having blue collar–type employment outside of the home. It has long been known that it takes longer to become pregnant at advanced maternal age. The association of blue collar work with taking longer to become pregnant may be due to less frequent coitus. In the CPS, women who had such employment usually had coitus only once a week during pregnancy whereas gravidas not working outside of their homes had coitus more frequently.

SPONTANEOUS ABORTION

A strong association has been reported between maternal cigarette smoking and spontaneous abortion.[1,27,29] The probability is strong that smoking is a major cause of abortions because chromosomal anomalies with major malformations are the basis for the majority of abortions before 10 weeks' gestation and a much smaller proportion of abortuses of smokers than of

TABLE 5–1.

Risk Factors for Poor Pregnancy Outcomes That Were Analyzed for Their Correlation With Cigarette Smoking During Pregnancy*

Socioeconomic and demographic
  Socioeconomic status
  Mother blue collar worker
  Sex of child male
  Child lost a parent
  Father of baby not living in home
  Unfavorable emotional environment in home
Prepregnancy factors
  High parity
  Mother: mental retardation
  Mother: mental illness during pregnancy
  Mother has congenital malformations
  Dysmenorrhea
  Mother unmarried
Maternal pregnancy factors
  Thin pregravid
  Age >35 yr
  Organic heart disease
  Urinary tract infection
  Asthma
  Psychosis or severe neurosis
  Alcoholism
  Hyperemesis
  Low pregnancy weight gain
  Few or no visits for prenatal medical care
  Seizures
  Pneumonia
  Hyperthyroidism
  Incompetent cervix
  Addiction to illicit drugs

Peptic ulcer
Acetonuria
Vaginal bleeding
Labor and delivery
  Breech presentation
  Induced onset of labor
  Arrested progress of active labor
  Abnormal fetal heart rate
  Used medium or high forceps
  Fetal aspiration
  Other malpresentation
  Used oxytocin
  Labor > 20 hr
  Vaginal bleeding
  Meconium in amniotic fluid
  Premature rupture of fetal membranes
Placenta and umbilical cord
  Single umbilical artery
  Umbilical cord prolapse
  Acute chorioamnionitis
  Tight knot in umbilical cord
  Abruptio placentae
  Placenta previa
Neonate
  Small for gestational age
  Congenital malformations
  Seizures
  Microcephaly
  Peak serum bilirubin value > 18 mg/DL
  Intracranial hemorrhage

*Factors shown in italics had a significant correlation with smoking.

TABLE 5–2.

Risk Factors for Requiring More Than 1 Year to Become Pregnant*

Risk Factors	Rate per 1,000 Births by Specified Risk Factors†	Relative Risks (95% Confidence Intervals)	Attributable Risks (95% Confidence Intervals)
All cases	187 (1125)		
Gravida: smoked cigarettes	**203** (360)‡	1.0 (0.9, 1.1)	.00 (−.01, .01)
Gravida: age >34 yr	**379** (100)§	**2.9** (2.0, 4.3)	**.07** (.04, .09)
Gravida: blue collar worker	**238** (585)§	**1.7** (1.4, 2.0)	**.19** (.13, .25)
Population attributable risk			**.26** (.22, .31)

*Significant values are in boldface.
†Numbers of cases are in parentheses.
‡P<.005 compared with value when risk factor was absent.
§P<.001 compared with value when risk factor was absent.

nonsmokers have chromosomal abnormalities.[1] In the CPS cigarette smokers had more spontaneous abortions than did nonsmokers. These were mainly late abortions because most of the women who entered the CPS did so after early abortions would have taken place.[46] The higher frequency of these late abortions in CPS smokers than in nonsmokers was independent of advanced maternal age and congenital malformations in the embryos, the only other factors in the CPS that had a strong association with abortions. Eleven percent of the abortions in the CPS could be attributed to cigarette smoking (Table 5–3).

FETAL HYPOXIA

There are several mechanisms by which maternal smoking during pregnancy might make a fetus hypoxic. Both the nicotine and the carbon monoxide that women absorb from cigarette smoke may reduce the delivery of oxygen to fetal tissues. Nicotine in cigarette smoke is presumed to be the reason why blood flow from the uterus to the placenta decreases for 5 to 15 minutes with each cigarette smoked.[31] Carbon monoxide from cigarette smoke produces substantial levels of carboxyhemoglobin in the fetal blood.[10]

These factors probably affect the fetus because hemoglobin values in full-term born neonates were more frequently greater than 20 mg/dL when their mothers had smoked than when they had not smoked during pregnancy (Table 5–4). This finding was independent of a number of other factors that are associated with both cigarette smoking and high hemoglobin values (see Table 5–4).

FETAL GROWTH RETARDATION

More than 50 published studies from many nations have found that birth weights are reduced owing to fetal growth retardation in the offspring of women who smoke cigarettes during pregnancy.[7,41,49] In the CPS the severity of the fetal growth retardation increased with the number of

TABLE 5–3.

Risk Factors for Spontaneous Abortion*

Risk Factors	Rate per 1,000 Births by Specified Risk Factors†	Relative Risks (95% Confidence Intervals)	Attributable Risks (95% Confidence Intervals)
All cases	7 (287)		
Gravida smoked cigarettes	**9** (101)‡	**1.5** (1.1, 2.0)	**.11** (.09, .14)
Gravida: age > 34 years	**19** (64), *P* < .001	**3.1** (2.2, 5.3)	**.13** (.09, .14)
Malformations in embryo	**500** (7), *P* < .001	**4.1** (1.0, 16.4)	**.03** (.00, .06)
Population attributable risk			**.27** (.24, .31)

Significant values are in boldface.
†*Numbers of cases are in parentheses.*
‡*P* < .01 compared with value when risk factor was absent.

TABLE 5–4.

Risk Factors for Neonates Having a Hemoglobin Value > 20 gm/DL*

Risk Factors	Rate per 1,000 Births by Specified Risk Factors†	Relative Risks (95% Confidence Intervals)	Attributable Risks (95% Confidence Intervals)
All cases	376 (6,017)		
Gravida smoked cigarettes	**405** (1,901)‡	**1.2** (1.1, 1.3)	**.07** (.04, .10)
Gravida: age > 34 yr	**419** (511)‡	**1.2** (1.1, 1.4)	**.02** (.01, .03)
< 5 visits for prenatal medical care	**420** (1,713)‡	**1.2** (1.1, 1.3)	**.05** (.03, .07)
Gravida: urinary tract infection	**448** (1,037)‡	**1.3** (1.2, 1.5)	**.05** (.03, .06)
Gravida: blue collar worker	**400** (3,148)‡	**1.1** (1.1, 1.2)	**.06** (.03, .09)
Father of baby not in home	**424** (1,362)‡	**1.2** (1.1, 1.3)	**.04** (.02, .05)
Population attributable risk			**.29** (.24, .34)

Significant values are in boldface.
†*Numbers of cases are in parentheses.*
‡*P* < .001 compared with value when risk factor was absent.

cigarettes smoked, but not with the number of years gravidas had smoked or with the number of cigarettes smoked before pregnancy (Fig 5–1).[7,13,28,49,57,59] Quitting smoking before the 30th week of gestation reportedly reduces this growth retardation.[33] Complete cessation of smoking is reportedly much more effective than partial cessation in increasing fetal growth.[21]

Speculations on the cause of the growth retardation include suboptimal maternal food intake, carboxyhemoglobin-induced fetal hypoxia, reductions in uteroplacental blood flow due to vasospasm in the uterus or to drops in maternal blood pressure, low fetoplacental blood flow, direct toxic effects of tobacco products on fetal organs, and genetic differences between smokers and nonsmokers.[32,36,41,44,47,51,59,60] The growth retardation could also be related to maternal pregravid body weight because as a group, mothers who smoke during pregnancy have lower prepregnancy body weights than nonsmokers,

and maternal pregravid body weight has a strong, positive influence on fetal growth.[44] Finally, it has been reported that the growth retardation associated with maternal smoking is related to a significant increase in fetoplacental vascular resistance.[36] Such an increase often accompanies the fetal growth retardation that is present with disorders that produce chronic low uteroplacental blood flow.[17] As previously noted, cigarette smoking reduces oxygen delivery to the placenta by reducing blood flow into the intervillous space.[31] Oxygen deprivation in turn initiates placental vasoconstriction, which increases placental vascular resistance.[22] This raises the possibility that some of the growth retardation associated with maternal cigarette smoking during pregnancy could be related to inadequate fetal blood flow into the placenta.

In the CPS, smoking-associated fetal growth retardation did not disappear when data were stratified by mothers' pregravid body weights and pregnancy

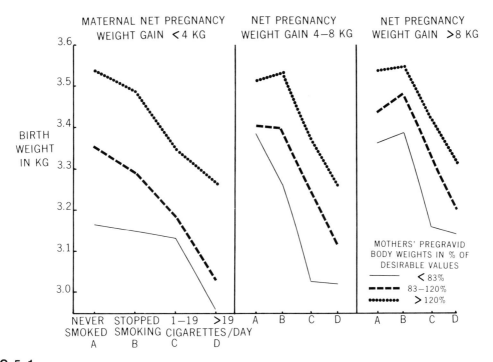

FIG 5–1.

In the CPS the low birth weights associated with maternal cigarette smoking during pregnancy were not abolished when the data were stratified by maternal pregravid body weights and pregnancy weight gains.

weight gains, so the growth retardation was not solely due to low maternal pre-gravid nutritional stores or to low food intake during pregnancy (see Fig 5–1). The growth retardation was present in intra-pair comparisons of siblings whose mothers smoked in one but not in the other of their two pregnancies, so the growth retardation was not likely due to genetic factors (Table 5–5). The growth retardation was not due to uterine vascular damage acquired before pregnancy because no growth retardation was present when mothers stopped smoking before or during early pregnancy. Finally, a strong, inverse correlation between smoking and low birth weight but not small head cir-cumference persisted after taking a number of other factors that affect fetal growth into consideration (Tables 5–6 and 5–7). This supports all of the previous reports that maternal cigarette smoking during pregnancy independently retards fetal growth.

Fetal hypoxia produced by smoking-generated carboxyhemoglobin may have little or no role in the growth retardation produced by cigarette smoking because previous studies have shown that oxygen transfer from the maternal to the fetal blood is little affected by maternal smok-ing.[16] In a study of erythroblastosis fetalis we found that fetal hypoxia, in the absence of low uteroplacental blood flow, had little

TABLE 5–5.

Intrapair Comparisons of Siblings Whose Mothers Smoked in One but Not in the Other of Consecutive Full-Term Pregnancies*

	Mean Measurements (N = 140)	
	Birth	7 Years of Age
Body weights		
Stopped smoking	3,341 ± 440 g ·	24.3 ± 4.6 kg
Continued smoking	2,898 ± 384,$P<.001$	22.9 ± 3.1 kg, $P<.001$
Body lengths (cm)		
Stopped smoking	50.9 ± 2.2	121.2 ± 5.0
Continued smoking	50.3 ± 2.4†	119.5 ± 4.6, $P<.001$
Head circumferences (cm)		
Stopped smoking	34.4 ± 1.2	51.6 ± 1.3
Continued smoking	33.8 ± 1.3, $P<.001$	51.4 ± 1.4
Placental weights (g)		
Stopped smoking	458 ± 88	
Continued smoking	431 ± 84, $P<.01$	

*All values ± 1 SD.
†$P<.02$ compared with value in stopped-smoking category.

TABLE 5–6.

Risk Factors for Fetal Growth Retardation (Birth Weight Percentiles 1–10)*

Risk Factors	Rate per 1,000 Births by Specified Risk Factors†	Relative Risks (95% Confidence Intervals)	Attributable Risks (95% Confidence Intervals)
All cases	99 (4,022)		
Gravida smoked cigarettes	**122** (1,354), $P<.001$	**1.7** (1.6, 1.9)	**.17** (.14, .20)
Fetus-congenital malformations	103 (295), $P<.01$	1.1 (1.0, 1.2)	.01 (.00, .02)
Gravida: thin pregravid	**106** (3,241), $P<.01$	**1.8** (1.6, 1.9)	**.24** (.20, .28)
Low pregnancy weight gain	103 (342)‡	1.2 (1.1, 1.3)	.03 (.01, .05)
Gravida: blue collar worker	**106** (2,269), $P<.01$	**1.4** (1.3, 1.6)	**.13** (.09, .17)
Population attributable risk			**.58** (.49, .66)

*Significant values are in boldface.
†Numbers of cases are in parentheses.
‡$P<.02$ compared with value when risk factor was absent.

effect on fetal growth.[37] In the CPS, a positive correlation existed between the birth weights and the hemoglobin levels in neonates of heavy smokers (Fig 5–2). High hemoglobin levels in neonates are a characteristic consequence of chronic fetal hypoxemia. If chronic hypoxia were the cause of smoking-generated fetal growth retardation, one would expect birth weights to have decreased with rising hemoglobin levels in neonates. Finding a reversed relationship is still another piece of evidence that hypoxia is not the cause of the fetal growth retardation associated with mothers' smoking during pregnancy.

There is a report that a large caffeine consumption potentiates the fetal growth retardation associated with cigarette smoking.[4] There are more than 4,000 chemical compounds in tobacco smoke, few of which have been tested for their effects on fetal growth. Perhaps one or more of these untested compounds is responsible for the growth retardation.

TABLE 5–7.

Risk Factors for Microcephaly at Birth (Head Circumference Percentiles 1–10)*

Risk Factors	Rate per 1,000 Births by Specified Risk Factors†	Relative Risks (95% Confidence Intervals)	Attributable Risks (95% Confidence Intervals)
All cases	99 (3,822)		
Gravida smoked cigarettes	**146** (1,533), P<.001	1.0 (0.8, 1.2)	.00 (−.01, .01)
Fetus: congenital malformations	**114** (284)‡	**1.1** (1.0, 1.2)	**.02** (.01, .03)
Gravida: thin pregravid	**104** (3,248), P<.001	**1.4** (1.2, 1.7)	**.22** (.17, .28)
Gravida: blue collar worker	**105** (2,134), P<.001	**1.1** (1.0, 1.3)	**.04** (.01, .07)
Population attributable risk			**.27** (.18, .37)

*Significant values are in boldface.
†Numbers of cases are in parentheses.
‡P<.005 compared with value when risk factor was absent.

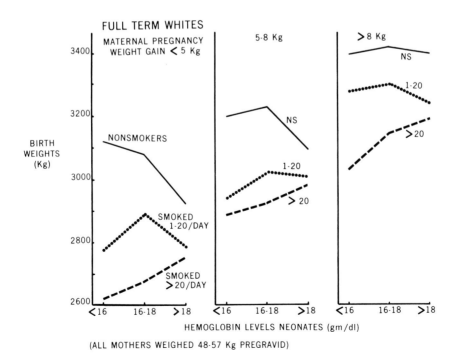

FIG 5–2.
In the children of heavy smokers neonatal hemoglobin values increased with birth weights. The reverse was true for the children of nonsmokers.

FETAL LUNG MATURATION AND LUNG GROWTH

In the CPS and in other studies fetal lungs matured more rapidly when women smoked than when they did not smoke during pregnancy.[14,44,50] This accelera-

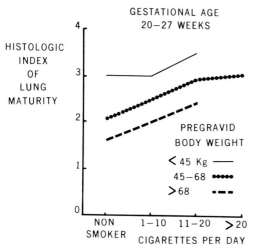

FIG 5–3.
Fetal lungs matured more rapidly when women smoked than when they did not smoke during pregnancy.

tion of fetal lung maturation increased with the number of cigarettes smoked and was independent of several other factors that accelerate lung maturation (Fig 5–3). As a result, the respiratory distress syndrome had a lower frequency at every preterm gestational age in the neonates of smokers than of nonsmokers (Fig 5–4). The greater the number of cigarettes smoked, the lower were the frequency and the case fatality rate of the neonatal respiratory distress syndrome. The result was a lower neonatal mortality rate due to the neonatal respiratory distress syndrome for infants born before 30 weeks to smokers than to nonsmokers (Fig 5–5). Low uteroplacental blood flow has been known for some years to accelerate fetal lung maturation. Since smoking reduces such flow, underperfusion is a possible explanation for the accelerated lung maturation.[18,50] Collins et al. and others have reported that maternal smoking during pregnancy can retard fetal lung growth and this growth retardation is perpetuated when children are passively exposed to cigarette smoke after birth.[12,56] The clinical significance of this growth retardation remains to be determined.

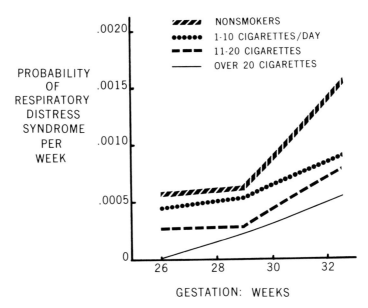

FIG 5–4.
In the CPS the probability of neonates developing the respiratory distress syndrome markedly decreased when their mothers had smoked during pregnancy.

PRETERM DELIVERY

Several investigators have claimed that smoking increases the frequency of preterm birth by as much as 50%.[5,30] Other investigators have failed to find such an effect.[20] We used the data from the CPS to investigate this issue. In the CPS cigarette smokers had a 1.05 relative risk of spontaneous preterm delivery before taking potentially confounding risk factors into consideration. After taking more than 20 of these risk factors into consideration the relative risk was reduced to 1.00, so smoking did not increase the risk of preterm birth in the CPS apart from its small roles in the genesis of abruptio placentae and premature rupture of the fetal membranes (Tables 5–8 through 5–10).

PERINATAL MORTALITY

There are many reports that women who smoke cigarettes have more stillbirths and neonatal deaths than nonsmokers.[2,7,26,35] Many have accepted these findings at face value because maternal cigarette smoking retards fetal growth and there is a well-established positive correlation between fetal growth retardation and perinatal mortality. Cigarette smoking is also widely accepted as a cause of perinatal death because there are many reports that maternal smoking increases the risk for both abruptio placentae and placenta previa.[38,40,44] Many years ago Yerushalmy found that the growth-retarded neonates of cigarette smokers had a better survival rate than the same-sized infants of nonsmokers.[61] In the CPS the uncorrected relative risk of maternal smoking for the death of fetuses and neonates was 1.22, which is close to the 1.28 value in the 1972 report of the British Perinatal Mortality Survey.[7] The British survey did not collect information on the other risk factors on which information is needed to do a credible study of the reasons why smoking increased the risk for perinatal death. Information on many of these other risk factors is available in

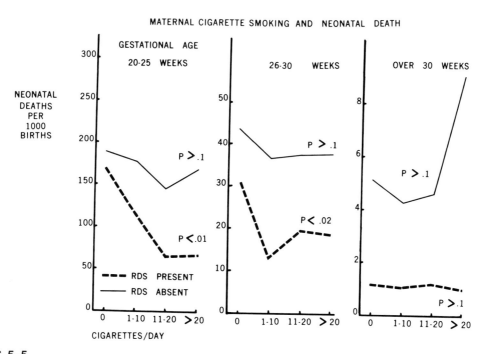

FIG 5–5.
For infants born before 30 weeks' gestation, death related to the neonatal respiratory distress syndrome *(RDS)* was less frequent when mothers had smoked than when they had not smoked during pregnancy.

TABLE 5–8.

Risk Factors for Spontaneous Preterm Birth*

Risk Factors	Rate per 1,000 Births by Specified Risk Factors†	Relative Risks (95% Confidence Intervals)	Attributable Risks (95% Confidence Intervals)
All cases	254 (12,225)		
Gravida smoked cigarettes	**260** (3,283)‡	1.0 (0.9, 1.1)	.00 (−.01, .01)
Gravida: unmarried	**313** (2,734)‡	**1.4** (1.3, 1.5)	**.05** (.04, .06)
Gravida: high parity	**258** (8,934)‡	1.1 (1.0, 1.2)	**.07** (.04, .10)
Urinary tract infection	**281** (2,035)‡	**1.1** (1.1, 1.2)	**.02** (.01, .03)
Incompetent cervix	**720** (152)‡	**5.9** (4.2, 8.2)	**.01** (.01, .02)
Acute chorioamnionitis	**483** (2,332)‡	**98** (64, 145)	**.19** (.18, .20)
Premature membrane rupture	**346** (2,797)‡	**1.5** (1.4, 1.6)	**.12** (.11, .13)
Gravida: blue collar worker	**273** (7,005)‡	**1.1** (1.1, 1.2)	**.05** (.03, .07)
Population attributable risk			*.62* (.59, .62)

Significant values are in boldface.
†Numbers of cases are in parentheses.
‡P < .001 compared with value when risk factor was absent.

TABLE 5–9.

Risk Estimates for Antecedents to the Development of Fresh Abruptio Placentae*

Risk Factors	No. of cases of Abruptio Placentae per 1,000 Cases With Risk Factor†	Relative Risks (95% Confidence Intervals)	Attributable Risks (95% Confidence Intervals)
All cases	21 (1,140)		
Maternal factors			
Smoked during pregnancy	**27** (295), P < .001	**1.5** (1.2, 1.9)	**.07** (.05, .09)
Preeclampsia, eclampsia	**35** (319), P < .001	**1.7** (1.4, 2.0)	**.09** (.06, .12)
Age ≥ 35 yr	**28** (91), P < .005	**1.8** (1.2, 2.6)	**.03** (.02, .04)
Fetal factor			
Major fetal malformations	**32** (160), P < .001	**1.6** (1.1, 2.2)	**.03** (.02, .04)
Placental factor			
Acute chorioamnionitis	**39** (269), P < .001	**1.9** (1.7, 2.2)	**.08** (.05, .11)
Markers for vigorous fetal motor activity			
Unusually long umbilical cord	**24** (517), P < .002	**1.6** (1.2, 2.0)	**.11** (.09, .13)
Other indicators			*.01* (.00, .02)
Population attributable risk			*.40* (.36, .45)

Significant values are in boldface.
†Numbers of cases are in parentheses.

the CPS. When these risk factors were taken into consideration, mothers' smoking during pregnancy was no longer a risk factor for fetal or neonatal death (Table 5–11). Based on these findings it cannot be taken for granted that persuading women to stop smoking during pregnancy will reduce perinatal mortality rates.

OTHER COMPLICATIONS OF PREGNANCY

In the CPS premature separation of the placenta from the wall of the uterus (abruptio placentae) increased in frequency with the number of cigarettes smoked (see Table 5–9).[38,39,44] This risk decreased to the level found in nonsmok-

TABLE 5–10.

Risk Estimates for Antecedents to the Development of Fetal Membrane Rupture 1–12 Hours Before Onset of Labor*

Risk Factors	No. of Cases of Premature Membrane Rupture per 1,000 Cases With Risk Factor†	Relative Risks (95% Confidence Intervals)	Attributable Risks (95% Confidence Intervals)
All cases	98 (5,829)		
Maternal factors			
Smoked during pregnancy	117 (1,325), *P*<.001	**1.3** (1.2, 1.4)	**.05** (.04, .06)
Age ≥ 35 yr	124 (448), *P*<.001	**1.3** (1.2, 1.5)	**.02** (.01, .02)
Incompetent cervix	201 (48), *P*<.001	**2.2** (1.2, 4.1)	**.01** (.00, .01)
Placental factor			
Acute chorioamnionitis	160 (1,349), *P*<.001	**1.9** (1.8, 2.1)	**.44** (.41, .47)
Markers for high fetal motor activity			
Diffuse subchorionic fibrin	109 (862), *P*<.001	**1.2** (1.1, 1.3)	**.04** (.03, .05)
Unusually long umbilical cord	111 (662), *P*<.01	**1.1** (1.0, 1.2)	**.02** (.01, .03)
Other indicators			**.02** (.00, .05)
Population attributable risk			***.59*** (.56, .63)

*Significant values are in boldface.
†Numbers of cases are in parentheses.

TABLE 5–11.

Risk Factors for Fetal or Neonatal Death*

Risk Factors	Rate per 1,000 Births by Specified Risk Factor†	Relative Risks (95% Confidence Intervals)	Attributable Risks (95% Confidence Intervals)
All cases	56 (3,265)		
Gravida: smoked cigarettes	61 (943), *P*<.001	1.0 (.09, 1.1)	.00 (−.01, .01)
Gravida: age >34 yr	98 (431), *P*<.001	**1.6** (1.0, 2.4)	**.01** (.00, .01)
Preterm birth	116 (1,366), *P*<.001	**2.4** (1.8, 3.2)	**.16** (.12, .19)
Acute chorioamnionitis	72 (719), *P*<.001	**2.1** (1.6, 2.7)	**.14** (.10, .18)
Breech presentation	228 (485), *P*<.001	**2.7** (1.6, 4.4)	**.04** (.02, .06)
Premature membrane rupture	61 (575), *P*<.001	**1.7** (1.4, 2.1)	**.02** (.00, .04)
Low pregnancy weight gain	65 (288)‡	**1.3** (1.0, 1.8)	**.05** (.03, .07)
Population attributable risk			***.41*** (.38, .45)

*Significant values are in boldface.
†Numbers of cases are in parentheses.
‡*P*<.02 compared with value when risk factor was absent.

ers after women stopped smoking during pregnancy. Necrosis of the decidua at the edge of the placenta and microinfarcts in the placenta, both of which are more frequent in smokers than in nonsmokers, are sometimes the nidus for placental abruptions.[39] Both of these antecedents of abruptions are likely the result of inadequate blood flow to the decidua. As mentioned, studies have shown that smoking a single cigarette reduces uteroplacental blood flow for 5 to 15 minutes, which on occasion might be long enough to produce decidual necrosis and small placental infarcts.[31] Premature rupture of the fetal membranes also increased in frequency with maternal cigarette smoking during pregnancy (see Table 5–10).

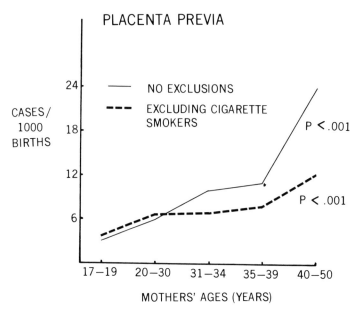

FIG 5–6.
In the CPS the frequency of placenta previa increased most rapidly with increasing maternal age when women had been cigarette smokers for many years.

Placenta previa increased in frequency in the CPS with the number of years a woman had smoked but not with her smoking in the pregnancy under analysis (Fig 5–6).[38,44] How might long-term smoking predispose to placenta previa? We have found that smoking accelerates the development of sclerotic lesions in the media of small uterine arteries and arterioles, which may reduce blood flow to many areas of the endometrium. Perhaps this uneven blood flow makes many sites in the endometrium unfavorable for implantation so that the fertilized ova more often implant low in the uterus where the placenta can impinge on the os.

DEVELOPMENTAL ABNORMALITIES IN CHILDREN

A number of studies have reported behavioral disorders, neurologic abnormalities, and impaired cognitive skills in children whose mothers smoked during pregnancy.[6,52] These findings have not been widely accepted as proof that smoking damages fetal brains because the studies that produced them controlled for only a few of the many genetic, maternal lifestyle, and environmental factors that influence children's psychomotor development.[6,52] None of these older studies took into consideration nonsmoking behavioral differences between women who smoke and women who do not smoke. For example, women who smoke reportedly drink more alcohol and coffee, are more anxious, and are less socially responsible than nonsmokers.[61] To at least partially avoid the effects of these and other potentially confounding variables we compared the psychomotor and sensory development of siblings born to mothers who smoked in only one of two pregnancies they had in the CPS.[43,44] To avoid the effects of birth order, an equal number of sibling pairs were analyzed in which women smoked in the first and in the second of the two pregnancies. Hyperactivity, hypersensitivity to sensory stimuli, short attention span, impulsive behavior, and retardation of some reading and writing skills were more frequent in the siblings produced by the pregnancy in which the mother smoked (Table 5–12).[43] The impairments in language, reading, and writing skills were very small and

TABLE 5–12.

A Comparison of Behavioral and Other Abnormalities in Siblings Whose Mothers Smoked During but One of Two Pregnancies

	Smoked During Pregnancy*	
	No	Yes
Age 1 yr		
Abnormal behavior control	57 (60)	80 (85), $P < .05$
Hypersensitive to sensory stimuli	2 (2)	12 (13), $P < .01$
Age 7 yr		
Hyperactivity	18 (5)	59 (16), $P < .05$
Easily distracted	7 (2)	48 (13), $P < .01$
Impulsive behavior	7 (2)	48 (13), $P < .01$
Short attention span	7 (2)	40 (11), $P < .05$
Achievement test results		
Speaking: mispronunciations	0.3 ± 1.1	0.9 ± 1.6, $P < .01$
Reading	37 ± 12†	35 ± 12, $P < .05$†
Writing from dictation	12 ± 2†	11 ± 2, $P < .01$†
Wide range achievement test	37 ± 12†	35 ± 12, $P < .05$†

Abnormality per 1,000 children. Numbers of cases are in parentheses.
†Mean scores.

probably not much of a problem for the affected children, parents, and teachers. Behavioral abnormalities, particularly hyperactivity, being impulsive, and having a short attention span, are more likely to have posed problems for the affected children and those who associate with them. Maternal smoking during pregnancy did not produce any impairments in the motor or sensory functions of the children in our analyses.[43]

Many studies have been conducted to try to determine if maternal smoking during pregnancy increases the frequency of fetal malformations.[20,58] Most of the findings have been negative, so smoking is probably either nonteratogenic or only weakly teratogenic.[58] There are reports that maternal smoking during pregnancy increases the risk of childhood cancer by about 50%.[55] Most of the increase is reportedly in the frequencies of lymphoma, acute lymphocytic leukemia, and Wilms' tumor.[25]

SUDDEN INFANT DEATH SYNDROME

The *sudden infant death syndrome (SIDS)* is usually defined as the sudden,

unexpected death of an apparently healthy infant for whom a routine autopsy fails to identify the cause of death. This definition reflects the unexpected nature of the deaths but not the chronic abnormalities that are present in several organs of more than half of the victims.[42] These abnormalities point to chronic damage in brainstem structures that regulate breathing, sucking, and several autonomic nervous system functions.[42] There is a large overlap between the antenatal risk factors for SIDS and the antenatal risk factors for long-term neurologic abnormalities in children.[42] This supports the possibility that SIDS has its roots in antenatal brain damage or maldevelopment. After taking other identified risk factors into account, maternal cigarette smoking during pregnancy accounted for 16% of the SIDS deaths in the CPS.[42]

REFERENCES

1. Alberman E, Creasy M, Elliott M: Maternal factors associated with fetal chromosomal anomalies in spontaneous abortions. *Br J Obstet Gynaecol* 1976; 83:621–627.

2. Andrews J, McGarry JM: A community study of smoking in pregnancy. *J Obstet Gynaecol Br Commonw* 1972; 79:1057–1073.

3. Baird DD, Wilcox AJ: Cigarette smoking associated with delayed conception. *JAMA* 1985; 253:2979–2983.

4. Beaulac-Baillargeon L, Desrosiers C: Caffeine-cigarette interaction on fetal growth. *Am J Obstet Gynecol* 1987; 157:1236–1240.

5. Berkowitz GS, Holford TR, Berkowitz RL: Effects of cigarette smoking, alcohol, coffee and tea consumption on preterm delivery. *Early Hum Dev* 1982; 7:239–250.

6. Butler NR, Goldstein H: Smoking in pregnancy and subsequent child development. *Br Med J* 1973; 4:573–575.·

7. Butler NR, Goldstein H, Ross EM: Cigarette smoking in pregnancy: Its influence on birth weight and perinatal mortality. *Br Med J* 1972; 2:127–130.

8. Bruzzi P, Green SB, Byar DP, Brinton LA, Schairer C: Estimating the population attributable risk for multiple risk factors using case-control data. *Am J Epidemiol* 1985; 122:904–914.

9. Chow WH, Daling JR, Weiss NS, Voight LF: Maternal cigarette smoking and tubal pregnancy. *Obstet Gynecol* 1988; 71:167–170.

10. Cole PV, Hawkins LH, Roberts D: Smoking during pregnancy and its effects on the fetus. *J Obstet Gynaecol Br Commonw* 1972; 79:782–787.

11. *The Collaborative Study on Cerebral Palsy, Mental Retardation and Other Neurological and Sensory Disorders of Infancy and Childhood Manual.* Bethesday, Md, US Department of Health, Education, and Welfare, 1966.

12. Collins MH, Moessinger AC, Kleinerman J, Bassi J, Rossa P, Collins AM, James LS, Blanc WA: Fetal lung hypoplasia associated with maternal smoking: A morphometric analysis. *Pediatr Res* 1985; 19:408–412.

13. Cope I, Lancaster P, Stevens L: Smoking in pregnancy. *Med J Aust* 1973; 1:673–677.

14. Curet LB, Rao AV, Zachman RD, Morrison J, Burkett G, Poole WK: Maternal smoking and respiratory distress syndrome. *Am J Obstet Gynecol* 1983; 147:446–450.

15. Daling JR, Weiss NS, Spadoni LR, Moore DE, Voight L: Cigarette smoking and primary tubal infertility, in Rosenberg MJ (ed): *Smoking and Reproductive Health*, Littleton, Mass, PSG Publishing Co, 1987, pp 40–46.

16. Denis P, Pasquis P, Duval C, Lefrancois R: P_{50} values of non smoker and smoker pregnant women. *Biomedicine* 1980; 33:49–51.

17. Fok RY, Pavlova Z, Benirschke K, Paul RH, Platt LD: The correlation of arterial lesions with umbilical artery Doppler velocimetry in the placentas of small-for-dates pregnancies. *Obstet Gynecol* 1990; 75:578–583.

18. Gluck L, Kulovich MV: Lecithin/sphingomyelin ratios in amniotic fluid in normal and abnormal pregnancy. *Am J Obstet Gynecol* 1973; 115:539–546.

19. Hastings RP (ed): *SUGI Supplemental Library User's Guide*, ed 5. Cary, NC, SAS Institute, 1986.

20. *The Health Consequences of Smoking for Women, a Report of the Surgeon General.* US Department of Health and Human Services, 1980.

21. Hebel JR, Fox NL, Sexton M: Dose-response of birth weight to various measures of maternal smoking during pregnancy. *J Clin Epidemiol* 1988; 41:483–489.

22. Howard RB, Hosokawa T, Maguire MH: Hypoxia-induced fetoplacental vasoconstriction in perfused human placental cotyledons. *Am J Obstet Gynecol* 1987; 157:1261–1266.

23. Howe G, Westhoff C, Vessey M, Yeates D: Effects of age, cigarette smoking and other factors on fertility: Findings in a large prospective study. *Br Med J* 1985; 290:1697–1700.

24. *James I (King of England 1603–25), A Counterblaste to Tobacco.* London, Rodale Press, 1954.

25. John EM, Savitz DA, Sandler DP: Prenatal exposure to parent's smoking and childhood cancer. *Am J Epidmiol* 1991; 133:123–132.

26. Kleinman JC, Pierre MB Jr, Madans JH, Land GH, Schramm WF: The effects of maternal smoking on fetal and infant mortality. *Am J Epidemiol* 1988; 127:274–282.

27. Kline J: Environmental exposures and spontaneous abortion, in Gold E (ed): *The Changing Risk of Disease in Women, American Epidemiological Approach.* Lexington, Mass, Collamore Press, 1984, pp 127–138.

28. Kline J, Stein Z, Hutzler M: Cigarettes, alcohol and marijuana: Varying associations with birthweight. *Int J Epidemiol* 1987; 16:44–51.

29. Kline J, Stein ZA, Susser M, Warburton D: Smoking: A risk factor for spontaneous abortion. *N Engl J Med* 1977; 297:793–796.

30. Kramer MS: Determinants of low birth weight: Methodological assessment and meta-analysis. *Bull WHO* 1987; 65:663–737.

31. Lehtovirta P, Forss M: The acute effect of smoking on intervillous blood flow of the placenta. *Br J Obstet Gynaecol* 1978; 85:729–731.

32. Longo LD: The biological effects of carbon monoxide on the pregnant woman, fetus and, newborn infant. *Am J Obstet Gynecol* 1977; 129:69–103.

33. MacArthur C, Knox EG: Smoking and pregnancy: Effects of stopping at different

stages. *Br J Obstet Gynaecol* 1988; 95:551–555.

34. Mattison DR: The effects of smoking on fertility from gametogenesis to implantation. *Environ Res* 1982; 28:410–433.

35. Meyer MB, Tonascia JA: Maternal smoking, pregnancy complications, and perinatal mortality. *Am J Obstet Gynecol* 1977; 128:494–502.

36. Morrow RJ, Ritchie JWK, Bull SB: Maternal cigarette smoking: The effects on umbilical and uterine blood flow velocity. *Am J Obstet Gynecol* 1988; 159:1069–1071.

37. Naeye RL: New observations in erythroblastosis fetalis. *JAMA* 1967; 200:281–286.

38. Naeye RL: The duration of maternal cigarette smoking, fetal and placental disorders. *Early Hum Dev* 1979; 3:229–237.

39. Naeye RL: Abruptio placentae and placenta previa: Frequency, perinatal mortality and cigarette smoking. *Obstet Gynecol* 1980; 55:701–704.

40. Naeye RL: Coitus and antepartum hemorrhage. *Br J Obstet Gynaecol* 1981; 88:765–770.

41. Naeye RL: Influences of maternal cigarette smoking during pregnancy on fetal and childhood growth. *Obstet Gynecol* 1981; 57:18–21.

42. Naeye RL: Sudden infant death syndrome, is the confusion ending? *Modern Pathol* 1988; 1:169–174.

43. Naeye RL, Peters EC: Mental development of children whose mothers smoked during pregnancy. *Obstet Gynecol* 1984; 64:601–607.

44. Naeye RL, Tafari N: *Risk Factors in Pregnancy and Diseases of the Fetus and Newborn.* Baltimore, Md, Williams & Wilkins Co, 1983.

45. Naeye RL, Peters EC, Bartholomew M, Landis JR: Origins of cerebral palsy. *Am J Dis Child* 1989; 143:1154–1161.

46. Niswander K, Gordon M: *The Women and Their Pregnancies*, Philadelphia, WB Saunders Co, 1972.

47. Papoz L, Eschwege E, Pequignot G, Barrat J, Schwartz D: Maternal smoking and birth weight in relation to dietary habits. *Am J Obstet Gynecol* 1982; 142:870–876.

48. Pettersson F, Fries H, Nillius SJ: Epidemiology of secondary amenorrhea. *Am J Obst Gynecol* 1973; 117:80–86.

49. *Reducing the Health Consequences of Smoking: 25 Years of Progress, A Report of the Surgeon General, US Department of Health and Human Services.* DHHS Publication No. (CDC), 1989, 89-8411.

50. Ross S, Naeye RL: Racial and environmental influences on fetal lung maturation. *Pediatrics* 1981; 68:790–795.

51. Rush D: Examination of the relationship between birthweight, cigarette smoking during pregnancy and maternal weight gain. *J Obstet Gynaecol Br Commonw* 1974; 81:746–752.

52. Saxton DW: The behavior of infants whose mothers smoke in pregnancy. *Early Hum Dev* 1978; 2:363–369.

53. Schneider NG, Houston JP: Smoking and anxiety. *Psychol Rep* 1970; 26:941–942.

54. Simpson WJ: A preliminary report on cigarette smoking and the incidence of prematurity. *Am J Obstet Gynecol* 1957; 73:808–815.

55. Stjernfeldt M, Berglund K, Lindsten J, Ludvigsson J: Maternal smoking during pregnancy and risk of childhood cancer. *Lancet* 1986; 1:1350–1352.

56. Tager IB, Weiss ST, Munoz A, Rosner B, Speizer FE: Longitudinal study of the effects of maternal smoking on pulmonary function in children. *N Engl J Med* 1983; 309:699–703.

57. Van den Berg C: Epidemiologic observations of prematurity: Effects of tobacco, coffee and alcohol, in Reed DM, Stanley FJ (eds): *Epidemiology of Prematurity.* Baltimore, Md, Urban & Schwarzenberg, 1977, pp 157–176.

58. Van Den Eeden SK, Karagas MR, Daling JR, Vaughan TL: A case-control study of maternal smoking and congenital malformations. *Pediatr Perinat Epidemiol* 1990; 4:147–155.

59. Visnjevac V, Mikov M: Smoking and carboxyhemoglobin concentrations in mothers and their newborn infants. *Hum Toxicol* 1986; 5:175–177.

60. Werler MM, Pober BR, Holmes LB: Smoking and pregnancy. *Teratology* 1985; 32:473–481.

61. Yerushalmy J: The relationship of parents' cigarette smoking to outcome of pregnancy: Implications as to the problem of inferring causation from observed associations. *Am J Epidemiol* 1971; 93:443–456.

CHAPTER 6

Disorders of the Umbilical Cord

SELECTING TISSUE FOR MICROSCOPIC EXAMINATION

At least three 3- to 4-cm-long segments of the umbilical cord should be fixed in buffered formalin. These segments should include grossly normal areas of the cord as well as any abnormal areas that are visible. Do not take cord tissue within 2 cm of the surface of the placenta for microscopic examination without recognizing that the two umbilical arteries often normally fuse at this site into a single vessel.

UMBILICAL CORD LENGTH

The length of the umbilical cord has long been recognized to have clinical significance. To get an accurate measurement, the length of cord segments cut out for blood gas analysis must be added to the lengths of segments that are attached to the placenta and to the baby. A cord length of less than 30 cm has occasionally delayed the completion of the second stage of labor, caused placental abruptions, an inversion of the uterus, cord herniation, and cord rupture. Unusually long cords (91st–100th percentiles) increase the frequencies of cord prolapse, cord knots, and nuchal cords, all of which increase the risk of cord compression. Long cords also predispose to the coiling of the cord around fetal parts, which occasionally arrests fetal descent. Fetal heart rate patterns that suggest cord compression have been reported with both abnormally long and abnormally short umbilical cords.[40,55] Cord prolapse and knots are particularly common with polyhydramnios, a setting in which the fetus can move freely within the uterus in late gestation and thereby acquire a long cord.

Both Miller et al.[41,42] and Moessinger et al.[45] have shown that tension applied to the umbilical cord by fetal movements greatly influences its length; the greater the movements, the longer the cord. The experimental production of oligohydramnios, and the administration to fetuses of drugs such as curare, alcohol, and β-blockers, which reduce fetal movements, have all produced short umbilical cords.[3,35,45] Placing the fetus outside of the uterus where it can move freely has produced an abnormally long cord. Short umbilical cords have been found at birth with conditions in which fetal movements were restricted. These include fetal limb dysfunction, oligohydramnios, uterine malformations, fetuses whose bodies were fixed to the uterine wall by amniotic bands, and maternal drugs that produced fetal lethargy.[35,55,59,68]

We analyzed umbilical cord length in 35,799 neonates from the Collaborative Perinatal Study (CPS) and found that increases in cord length slowed after the 28th week of gestation but did not stop until term was reached (Fig 6–1).[46] This late gestational slowing was presumably the result of fetal movements being constrained by the growing fetus filling most of the available space in the uterus. The following additional factors had a positive correlation with umbilical cord length: maternal pregravid body weight, maternal pregnancy weight gain, fetus being male, high family socioeconomic status, and maternal height.[46] Race, disorders that reduce uteroplacental blood flow, maternal mental retardation, maternal alcoholism, narcotic addiction, and cigarette smoking had no effect on cord length. Cords were abnormally short with oligohydramnios and abnormally long with hydramnios (Fig 6–2). Hypotonic neonates born before 34 weeks' gestation had an increased frequency of short umbilical cords which suggests that their hypotonia was sometimes of antenatal origin (Fig 6–3).

In the CPS short umbilical cords were associated with fetal growth retardation,

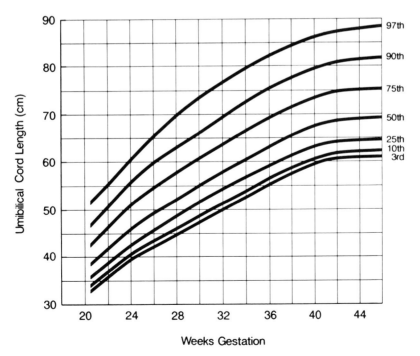

FIG 6–1.
Umbilical cord length percentiles at various gestational ages.

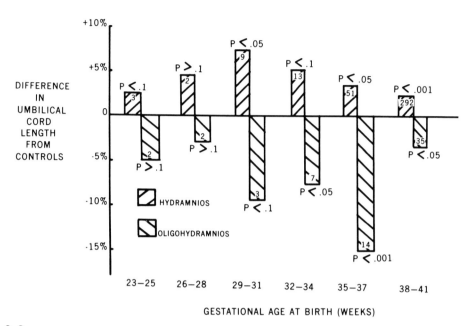

FIG 6–2.
In the CPS umbilical cords were abnormally short with oligohydamnios and abnormally long with hydramnios.

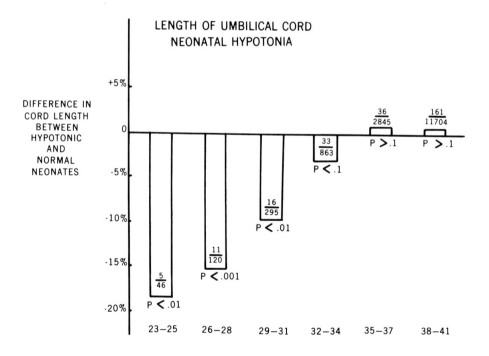

FIG 6–3.
Children born before 34 weeks' gestation who were hypotonic in the neonatal period had an increased frequency of abnormally short umbilical cords.

TABLE 6–1.

Disorders of Umbilical Cord Length in Full-Term Gestations*

	Frequencies of Long and Short Cords	Perinatal Mortality Rate	Fetal Growth Retardation	Neurologic Abnormalities at 7 Years
All cases		*15 (686)*	*88 (4,089)*	*29 (1,355)*
Short cord (<35 cm at term)	16 (768)	50 (42), *P* < .001	168 (129), *P* < .001	44 (33)
Relative risks†		1.2, *P* < .05	2.1, *P* < .001	1.3, *P* < .05
Long cord (>70 cm at term)	154 (7,172)	5 (33), *P* < .001	64 (459), *P* < .001	32 (229)
Relative risks†		0.3, *P* < .001	0.7, *P* < .001	1.1

*Frequencies per 1,000 births. Numbers of cases are in parentheses.
†Relative risk values have been calculated to take the following possible confounding variables into consideration: major congenital malformations, acute chorioamnionitis, disorders of low uteroplacental blood flow, and, when appropriate, gestational age at birth.

high fetal and neonatal mortality rates, and an increased frequency of long-term neurologic abnormalities after disorders that commonly retard fetal growth and cause perinatal death were taken into consideration (Table 6–1). Unusually long umbilical cords were associated with lower-than-expected frequencies of fetal growth retardation and perinatal death (see Table 6–1). This raises the possibility that children who are physically very active before birth have an intrinsic vigor that enhances their chances of being born alive and surviving through the neonatal period. In a study of 1,000 spontaneous abortions an elongated umbilical cord with loops around the neck or extremities was present in 13.4% of the cases.[33] Vigorous motor activity was often observed in the embryos with unusually long cords.

In the CPS umbilical cord length correlated with a child's mental and motor development. IQ values of less than 80 were 25% more frequent and cerebral palsy three times as frequent when umbilical cords were unusually short as when they were normal in length (Figs 6–4 and 6–5).[46] The psychomotor development of same-sex siblings was compared when one had an umbilical cord more than 20 cm longer than the other. The siblings who had the shorter cords had a 2.2-fold greater frequency of IQ values less than 80 and a 1.8-fold greater frequency of motor abnormalities than their siblings with the longer cords.[46] In the CPS, short umbilical cords were associated with seizure disorders and hyperactive behavior (Figs 6–4 and 6–6). Abnormally long cords had a positive correlation with abnormal behavior control and hyperactive behavior at 1 year of age (see Figs 6–5 and 6–6). These associations with cord length suggest that the abnormal behavior sometimes originated before birth.[46]

Breech presentation is often associated with infrequent or weak fetal movements, so it is not surprising that in the CPS umbilical cord lengths were shorter with breech than with vertex presentations.[46,65] Twins have shorter umbilical cords than single-born infants, presumably because the presence of two babies crowds the available intrauterine space and thereby limits fetal movements.[66]

UMBILICAL CORD TWIST

The twist of the umbilical cord, often called its spiral or its helix, is present as early as the 42nd day of gestation and is well established by 9 weeks' gestation (Fig 6–7).[14,38] Left twists outnumbered right twists by 7 to 1, perhaps because the right umbilical artery is usually larger than the left and the torque resulting from the differing blood flows causes the cord to twist to the left.[38] The credibility of this explanation is strengthened by the absence of twist in many cords that have only one umbilical artery.[38] Long cords tend to have more spiraling, which Benirschke and Kaufmann cite as evidence that unusually long cords are the result of in-

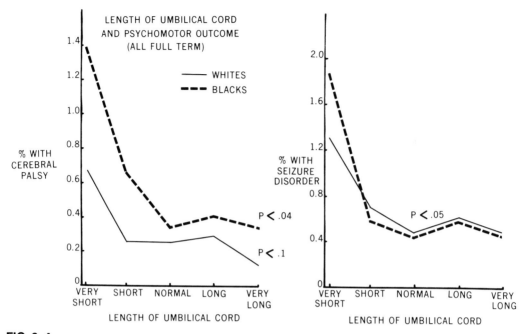

FIG 6–4.
Children born in the CPS with short umbilical cords subsequently had increased frequencies of cerebral palsy and chronic nonfebrile seizure disorders.

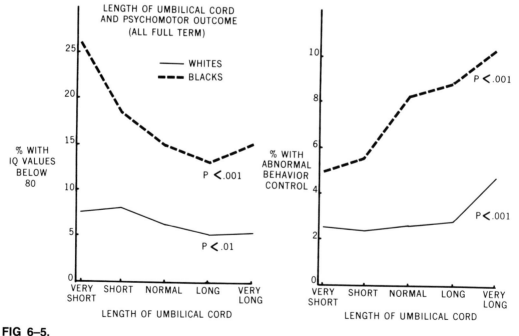

FIG 6–5.
Short umbilical cords in the CPS had a positive correlation with low IQ values at 4 years of age. Abnormal behavior control at 1 year of age was more frequent with long than with short umbilical cords.

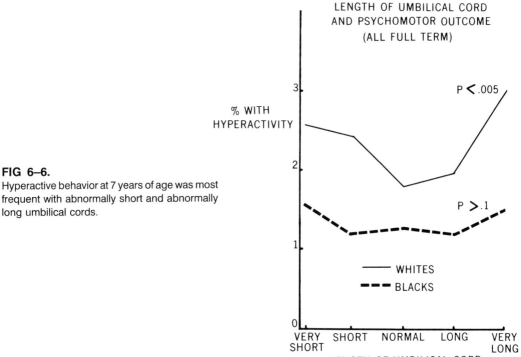

LENGTH OF UMBILICAL CORD
AND PSYCHOMOTOR OUTCOME
(ALL FULL TERM)

FIG 6–6.
Hyperactive behavior at 7 years of age was most frequent with abnormally short and abnormally long umbilical cords.

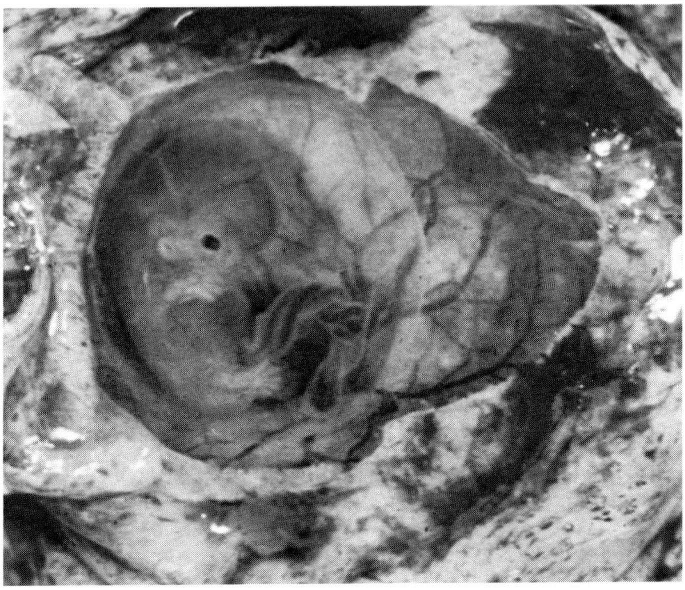

FIG 6–7.
A twist is present in the umbilical cord of this very early embryo.

creased fetal movements.[7] Twist is sometimes absent in settings in which fetal movements were restricted, including cases in which fetuses are fixed to the uterine wall by amniotic bands.[68] An increased fetal mortality has been reported with excessive spiraling, presumably because such spiraling occasionally leads to constrictions that compress the vessels in the cord (Fig 6–8).[7] Bender et al.

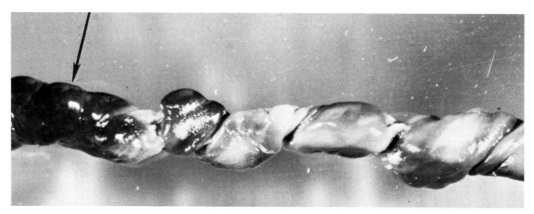

FIG 6–8.
The marked spiraling of this umbilical cord has led to severe constrictions. Note the marked congestion of the cord behind the constrictions *(arrow).*

TABLE 6–2.

Risk Estimates for Antecedents to the Development of a Narrow Umbilical Cord*

Risk Factors	No. of Cases of Narrow Umbilical Cord per 1,000 Cases With Risk Factor†	Relative Risks (95% Confidence Intervals)	Attributable Risks (95% Confidence Intervals)
All cases	2 *(78)*		
Maternal factor			
Smoked during pregnancy	**4** *(36), P<.001*	**3.2** (2.0, 4.9)	**.26** (.19, .33)
Fetal factors			
Infant dysmature at birth	**7** *(19), P<.001*	**4.1** (2.4, 6.9)	**.14** (.07, .21)
Major fetal malformations	**3** *(13), P<.05*	**3.7** (1.0, 14.9)	**.01** (.00, .01)
Placental and cord factors			
Unevenly accelerated maturation	**4** *(41), P<.001*	**3.5** (2.2, 5.5)	**.31** (.24, .38)
Placental growth retardation	**5** *(15), P<.001*	**3.0** (2.2, 3.8)	**.17** (.10, .24)
Population attributable risk			**.87** *(.80, .94)*
Pregnancy outcomes			
Preterm birth	1 *(14), P>.1*	0.8 (0.3, 1.6)	
Fetal growth retardation	**6** *(24), P<.001*	**3.2** (1.9, 5.3)	
Stillbirth	1 *(1)*		
Neonatal death	4 *(3), P>.1*	2.1 (0.7, 2.1)	
Neurologic abnormalities at 7 yr	3 *(4), P>.1*	1.6 (0.5, 2.8)	

*Significant values are in boldface.
†Numbers of cases are in parentheses.

have reported that the more a cord spirals, the better the pregnancy outcome.[4] This would be expected if many spirals are a reflection of vigorous fetal movements because other evidence of vigorous fetal motor activity, such as a long umbilical cord, are associated with a low perinatal mortality rate (Table 6–1).

NARROW UMBILICAL CORD

The umbilical cord was recorded as very narrow in 0.2% of the neonates in the CPS (Table 6–2). All of the risk factors for the cord being very narrow are factors that are associated with fetal growth retardation. These include maternal cigarette smoking during pregnancy; unevenly accelerated placental maturation, which is a characteristic consequence of low uteroplacental blood flow; major fetal malformations; dysmature fetal growth; and a growth-retarded placenta (see Table 6–2). After taking all of these risk factors into consideration, a very narrow umbilical cord was not associated with any unfavorable pregnancy outcome (see Table 6–2). Umbilical cord circumference has been related to the amount of Wharton's jelly that is present, which in turn has a positive correlation with the water content of the cord.[63] There is a reported tendency for amniotic fluid volume to be low when the cord is thin.[61] This would be expected since unevenly accelerated placental maturation, a marker for both chronically low uteroplacental blood flow and a low amniotic fluid volume, was a major risk factor for a very narrow umbilical cord.

Many have speculated that cord compression is more frequent when the cord is thin. This was confirmed by findings in the CPS. Cord prolapse was 3.2-fold more frequent with a narrow than with a normally thick cord ($P < .001$). When the cord prolapsed, fetal or neonatal death was 3.1-fold more frequent with a narrow than with a normally thick cord ($P < .02$). When the cord did not prolapse, a very narrow cord did not increase the risk for fetal or neonatal death.

MARGINAL INSERTION OF THE UMBILICAL CORD (BATTLEDORE PLACENTA)

Insertion of the umbilical cord into the edge of the placenta was recorded in 2.7% of the placentas in the CPS (Fig 6–9). This is a somewhat lower figure than has been reported by some other investigators.[7] Risk factors were identified for 21% of these marginal insertions (Table 6–3). These antecedents were unevenly accelerated placental maturation, being a twin, placental growth retardation, major congenital fetal malformations, maternal di-

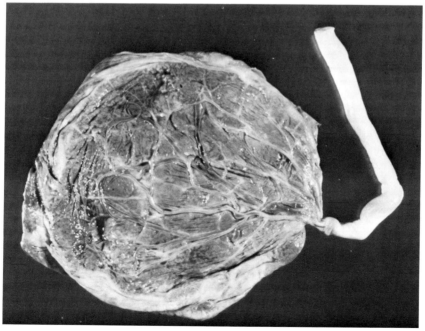

FIG 6–9.
Marginal insertion of the umbilical cord. In the British literature this is known as a "battledore placenta."

TABLE 6–3.

Risk Estimates for Antecedents to the Development of Marginal Insertion of Umbilical Cord*

Risk Factors	No. of Marginal Insertions of Cords per 1000 Cases With Risk Factor†	Relative Risks (95% Confidence Intervals)	Attributable Risks (95% Confidence Intervals)
All cases	27 *(1,314)*		
Maternal factors			
Acetonuria during 1st trimester	**66** (87), *P* < .005	**1.3** (1.1, 1.7)	**.02** (.01, .02)
Diabetes mellitus	**41** (23), *P* < .05	**1.5** (1.0, 2.1)	**.01** (.00, .01)
Fetal factors			
Twins	**74** *(74), P* < .001	**3.0** (2.8, 3.2)	**.04** (.03, .05)
Major fetal malformations	**33** *(141), P* < .001	**1.2** (1.0, 1.4)	**.02** (.01, .02)
Placental factors			
Unevenly accelerated maturation	**35** *(279), P* < .001	**1.3** (1.0, 1.7)	**.07** (.04, .10)
Placental growth retardation	**38** *(119), P* < .001	**1.5** (1.1, 2.0)	**.05** (0.3, .07)
Population attributable risk			**.21** *(.19, .24)*
Pregnancy outcomes			
Preterm birth	32 *(326), P* > .1	1.2 (0.9, 1.6)	
Fetal growth retardation	**43** *(167), P* < .001	1.2 (0.9, 1.6)	
Stillbirth	**46** *(38) P* < .001	1.1 (0.8, 1.4)	
Neonatal death	**45** *(39), P* < .001	1.0 (0.7, 1.4)	
Neurologic abnormalities at 7 yr	25 *(37), P* > .1	0.9 (0.8, 1.1)	

*Significant values are in boldface.
†Numbers of cases are in parentheses.

abetes mellitus, and first-trimester maternal acetonuria in the absence of diabetes mellitus. Fox has reported that marginal insertion of the umbilical cord is not associated with fetal abnormalities or with other unfavorable pregnancy outcomes.[19] This was not true in the CPS. Marginal insertion of the cord was associated with increased frequencies of fetal growth retardation, stillbirth, and neonatal death (see Table 6–3). All of these unfavorable outcomes disappeared when unevenly accelerated placental maturation, a characteristic consequence of low uteroplacental blood flow, was taken into consideration. Thus, marginal insertion of the umbilical cord, in the absence of presumed low uteroplacental blood flow, did not have any unfavorable fetal or neonatal consequences.

VELAMENTOUS INSERTION OF THE UMBILICAL CORD

Velamentous insertion of the umbilical cord is present when umbilical vessels traverse the fetal membranes, unsupported by either the umbilical cord or by placental tissue (Fig 6–10). It was recorded in 0.3% of the placentas in the CPS (Table 6–4). This is a somewhat lower frequency than has been reported by some previous investigators.[7] Benirschke and Driscoll postulated that velamentous insertion originates when the cord becomes stranded as the result of a unidirectional lateral growth of the chorion frondosum.[6] What causes such unidirectional growth? In the CPS, antecedents or risk factors were identified for 30% of the velamentous cord insertions. These included maternal cigarette smoking during pregnancy, advanced maternal age, maternal diabetes mellitus, a congenital syndrome in the fetus, and placental growth retardation (see Table 6–4). After taking all of these risk factors into consideration, velamentous insertion of the umbilical cord was not associated with any unfavorable pregnancy outcome except for a doubling of the risk for neurologic abnormalities at 7 years of age (see Table 6–4). All of this latter

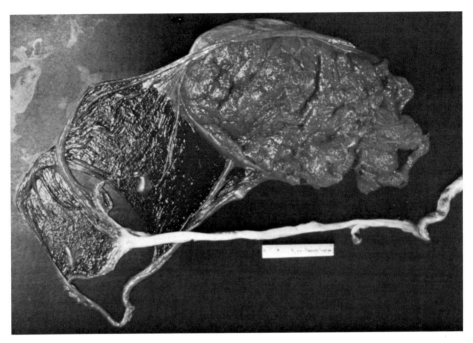

FIG 6–10.
Velamentous (membranous) insertion of the umbilical cord.

TABLE 6–4.
Risk Estimates for Antecedents of the Development of a Velamentous Insertion of the Umbilical Cord into the Fetal Membranes*

Risk Factors	No. of Cases of Velamentous Insertion per 1000 Cases With Risk Factor†	Relative Risks (95% Confidence Intervals)	Attributable Risks (95% Confidence Intervals)
All cases	3 *(127)*		
Maternal factors			
Smoked during pregnancy	**4** *(37), P* < .01	**1.6** (1.1, 2.4)	**.12** (.09, .14)
Age ≥ 35 yr	**6** *(17), P* < .001	**2.3** (1.4, 3.9)	**.08** (.06, .10)
Diabetes mellitus	**12** *(7), P* < .001	**4.2** (1.9, 9.2)	**.04** (.01, .07)
Fetal factors			
Congenital syndromes	**11** *(3), P* < .01	**3.8** (1.2, 12.4)	**.01** (.00, .01)
Placental factor			
Placental growth retardation	**4** *(17), P* < .05	**1.6** (1.1, 2.2)	**.06** (.02, .11)
Population attributable risk			**.30** *(.25, .34)*
Pregnancy outcomes			
Preterm birth	**3** *(31), P* < .001	1.1 (0.6, 1.7)	
Fetal growth retardation	3 (11), P > .1	1.0 (0.6, 1.7)	
Stillbirth	2 (2) P > .1	1.0 (0.3, 1.9)	
Neonatal death	2 (2), P > .1	0.8 (0.1, 2.1)	
Neurologic abnormalities at 7 yr	**6** *(12), P* < .05	**1.7** (1.0, 2.7)	
Hyperactivity syndromes		**2.6** (1.4, 5.2)	

*Significant values are in boldface.
†Numbers of cases are in parentheses.

increase was in a single category, hyperactivity syndromes.

Most authors who write about velamentous insertion of the umbilical cord emphasize the risk of tearing the unsupported vessels during delivery with resultant fetal blood loss.[37,71] Fetal or neonatal death occurs with at least half of such tears.[56] The risk of such tearing is greatest when the unsupported vessels cross the cervical os *(vasa previa)*. Vessel rupture can take place before the onset of labor, at the time the membranes rupture, or at any subsequent time before the umbilical cord is clamped.[9] Hemorrhage is most frequent when the membranes are prematurely ruptured or when the descending head of the fetus tears the vessels.[54] When such a rupture is suspected, a low hemoglobin value in fetal scalp blood will help to confirm the blood loss if enough time has passed for hemodilution to have taken place. If a large blood loss has occurred, rapid delivery and prompt transfusion can save an infant's life.[44] There have been many claims that velamentous insertion of the cord is more frequent in preterm than in full-term born infants.[19] This was not the case in the CPS after confounding risk factors had been taken into consideration (see Table 6–4).

UMBILICAL CORD KNOTS

Umbilical cord knots fall into two categories, false and true. False knots appear as nodular swellings of the cord that are caused by local accumulations of Wharton's jelly, redundancies of local vessels, or vascular dilatation (Fig 6–11). These false knots have no clinical significance.

True knots in the umbilical cord have been reported in from 0.1% to 1.0% of deliveries and to have a perinatal mortality rate of 8% to 11% (Fig 6–12).[19] Knots must be very tight to obstruct blood flow in the umbilical vein.[12] The vein sometimes thromboses at the site of the knot, and vein dilatation is typically present between the knot and the placenta.[7]

True knots were present in 1% of the umbilical cords in the CPS (Table 6–5). They were strongly associated with unusually long (91st–100th percentile) umbilical cords and with diffuse fibrin beneath the chorionic (fetal) plate of the placenta. Both unusually long umbilical cords and diffuse subchorionic fibrin are markers of vigorous fetal motor activity, so their association with cord knots supports the possibility that knots are often the consequence of vigorous movements.[46,48] In the

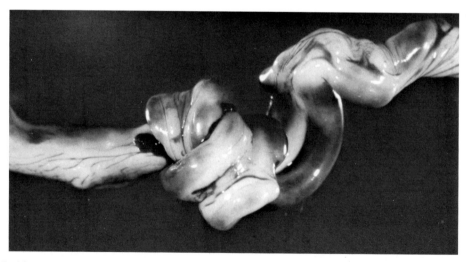

FIG 6–11.
A "false" knot in an umbilical cord. It is comprised of redundant blood vessels.

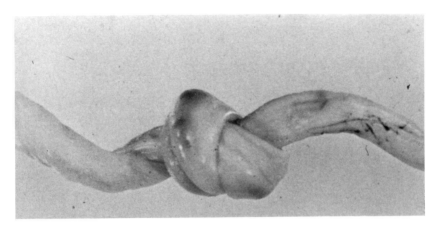

FIG 6–12.
Tight knot in the umbilical cord that was responsible for a stillbirth.

CPS umbilical cord knots increased the risk for stillbirth but not for neonatal death after the antecedent risk factors for such knots had been taken into consideration (see Table 6–5). There were no other unfavorable clinical consequences of umbilical knots when these antecedent risk factors were taken into account (see Table 6–5).

Since umbilical cord knots are capable of obstructing blood flow, why do they so seldom have serious clinical conse-

quences? In many cases the physical characteristics of Wharton's jelly probably prevents umbilical cord blood vessel compression by diffusing the pressure exerted by knots. In addition, the outer surface of the umbilical cord is very slippery, so that it is difficult for knots to maintain a tight hold. In the CPS tight umbilical cord knots were not associated with an increase in long-term neurologic abnormalities. This suggests that if periodic tightening of the knots takes place, the tightening rarely

TABLE 6–5.
Risk Estimates for Antecedents to Development of a Tight Knot in the Umbilical Cord*

Risk Factors	No. of Cords With Knots per 1,000 Cases With Risk Factor†	Relative Risks (95% Confidence Intervals)	Attributable Risks (95% Confidence Intervals)
All cases	10 *(563)*		
Maternal factor			
Preeclampsia, eclampsia	**13** *(122)*, P < .05	**1.2** (1.0, 1.4)	**.04** (.01, .07)
Fetal factor			
Sex = male	**13** *(344)*, P < .001	**1.5** (1.2, 1.4)	**.17** (.15, .19)
Markers for high fetal motor activity			
Unusually long umbilical cord	**19** *(403)*, P < .001	**4.2** (3.4, 5.1)	**.46** (.43, .49)
Diffuse subchorionic fibrin	**10** *(199)*, P < .05	**1.2** (1.1, 1.4)	**.03** (.02, .04)
Other indicators			**.05** (0.3, .08)
Population attributable risk			**.73** *(.69, .77)*
Pregnancy outcomes			
Preterm birth	9 *(102)*, P > .1	0.9 (0.7, 1.2)	
Fetal growth retardation	10 *(45)*, P > .1	1.0 (0.9, 1.2)	
Stillbirth	**22** *(19)* P < .001	**19.1** (9.9, 29.4)	
Neonatal death	8 *(8)*, P > .1	0.8 (0.5, 1.3)	
Neurologic abnormalities at 7 yr	7 *(12)*, P > .1	0.7 (0.4, 1.1)	

*Significant values are in boldface.
†Numbers of cases are in parentheses.

persists long enough to cause brain damage, or if such brain damage occurs, the fetus dies.[47,48,69] If there is uncertainty about whether a knot was tight enough to obstruct blood flow, look for focal grooving, narrowing, edema, or thrombosis in the cord or a marked congestion of the cord between the knot and the placenta. All are indications that a knot could have been tight enough to obstruct blood flow.

ENTANGLEMENT OF UMBILICAL CORD

An entangled umbilical cord is a rare cause of stillbirth or neonatal death in single-born infants. A cord entangled around a body part sometimes leaves easily recognized grooves on the skin. Such entanglements around arms, legs, or the trunk were not associated in the CPS with an increased risk of stillbirth, neonatal death, or long-term neurologic abnormalities in single-born infants. Vascular congestion and edema on one side of an obstruction, a hemorrhage into Wharton's jelly, or vascular thrombosis in the cord helps to confirm that an entanglement was present before delivery. Umbilical cord entanglement is a frequent occurrence when there is no dividing membrane between the twins. In the CPS 20% of such monoamnionic, monochorionic twins were stillborn as the result of their entangled cords obstructing umbilical cord blood flow. Such fatal entanglements are most frequent in the first two trimesters of pregnancy when the two fetuses are still small enough to be able to move about freely within the uterine cavity.[7]

UMBILICAL CORD TORSION AND STRANGULATION

Umbilical cord torsion is a rare cause of fetal death. It is usually seen within 1 to 3 cm of the fetal end of the cord.[22,23] Strangulation of the umbilical cord by an amniotic band has been present in about 10% of the reported cases of the amniotic band syndrome.[26]

UMBILICAL CORD TIGHT AROUND THE NECK

In the CPS 735 children were born with two or more coils of umbilical cord tight around their necks (Table 6–6). This was 1.4% of all the children born in the study. The major antecedents of these nuchal cords were an unusually long (91st–100th percentile) umbilical cord and being male. A long umbilical cord is strongly associated with multiple evidences of a hyperactive fetus so its association with a tight nuchal cord supports the possibility that nuchal cords are sometimes the result of vigorous fetal motor movements.[46] Apart from rare cases of strangulation, children in the CPS born with nuchal cords were intrinsically healthy because they had a much lower neonatal mortality rate than infants in the study as a whole (see Table 6–6). Infants who had their umbilical cords loosely arranged around their necks at birth also had a very low neonatal mortality rate. Their relative risk for neonatal death was significantly lower 0.8 (95% confidence intervals 0.6, 1.0) than the risk of neonatal death in the CPS as a whole.

Whether loose or tight around the neck at birth, a nuchal cord did not increase the risk for long-term neurologic abnormalities (see Table 6–6). This suggests that if cord compression took place it did not persist long enough to damage the fetal brain, or else the damage led to stillbirth. A few such stillbirths probably occurred because the relative risk for stillbirth was much lower when the umbilical cord was loose (0.1 [0.0, .02]) than when it was tight around the neck (1.1 [0.8, 1.4]). The very low risk of stillbirth and neonatal death with a loose nuchal cord raises the possibility that physically very active fetuses are intrinsically very healthy and better able to survive fetal and neonatal stress than children who are less active before birth.

TABLE 6–6.

Risk Estimates for Antecedents to the Development of Umbilical Cord Tight Around the Neck of the Fetus Two or More Times*

Risk Factors	No. of Cases With Umbilical Cord Tight Around Neck Two or More Times per 1,000 Cases With Risk Factor†	Relative Risks (95% Confidence Intervals)	Attributable Risks (95% Confidence Intervals)
All cases	14 *(735)*		
Fetal factors			
Race = white	**17** *(402), P < .001*	**1.2** (1.0, 1.4)	**.04** (.02, .06)
Sex = male	**16** *(342), P < .05*	**1.1** (1.0, 1.2)	**.06** (.04, .07)
Marker for high fetal motor activity			
Unusually long umbilical cord	**36** *(221), P < .001*	**3.2** (2.4, 4.1)	**.26** (.22, .31)
Population attributable risk			**.36** (.33, .39)
Pregnancy outcomes			
Preterm birth	**11** *(127), P < .02*	1.0 (0.8, 1.3)	
Fetal growth retardation	**20** *(89), P < .001*	**1.8** (1.4, 2.3)	
Stillbirth	**26** *(19) P < .02*	1.1 (0.8, 1.4)	
Neonatal death	10 *(7), P > .1*	**0.6** (0.2, 1.0)	
Neurologic abnormalities at 7 yr	14 *(24), P > .1*	1.1 (0.6, 1.6)	

*Significant values are in boldface.
†Numbers of cases are in parentheses.

Thus the risk for stillbirth posed by a nuchal cord appears to be more than balanced by the intrinsic vigor and good health of the associated fetuses. This counterbalancing good health and vigor is the reason why many have concluded that nuchal cords do not increase perinatal mortality despite the many cases in which a tight nuchal cord caused stillbirth.[17,34,62]

Children born with the cord around their necks reportedly have increased frequencies of variable fetal heart rate decelerations during labor and acidemia in their umbilical cord blood.[24] Shepard et al. found that newborns with nuchal cords were more often anemic than controls, presumably because venous return from the placenta was reduced as the result of compression of the umbilical vein.[60]

UMBILICAL CORD PROLAPSE

Umbilical cord prolapse was recorded in 1% of the deliveries in the CPS (Table 6–7). Antecedent risk factors were identified for 75% of the cord prolapses. These antecedents were breech presentation, preterm birth, multiparity, major fetal malformations, twins, an unusually long umbilical cord (91st–100th percentile), acute chorioamnionitis, premature rupture of the fetal membranes, and incompetent cervix (see Table 6–7). Most of these factors predisposed to cord prolapse because the fetus had not rotated to a vertex presentation. After such rotation the fetal head fills the pelvic outlet so the cord cannot easily slip by and become compressed between the fetal head and the pelvic bones. Most of the risk factors for cord prolapse independently increase the risk for stillbirth, so how much of the high perinatal mortality associated with cord prolapse is due to the prolapse itself and how much is due to its antecedents? In the CPS cord prolapse had a high frequency of stillbirth and neonatal death independent of its antecedent risk factors (see Table 6–7). This high mortality has been reported many times in the past.[72] These deaths are the result of the fetal head or other body part compressing the umbilical cord against the pelvic wall, which obstructs blood flow in the cord. After taking antecedent risk factors into consideration,

TABLE 6–7.

Risk Estimates for Antecedents to an Umbilical Cord Prolapse*

Risk Factors	No. of Cases With an Umbilical Cord Prolapse per 1,000 Cases With Risk Factor†	Relative Risks (95% Confidence Intervals)	Attributable Risks (95% Confidence Intervals)
All cases	10 (567)		
Maternal factors			
Multigravida	**11** (333), P < .001	**1.3** (1.1, 1.6)	**.13** (.11, .14)
Podalic version	**450** (9), P < .001	**29.8** (2.4, 90.3)	**.02** (.01, .03)
Premature membrane rupture	**11** (175), P < .001	**1.1** (1.0, 1.2)	**.01** (.00, .01)
Incompetent cervix	**59** (14), P < .001	**3.0** (1.6, 5.4)	**.01** (.01, .02)
Fetal factors			
Breech presentation	**94** (177), P < .001	**12.8** (10.6, 15.5)	**.25** (.21, .28)
Preterm birth	**20** (247), P < .001	**2.2** (1.8, 2.7)	**.16** (.14, .18)
Major fetal malformations	**18** (89), P < .001	**1.7** (1.4, 2.2)	**.06** (.05, .07)
Twins	**44** (55), P < .001	**3.9** (2.9, 5.3)	**.06** (.05, .08)
Placental factor			
Acute chorioamnionitis	**13** (123), P < .001	**1.4** (1.1, 1.7)	**.05** (.04, .06)
Marker for high fetal motor activity			
Unusually long umbilical cord	**13** (253), P < .001	**1.2** (1.1, 1.4)	**.04** (0.3, .06)
Population attributable risk			**.75** (.73, .77)
Pregnancy outcomes			
Fetal growth retardation	**15** (67), P < .001	1.2 (0.9, 1.7)	
Stillbirth	**37** (80), P < .001	**2.9** (1.6, 4.5)	
Neonatal death	**49** (52), P < .001	**1.9** (1.1, 3.2)	
Neurologic abnormalities at 7 yr	7 (12), P > .1	0.7 (0.4, 1.2)	

*Significant values are in boldface.
†Numbers of cases are in parentheses.

umbilical cord prolapse was not associated with an increased frequency of long-term neurologic abnormalities. This absence of long-term neurologic abnormalities has been noted in previous follow-up studies of umbilical cord prolapse.[47] The reason appears to be that acute antenatal hypoxia severe enough to damage the fetal brain before birth is almost always fatal.[51]

GROSS EDEMA OF THE UMBILICAL CORD

Gross edema of the umbilical cord was identified in 2.7% of the deliveries in the CPS (Fig 6–13). Its antecedent risk factors were preeclampsia and eclampsia, which cause low uteroplacental blood flow; preterm birth; the fetus being male; diffuse fibrin beneath the chorionic (fetal) plate of the placenta; and acute chorioamnionitis (Table 6–8). The association of umbilical cord edema with acute chorioamnionitis

is easy to understand because acute chorioamnionitis is an infectious process that often affects the umbilical cord and manifests as acute funisitis. There is a tendency for Wharton's jelly to decrease with age, so it is not surprising that the cords of preterm born infants more often give the gross appearance of edema than do the cords of full-term infants. The association of presumed low uteroplacental blood flow with umbilical cord edema might relate to the systemic hypertension and heart failure that sometimes develop in a fetus when gravidas are preeclamptic or eclamptic.[8,31] After taking all of the antecedent risk factors into account, an edematous cord was associated with an increased risk of stillbirth (see Table 6–8).

SINGLE UMBILICAL ARTERY

A single umbilical artery was present in 0.7% of the umbilical cords in the CPS

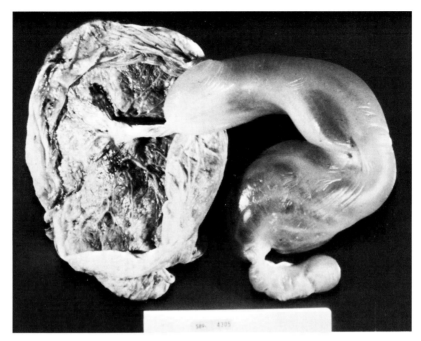

FIG 6–13.
Marked edema in the umbilical cord.

(Table 6–9 and Fig 6–14). This diagnosis must be confirmed from a cord segment that is far distant from the placental surface because the two arteries sometimes fuse into a single vessel within 2 cm of the placenta and occasionally this fusing occurs at distances greater than 2 cm from the placental surface.[2,19,36] A single umbilical artery can occasionally represent a failure of development, particularly

TABLE 6–8.

Risk Estimates for Antecedents to the Development of a Grossly Edematous Umbilical Cord*

Risk Factors	No. of Cases of Edematous Cord per 1,000 Cases With Risk Factor†	Relative Risks (95% Confidence Intervals)	Attributable Risks (95% Confidence Intervals)
All cases	27 *(1,311)*		
Maternal factor			
Preeclampsia, eclampsia	37 (320), *P* < .001	**1.7** (1.2, 2.2)	**.15** (.08, .23)
Fetal factors			
Sex: male	**31** *(764)*, *P* < .001	**1.4** (1.2, 1.6)	**.15** (.13, .16)
Birth asphyxial disorder	**72** *(7)*, *P* < .005	**1.7** (2.0, 3.6)	.00
Placental factors			
Diffuse subchorionic fibrin	**37** *(316)*, *P* < .001	**1.6** (1.4, 1.9)	**.12** (.10, .13)
Acute chorioamnionitis	**35** *(315)*, *P* < .001	**1.4** (1.2, 1.6)	**.07** (.06, .08)
Population attributable risk			**.48** *(.45, .50)*
Pregnancy outcomes			
Preterm birth	**43** *(445)*, *P* < .001	**1.8** (1.6, 2.1)	
Fetal growth retardation	**19** *(77)*, *P* < .001	**0.7** (0.6, 1.0)	
Stillbirth	**87** *(72) P* < .001	**2.4** (1.3, 3.8)	
Neonatal death	**53** *(47)*, *P* < .001	1.4 (0.5, 4.2)	
Neurologic abnormalities at 7 yr	25 *(38)*, *P* > .1	1.0 (0.8, 1.2)	

*Significant values are in boldface.
†Numbers of cases are in parentheses.

TABLE 6–9.

Risk Estimates for Antecedents to the Development of a Single Umbilical Artery*

Risk Factors	No. of Cases of Single Umbilical Arteries per 1,000 Cases With Risk Factor†	Relative Risks (95% Confidence Intervals)	Attributable Risks (95% Confidence Intervals)
All cases	7 *(364)*		
Maternal factor			
Smoked during 1st trimester	**11** *(104), P < .001*	**1.6** (1.3, 2.0)	**.11** (.09, .13)
Maternal diabetes mellitus	**16** *(10), P < .01*	**1.9** (1.0, 3.7)	**.01** (.00, .02)
Fetal factors			
Major fetal malformations	**17** *(77), P < .005*	**2.3** (1.7, 3.1)	**.11** (.09, .14)
Minor fetal malformations	**14** *(39), P < .001*	**1.2** (1.0, 1.5)	**.01** (.00, .02)
Placental factors			
Placental growth retardation	**12** *(39), P < .001*	**1.8** (1.3, 2.4)	**.08** (.04, .12)
Marginal insertion of cord	**14** *(17), P < .01*	**1.8** (1.1, 3.0)	**.02** (.01, .02)
Abnormally short umbilical cord	**12** *(14), P < .05*	**1.6** (1.2, 2.1)	**.02** (.00, .04)
Population attributable risk			***.35** (.29, .33)*
Pregnancy outcomes			
Preterm birth	**9** *(132), P < .05*	**1.2** (1.0, 1.4)	
Fetal growth retardation	**11** *(46), P < .001*	**1.7** (1.3, 2.4)	
Stillbirth	**28** *(24) P < .001*	**4.0** (2.7, 5.2)	
Neonatal death	**15** *(13), P < .01*	**1.7** (1.0, 3.1)	
Neurologic abnormalities at 7 yr	**10** *(15), P < .05*	1.1 (0.6, 1.8)	

*Significant values are in boldface.
†Numbers of cases are in parentheses.

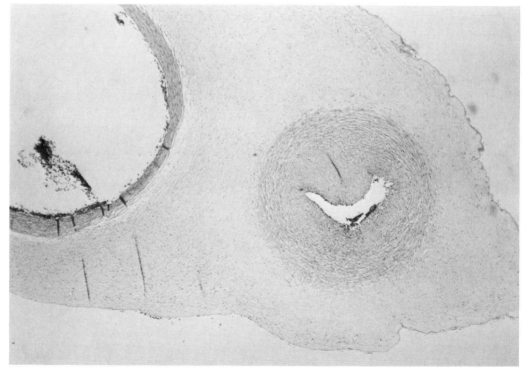

FIG 6–14.
A single umbilical artery.

when it is associated with fetal malformations. More often it appears to be the result of one artery being obliterated by thrombosis or by remodeling. In the case of remodeling a rudimentary second artery is sometimes visible at delivery. The frequency of fetal malformations is reported to be about the same with the primary absence and the secondary atrophy of an umbilical artery.[1] A microscopic examination is necessary to confirm the diagnosis of a single umbilical artery because one artery can be too small to be seen readily without the aid of a microscope.[20] A rudimentary vessel of this type is not always the remnant of an umbilical artery. Sometimes it is the remnant of an allantoic vessel.

In large studies the presence of a single umbilical artery has been associated with autosomal trisomies, the Zellweger syndrome, nonchromosomal fetal malformations, twins, preterm delivery, fetal growth retardation, maternal diabetes mellitus, seizure disorders, toxemia of pregnancy, antepartum hemorrhage, hydramnios, and oligohydramnios.[5,10,39,53,64,67] A single umbilical artery has been associated with more than 100 different fetal malformations and no two studies agree on which malformations predominate. Among twins a single umbilical artery is usually present in only one member, most often the smaller member of the pair.[39]

Antecedent risk factors were identified for 35% of the single umbilical arteries in the CPS (see Table 6–9). The risk factors were maternal cigarette smoking during early pregnancy, malformations in the fetus, a growth-retarded placenta, marginal insertion of the umbilical cord, a very short umbilical cord, and maternal diabetes mellitus (see Table 6–9). The teratogenic nature of diabetes mellitus is the presumed reason for its association with a single umbilical artery.[25] Cigarette smoking during pregnancy reportedly damages the endothelial cells that line the umbilical arteries, so it may be that this damage disposes to the thrombotic obliteration of some arteries. It has long been

known that a single umbilical artery is more frequent when fetal malformations are present, so single arteries appear to be another manifestation of this teratogenesis.[5] The malformations in some of these children are not detected until long after birth.[11] In the CPS 22% of the children who had major congenital malformations had a single umbilical artery.

In the CPS fetal growth retardation was increased 1.7-fold when a single umbilical artery was present (see Table 6–9). A single umbilical artery increased the risk for stillbirth four-fold and the risk for neonatal death 1.7-fold, after antecedent risk factors for a single artery had been taken into consideration (see Table 6–9). All of this mortality excess was in infants who were also growth-retarded at birth. This finding was independent of fetal malformations and the disorders that produce chronic low uteroplacental blood flow, the two most frequent causes of fetal growth retardation. Insufficient placental tissue related to the loss of one perfusing artery is a possible explanation for this excessive mortality because an undersized placenta was prominently associated with a single umbilical artery (see Table 6–9). Each umbilical artery serves part of the placenta, and if one artery did not develop, or if it disappeared early in gestation, the part of the placenta that it would have served might never have developed or it might have undergone a secondary atrophy.[7,30]

UMBILICAL CORD BLOOD VESSEL THROMBOSIS

Claimed causes of umbilical cord vessel thrombosis include velamentous insertion of the cord, acute inflammation, cord vessel varices, entangled cords, intravascular exchange transfusions, and fetal protein C deficiency.[7,58,73] Umbilical cord blood vessel thrombosis was an uncommon occurence (7/1,000) in the CPS (Table 6–10). Acute chorioamnionitis and markers for vigorous fetal motor activity were the only identified risk factors for the

TABLE 6–10.

Risk Estimates for Antecedents to the Development of Thrombosis of a Vessel in the Umbilical Cord*

Risk Factors	No. of Cases of Cord Vessel Thrombosis per 1,000 Cases With Risk Factor†	Relative Risks (95% Confidence Intervals)	Attributable Risks (95% Confidence Intervals)
All cases	7 *(289)*		
Placental factors			
Acute chorioamnionitis	**15** *(137)*, *P* < .001	**2.1** (1.6, 2.7)	**.22** (.19, .26)
Markers for vigorous fetal motor activity			
Diffuse subchorionic fibrin	**11** *(83)*, *P* < .05	**1.3** (1.0, 1.8)	**.10** (.07, .13)
Tight knot in umbilical cord	**22** *(7)*, *P* < .01	**3.3** (1.5, 7.2)	**.02** (.00, .03)
Other indicators			**.02** (.01, .04)
Population attributable risk			**.35** *(.32, .37)*
Pregnancy outcomes			
Preterm birth	**12** *(79)*, *P* < .005	**1.4** (1.1, 1.9)	
Fetal growth retardation	8 *(21)*, *P* > .1	0.8 (0.4, 1.4)	
Stillbirth	**43** *(20)*, *P* < .001	**2.8** (1.4, 4.4)	
Neonatal death	**19** *(10)*, *P* < .02	**2.8** (2.0, 3.6)	
Neurologic abnormalities at 7 yr	10 *(10)*, *P* > .1	1.1 (0.8, 1.5)	

*Significant values are in boldface.
†Numbers of cases are in parentheses.

disorder (see Table 6–10). Funisitis is a characteristic feature of acute chorioamnionitis, and vessel inflammation is a well-known cause of thrombosis. The presence of markers of vigorous fetal motor activity as risk factors for umbilical cord vessel thrombosis suggests that trauma to the cord by fetal movements caused some thromboses (see Table 6–10). Vigorous movements by the fetus sometimes traumatize the placenta, so it is reasonable to postulate that they sometimes traumatize the umbilical cord as well. A tight knot in the umbilical cord presumably predisposes to thrombosis by compressing blood vessels.

A high mortality has been associated in the literature with umbilical cord vessel thrombus.[18,29,73] In the CPS such thrombosis was a high risk for both stillbirth and neonatal death, independent of antecedent risk factors for the thrombosis (see Table 6–10). The perinatal mortality rate was particularly high (245/1,000) when thrombosis was associated with a tight knot in the cord. When cord knots were absent, umbilical vessel thrombosis increased the perinatal mortality rate only 2.8-fold. This supports the claim of Heifetz

that umbilical blood vessel thrombosis is mainly the result of other disorders and it is these other disorders, rather than the thrombosis, that are responsible for fetal death.[27] Umbilical cord vessel thrombosis can cause cerebral palsy.[7,29,50]

UMBILICAL CORD HEMATOMA

To make this diagnosis the hemorrhage should be identified before the cord is clamped because many of the hemorrhages seen by the pathologist are the result of cord clamping at the time of delivery (Fig 6–15). Benirschke and Kaufmann report that umbilical cord hematomas are related to abnormally short cords, trauma, and cord entanglements.[7] Umbilical cord hematomas were rarely recorded (1/1,000) in the CPS (Table 6–11). Seventy percent of the hematomas were associated with unusually long umbilical cords (91st–100th percentile), diffuse fibrin beneath the chorionic (fetal) plate of the placenta, or other indicators of vigorous fetal motor activity including cord knots, nuchal cords, and intervillous thrombi (see Table 6–11). A long umbilical

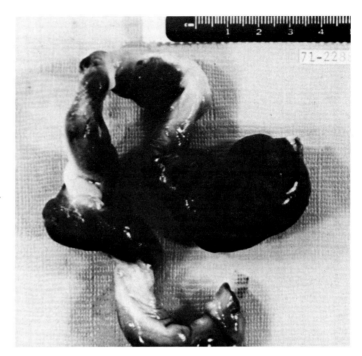

FIG 6–15.
A severe umbilical cord hematoma.

cord is often an indication that vigorous fetal movements placed tension on the cord and diffuse subchorionic fibrin appears to often be the consequence of fetal movements that traumatized the fetal surface of the placenta.[46,48] In the CPS umbilical cord hematomas were associated with a high rate of stillbirths after taking the just-mentioned antecedent risk factors for these hematomas into consid-

TABLE 6–11.

Risk Estimates for Antecedents to the Development of an Umbilical Cord Hematoma*

Risk Factors	No. of Cases of Umbilical Cord Hematoma per 1,000 Cases With Risk Factor†	Relative Risks (95% Confidence Intervals)	Attributable Risks (95% Confidence Intervals)
All cases	1 *(57)*		
Fetal factor			
Major congenital malformations	**2** *(8), P<.02*	**2.2** (1.2, 3.4)	**.09** (.05, .14)
Placental factor			
Acute chorioamnionitis	**2** *(13), P<.05*	**1.4** (1.0, 1.8)	**.10** (.06, .14)
Markers for high fetal motor activity			
Unusually long umbilical cord	**2** *(33), P<.005*	**2.1** (1.1, 3.8)	**.25** (.18, .31)
Diffuse subchorionic fibrin	**2** *(20), P<.05*	**1.7** (1.0, 3.3)	**.13** (.07, .18)
Other indicators			**.32** (.27, .37)
Population attributable risk			***.88** (.82, .94)*
Pregnancy outcomes			
Preterm birth	1 *(12), P>.1*	0.9 (0.6, 1.3)	
Fetal growth retardation	1 *(5), P>.1*	1.0 (0.8, 1.2)	
Stillbirth	**8** *(7) P<.01*	**7.4** (6.0, 9.0)	
Neonatal death	1 *(1), P>.1*	0.9 (0.6, 1.2)	
Neurologic abnormalities at 7 yr	1 *(1), P>.1*	0.6 (0.2, 1.1)	

*Significant values are in boldface.
†Numbers of cases are in parentheses.

eration (see Table 6–11). Fourteen percent of the fetuses and neonates with cord hematomas in the CPS died. In most published studies about half of the infants died.[16,57,70]

Thirty-three of the 36 hematomas in published studies originated from the umbilical vein.[16] Injection studies are useful in determining the origin of such hemorrhages. In recent years amniocentesis and percutaneous umbilical cord sampling have caused a few umbilical cord hematomas with resulting fetal death.[13,15,21,32]

EMBRYONIC REMNANTS IN THE UMBILICAL CORD

Embryonic remnants are present in 20% or more of umbilical cords. None of these remnants were associated in the CPS with an increase in perinatal mortality. These remnants fall into three categories: hemangiomas, teratomas, and cysts. Both *hemangiomas* and *teratomas* are noninvasive. Eighteen umbilical cord hemangiomas were reported in the literature up until 1987.[43] A few have been so

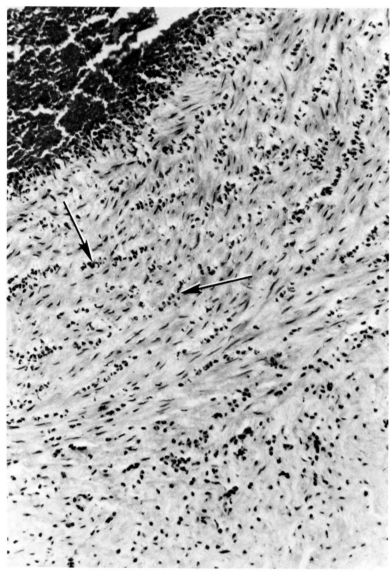

FIG 6–16.
Acute funisitis. *Arrows* point to acute inflammatory cells.

large that they interfered with delivery.[28] The largest was 17 cm in diameter. They appear as local swellings comprised of thin-walled capillaries lined by normal-appearing endothelial cells embedded in a myxoid stroma. None have had arterio-venous shunts large enough to produce fetal heart failure or to trap large numbers of platelets. Their presence has been iden-tified by ultrasonography as early as the tenth week of gestation.

Other embryonic residuals in the um-bilical cord include remnants of the allan-toic duct (urachus), the vitelline duct, and embryonic vessels. *Allantoic duct rem-nants* appear either as canalicular struc-tures lined by flattened epithelium and surrounded by concentric layers of con-nective tissue or as a mass of large packed cells. They are usually located between the two umbilical arteries. *Vitelline duct rem-nants* are most commonly situated at the margin of the cord and are lined by columnar or cuboidal epithelium which sometimes contains a small amount of mucus. At times these duct remnants have a surrounding coat of muscle. *Embryonic vascular remnants* usually appear as thin-walled vessels at the fetal end of the umbilical cord. Allantoic duct, vitelline duct, and embryonic vascular remnants do not appear to have any clinical signif-icance. We have not found them to be associated with major or minor malfor-mations in the newborn.

ACUTE FUNISITIS

Acute inflammation of the cord, known as *funisitis*, is a common disorder. It is the result of bacteria or mycoplasmas in the amniotic fluid attracting fetal neutrophils to migrate out of the umbilical blood vessels.[51] Rarely, maternal neutrophils in the amniotic fluid migrate into the cord. Usually acute funisitis passes through three stages. In the first, polymorphonu-clear leukocytes marginate on the surface of the endothelial cells that line the um-

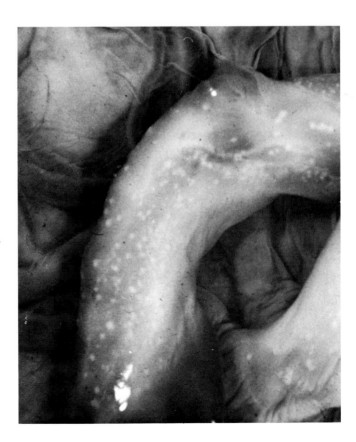

FIG 6–17.
Candidiasis of the umbilical cord.

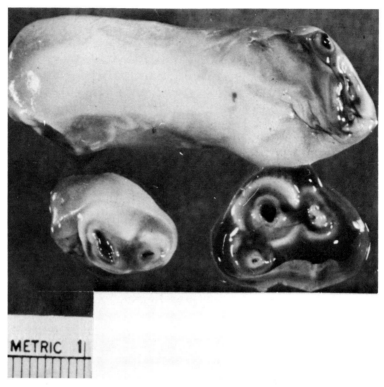

FIG 6–18.
Necrotizing funisitis.

bilical vein. Next, these fetal neutrophils begin to migrate through the walls of the vein. In this invasion the neutrophils occupy interstitial spaces, so that a thin rim of open space is usually visible about each neutrophil (Fig 6–16). This open space around the neutrophil helps to distinguish neutrophils from the folded nuclei of smooth muscle cells in the vessel's wall. In the third stage the neutrophils migrate beyond the wall of the vein to penetrate Wharton's jelly. In about half of the cases this process also involves one or both umbilical arteries. In this latter case the process is usually less advanced in the arteries than it is in the vein. The association of necrosis with neutrophils in Wharton's jelly is probably an indication that the inflammatory process was present for some time because inflammatory debris is not quickly mobilized from Wharton's jelly. The clinical significance of acute funisitis is discussed in Chapter 7.

A variant of acute funisitis is the presence of acute inflammatory cells in small clusters just beneath the amnionic covering of the umbilical cord. This is often a manifestation of infection by *Candida albicans* (Fig 6–17). If this organism is not visible in the sections initially examined, additional sections cut from the same block will usually reveal the mycelia.

Necrotizing funisitis manifests as a severe chronic inflammatory process in the umbilical cord with necrosis and sometimes calcium deposits (Fig 6–18). It has been reported in cases of congenital syphilis and herpes infections. Benirschke and Kaufmann think that it may represent an immune reaction to several different antigens.[7] It is not diagnostic for any single disorder.

REFERENCES

1. Altshuler G, Tsang RC, Ermocilla R: Single umbilical artery: Correlation of clinical status and umbilical cord histology. *Am J Dis Child* 1975; 129:697–700.

2. Arts NFT: Investigations on the vascular system of the placenta. I. General introduction and the fetal vascular system. *Am J Obstet Gynecol* 1961; 82:147–158.

3. Barron S, Riley EP, Smotherman WP, Kotch LE: Umbilical cord length in rats is altered by prenatal alcohol exposure. *Teratology* 1985; 31:49A–50A.

4. Bender HG, Werner C, Karsten C: Zum Einfluss der Nabelschnurstruktur auf Schwangerschafts und Geburtsverlauf. *Arch Gynakol* 1978; 225:347–362.

5. Benirschke K, Brown WH: A vascular anomaly of the umbilical cord: The absence of one umbilical artery in the umbilical cords of normal and abnormal fetuses. *Obstet Gynecol* 1955; 6:399–404.

6. Benirschke K, Driscoll SG: *The Pathology of the Human Placenta.* New York, Springer-Verlag, 1967, pp 205, 232–236.

7. Benirschke K, Kaufmann P: *Pathology of the Human Placenta.* New York, Springer-Verlag, 1990.

8. Berkowitz GS, Mehalek KE, Chitkara U, Rosenberg J, Cogswell C, Berkowitz RL: Doppler umbilical velocimetry in the prediction of adverse outcome in pregnancies at risk for intrauterine growth retardation. *Obstet Gynecol* 1988; 71:742–746.

9. Bilek K, Roth K, Piskazeck K: Insertio-velamentosa-Blutung vor dem Blasensprung. *Zentralbl Gynakol* 1962; 84:1536–1541.

10. Bjoro K Jr, Vascular anomalies of the umbilical cord: I. Obstetric implications. *Early Hum Dev* 1983; 8:119–127.

11. Bryan EM, Kohler HG. The missing umbilical artery. II. Paediatric follow-up. *Arch Dis Child* 1975; 50:714–718.

12. Chasnoff IJ, Fletcher MA: True knot of the umbilical cord. *Am J Obstet Gynecol* 1977; 127:425–427.

13. Chenard E, Bastide A, Fraser WD: Umbilical cord hematoma following diagnostic funipuncture. *Obstet Gynecol* 1990; 76:994–996.

14. Cullen TS: *Embryology, Anatomy and Diseases of the Umbilicus, Together with Diseases of the Urachus.* Philadelphia, WB Saunders Co, 1966.

15. DeSa DJ: Diseases of the umbilical cord, in Perrin EVDK (ed): *Pathology of the Placenta.* New York, Churchill Livingston Inc, 1984, p 121.

16. Dippel AL: Hematomas of the umbilical cord. *Surg Gynecol Obstet* 1940; 70:51–57.

17. Dippel AL: Maligned umbilical cord entanglements. *Am J Obstet Gynecol* 1964; 88:1012–1019.

18. Eggens JH, Bruinse HW: An unusual case of fetal distress. *Am J Obstet Gynecol* 1984; 148:219–220.

19. Fox H: *Pathology of the Placenta.* Philadelphia, WB Saunders Co, 1978.

20. Fujikura T: Single umbilical artery and congenital malformations. *Am J Obstet Gynecol* 1964; 88:829–830.

21. Gassner CB, Paul RH: Laceration of umbilical cord vessels secondary to amniocentesis. *Obstet Gynecol* 1976; 48:627–630.

22. Ghosh A, Woo JSK, MacHenry C, Wan CW, Ohoy KM, Ma HK: Fetal loss from umbilical cord abnormalities. A difficult case for prevention. *Eur J Obstet Gynec Reprod Biol* 1984; 18:183–198.

23. Gilbert EF, Zugibe FT: Torsion and constriction of the umbilical cord: A cause of fetal death. *Arch Pathol* 1974; 97:58–59.

24. Hankins GDV, Snyder RR, Hauth JC, Gilstrap LC III, Hammond T: Nuchal cords and neonatal outcome. *Obstet Gynecol* 1987; 70:687–691.

25. Haust MD: Maternal diabetes mellitus, effects on the fetus and placenta. *Monog Pathol* 1981; 22:201–285.

26. Heifetz SA: Strangulation of the umbilical cord by amniotic bands: Report of 6 cases and literature review. *Pediatr Pathol* 1984; 2:285–304.

27. Heifetz SA: Thrombosis of the umbilical cord, analysis of 52 cases and literature review. *Pediatr Pathol* 1988; 6:37–54.

28. Heifetz SA, Rueda-Pedraza ME: Hemangiomas of the umbilical cord. *Pediatr Pathol* 1983; 1:385–393.

29. Hoag RW: Fetomaternal hemorrhage associated with umbilical vein thrombosis. Case report. *Am J Obstet Gynecol* 1986; 154: 1271–1274.

30. Hobel CJ, Emmanouilides GC, Townsend DE, Yashiro K: Ligation of one umbilical artery in the fetal lamb: Experimental production of fetal malnutrition. *Obstet Gynecol* 1970; 36:582–588.

31. Howard RB, Hosokawa T, Maguire MH: Hypoxia-induced fetoplacental vasoconstriction in perfused human placental cotyledons. *Am J Obstet Gynecol* 1987; 157:1261–1266.

32. Jauniaux E, Donner C, Simon P, Vanesse M, Hustin J, Rodesch F: Pathologic aspects of the umbilical cord after percutaneous umbilical blood sampling. *Obstet Gynecol* 1989; 73:215–218.

33. Javert CT, Barton B: Congenital and acquired lesions of the umbilical cord and spontaneous abortion. *Am J Obstet Gynecol* 1952; 63:1065–1077.

34. Kan PS, Eastman NJ: Coiling of the umbilical cord around the foetal neck. *J Obstet Gynaecol Br Emp* 1957; 64:227–228.

35. Katz V, Blanchard G, Dingman C, Bowes WA Jr, Cefalo RC: Atenolol and short umbilical cords. *Am J Obstet Gynecol* 1987; 156:1271–1272.

36. Kelber R: Gespaltene "solitäre" Nabelschnur-arterie. *Arch Gynakol* 1976; 220:319–323.

37. Kouyoumdjian A: Velamentous insertion of the umbilical cord. *Obstet Gynecol* 1980; 56:737–742.

38. Lacro RV, Jones KL, Benirschke K: The umbilical cord twist: Origin, direction, and relevance. *Am J Obstet Gynecol* 1987; 157:833–838.

39. Leung AKC, Robson WLM: Single umbilical artery, a report of 159 cases. *Am J Dis Child* 1989; 143:108–111.

40. Leveno KJ, Quirk JG, Cunningham EG, Nelson SD, Santos-Ramos R, Tofanian A, DePalma RT: Prolonged pregnancy: I. Observations concerning the causes of fetal distress. *Am J Obstet Gynecol* 1984; 150:465–473.

41. Miller ME, Higginbottom M, Smith DW: Short umbilical cord, its origin and relevance. *Pediatrics* 1981; 67:618–621.

42. Miller ME, Jones MC, Smith DW: Tension: The basis of umbilical cord growth. *J Pediatr* 1982; 101:844.

43. Mishriki YY, Vanyshelbaum Y, Epstein H, Blanc W: Hemangioma of the umbilical cord. *Pediatr Pathol* 1987; 7:43–49.

44. Mitchell APB, Anderson GS, Russell JK: Perinatal death from foetal exsanguination. *Br Med J* 1957; 1:611–614.

45. Moessinger AC, Blanc WA, Marone PA, Polsen DC: Umbilical cord length as an index of fetal activity: Experimental study and clinical implications. *Pediatr Res* 1982; 16:109–112.

46. Naeye RL: Umbilical cord length: Clinical significance. *J Pediatr* 1985; 107:278–282.

47. Naeye RL: When and how does antenatal brain damage occur? in Iffy L (ed): *Second Perinatal Practice and Malpractice Symposium.* New York, Healthmark Communications, 1986, p 125.

48. Naeye RL: The clinical significance of absent subchorionic fibrin in the placenta. *Am J Clin Pathol* 1990; 94:196–198.

49. Naeye RL, Peters EC: Antenatal hypoxia and low IQ values. *Am J Dis Child* 1987; 141:50–54.

50. Naeye RL, Peters EC, Bartholomew M, Landis JR: Origins of cerebral palsy. *Am J Dis Child* 1989; 143:1154–1161.

51. Naeye RL, Tafari N: *Risk Factors in Pregnancy and Diseases of the Fetus and Newborn.* Baltimore, Williams & Wilkins Co, 1983.

52. Niswander KR: Asphyxia in the fetus and cerebral palsy, in Pitkin RM, Zlatnik FJ (eds): *Year Book of Obstetrics and Gynecology.* Chicago, Year Book Medical Publishers, Inc, 1983, p 107.

53. Peckham CH, Yerushalmy J: Aplasia of one umbilical artery: Incidence by race and certain obstetric factors. *Obstet Gynecol* 1965; 26:359–366.

54. Quek SP, Tan KL: Vasa previa. *Aust NZ J Obstet Gynaecol* 1972; 12:206–209.

55. Rayburn WF, Beynen A, Brinkman DL: Umbilical cord length and intrapartum complications. *Obstet Gynecol* 1981; 57:450–452.

56. Rucker MP, Tureman GR: Vasa previa. *Va Med Monthly* 1945; 72:202–207.

57. Ruvinsky ED, Wiley TL, Morrison JC, Blake PG: In utero diagnosis of umbilical cord hematoma by ultrasonography. *Am J Obstet Gynecol* 1981; 140:833–834.

58. Seeds JW, Chescheir NC, Bowes WA Jr, Owl-Smith FA: Fetal death as a complication of intrauterine intravascular transfusion. *Obstet Gynecol* 1989; 74:461–463.

59. Shenker L, Reed K, Anderson C, Hauck L, Spark R: Syndrome of camptodactyly, ankyloses, facial anomalies, and pulmonary hypoplasia (Pena-Shokeir syndrome): Obstetric and ultrasound aspects. *Am J Obstet Gynecol* 1985; 152:303–307.

60. Sheperd AJ, Richardson CJ, Brown JP: Nuchal cord as a cause of neonatal anemia. *Am J Dis Child* 1985; 139:71–73.

61. Silver RK, Dooley SL, Tamura RK, Depp R: Umbilical cord size and amniotic fluid volume in prolonged pregnancy. *Am J Obstet Gynecol* 1987; 157:716–720.

62. Sinnathuray TA: The nuchal cord incidence and significance. *J Obstet Gynaecol Br Commonwealth* 1966; 73:226–231.

63. Sloper KS, Brown RS, Baum JD: The water content of the human umbilical cord. *Early Hum Dev* 1979; 3:205–210.

64. Smith DW: Recognizable patterns of human malformation, in *Major Problems in Clinical Paediatrics*, vol 7. London, WB Saunders Co, 1982.

65. Soernes T, Bakke T: The length of the human umbilical cord in vertex and breech presentations. *Am J Obstet Gynecol* 1986; 154:1086–1087.

66. Soernes T, Bakke T: The length of the human umbilical cord in twin pregnancies. *Am J Obstet Gynecol* 1987; 157:1229–1230.

67. Some H: Single umbilical artery with congenital malformations. *Curr Top Pathol* 1979; 66:159–173.

68. Spatz WB, Nabelschnur-Längen bei Insektivoren und Primaten. *Z Saugetierk* 1968; 33:226–229.

69. Spellacy WN, Gravem H, Fisch RO: The umbilical cord complications of true knots, nuchal coils, and cords around the body. *Am J Obstet Gynecol* 1966; 94:1136–1142.

70. Summerville JW, Powar JS, Ueland K: Umbilical cord hematoma resulting in intrauterine fetal demise, a case report. *J Reprod Med* 1987; 32:213–216.

71. Uyanwah-Akpom P, Fox H: The clinical significance of marginal and velamentous insertion of the cord. *Br J Obstet Gynaecol* 1977; 84:941–943.

72. Widholm O, Nieminen U: Prolapse of the umbilical cord. *Acta Obstet Gynecol* 1963; 42:21–29.

73. Wolfman WL, Purohit DM, Self SE: Umbilical vein thrombosis at 32 weeks' gestation with delivery of a living infant. *Am J Obstet Gynecol* 1983; 146:468–470.

CHAPTER 7

Disorders of the Placenta and Decidua

THE DEVELOPMENT OF THE PLACENTA

Knowledge about the normal development of the placenta aids the recognition and interpretation of abnormalities in the organ.

Early Development

The first structure in the placenta to develop is the chorion, which evolves from the wall of the primitive blastocyst. Implantation is usually complete by about the 11th day after conception, at which time the primitive trophoblast has already differentiated into cytotrophoblastic and syncytiotrophoblastic cellular layers. The primitive villi are then formed when mesenchyme from the extraembryonic meso-derm invades the mass of trophoblastic cells. The columns of cytotrophoblastic cells then expand and fuse with their neighbors to complete the formation of an enclosed lacunar space, which is the intervillous space. Blood vessels invade the primitive villi, which thereafter become the stem villi. By this means the primary placental circulation is established by about the 17th day after conception.

Subsequent Development

Initially, the primary villi cover the entire surface of the implanted blastocyst. As the embryo grows the villi that are orientated toward the uterine cavity atrophy. This process is complete by the fourth month, after which villi are restricted to the definitive placenta. During this period villi continue to branch off the stem villi to form placental lobules.

Subsequently, there are two successive invasions of the uterine wall by trophoblastic cells. In the first, trophoblastic cells spread through the transformed endometrium, now known as the decidua basalis, and invade the inner myometrium for several millimeters, at which point the invasion stops (Figs 7–1 and 7–2).[276] As pregnancy advances these trophoblastic cells convert to the syncytial giant cells that are normally seen in the interstitium of the innermost myometrium. A second invasion of trophoblastic cells takes place inside the walls of the uterine spiral arteries. This remodels these arteries so they can expand and accommodate the large blood flow which the uterus supplies to the intervillous space during the remainder of pregnancy.[149,276] This invasion by trophoblastic cells inside the walls of the spiral arteries normally stops at the point where the spiral arteries join the radial arteries.

EVOLUTIONARY DEVELOPMENT OF THE VILLI

Stem villi are simple structures that have a core of loosely arranged mesen-

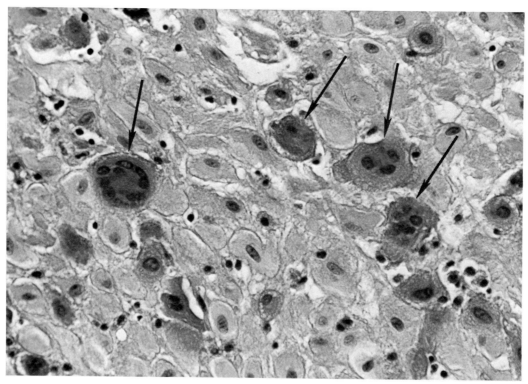

FIG 7–1.
Arrows point to syncytiotrophoblastic cells in the decidua basalis. Hematoxylin-eosin (HE) stain, ×1,200.

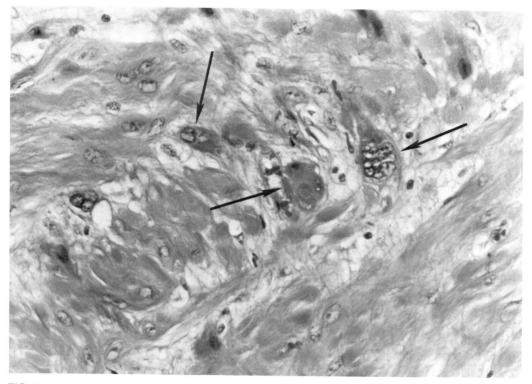

FIG 7–2.
Arrows point to syncytiotrophoblastic cells in the superficial myometrium. HE stain, ×1,200.

chyme covered by a double layer of trophoblastic cells. Hofbauer cells (macrophages) are scattered within the mesenchyme. The inner layer of the trophoblast is made up of cuboidal cells with large pale nuclei (Fig 7–3). This is termed the *cytotrophoblast*, and the cells are known as *Langhans' cells*. The outer layer of trophoblastic cells is termed the *syncytiotrophoblast*. It is comprised of flattened cells with small, darker-staining nuclei. Most villi normally have these two covering layers of trophoblastic cells during the first 20 weeks of gestation.

The placenta continues to grow until late in pregnancy by the repeated formation of trophoblastic buds from the stem villi. In the mature placenta the number of cotyledons is defined by the number of stem villi. With each branching the diameter of newly formed villi gets smaller while the volume of ingrowing capillaries

remains about the same, so an ever larger proportion of the villi become comprised of capillaries. In this process the ratio of large to small villi decreases, the number of cells inside the villi decreases, syncytial knots increase in size and number, and the cytotropholastic layer disappears except for a few cells. The walls of arteries become thicker in stem villi as smooth muscle is replaced by collagen.

Between 20 and 40 weeks of gestation the process of forming new villi increases the surface area of the villi sixfold.[3] As time passes the capillaries move closer to the trophoblastic layer, which facilitates gas and nutrient exchange with maternal blood in the intervillous space. As gestation advances fibroblasts lay down collagen in the stem villi, and arteries and veins within these villi develop smooth muscle in their walls.

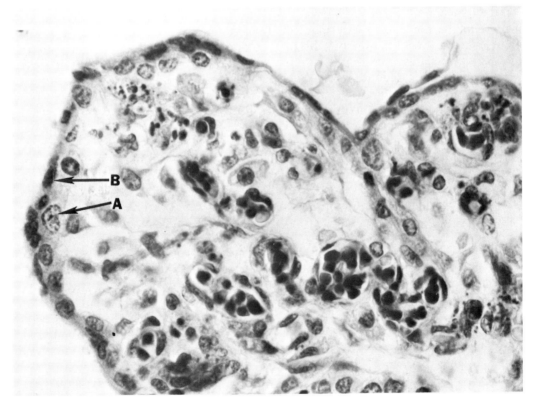

FIG 7–3.
A double layer of cytotrophoblastic *(A)* and syncytiotrophoblastic *(B)* cells cover the villi in the first half of gestation. HE stain, ×1,200.

Subsequent Development

Portions of the cytotrophoblast (Langhans' layer) are normally easily visible until about the 28th week of gestation. After the 28th week the cytotrophoblast progressively disappears, and the syncytiotrophoblast flattens. Nuclei become scarce in the syncytiotrophoblast except at intervals where they proliferate in large numbers to form multinucleated syncytial knots (Fig 7–4). After the 28th week the capillaries within villi become ever more prominent and many of the most peripheral villi become very small. Collagen continues to be deposited in the stem villi and the deposition extends variably into the terminal villi.

EXAMINING THE PLACENTA

Which Placentas Should Be Examined?

There are diagnostic, prognostic, investigative, educational, and legal reasons for examining the placenta. Every placenta should have a gross examination by the clinician performing the delivery. The results of this examination should be recorded and the resulting report should include the length of the umbilical cord, the location of the placenta in the uterus if it is known, and any other information that would not be obvious to individuals subsequently examining the placenta. All placentas should be referred to a central laboratory for examination by a pathologist or specially trained technician. There are several reasons for this. First, the accoucheur is sometimes too busy with the delivery to give the placenta, umbilical cord, and fetal membranes a thorough gross examination. Second, it is often desirable to store parts of each placenta in paraffin blocks, even when slides are not prepared for microscopic examination. Such storage is often undertaken because it is impossible to identify at the time of delivery all cases that may eventually be the subject of litigation.

Microscopic Examination

Placentas should be examined microscopically when there has been any abnormality in pregnancy, delivery, or the clinical condition of the neonate or mother. Microscopic examination is also important when there is gross abnormality in the placenta, umbilical cord, or fetal membranes. A partial list of gestational abnormalities that should lead to a placental examination include maternal diabetes mellitus or gestational glucose intolerance, any type of maternal hypertension, delivery before 38 weeks or after 42 weeks of gestation, oligohydramnios or polyhydramnios, fever or any other indication of maternal infection, a history or strong suspicion of maternal substance abuse, placenta previa, abruptio placentae, and any maternal bleeding during pregnancy apart from spotting early in the first trimester. A partial list of fetal and neonatal conditions which should lead to a microscopic examination of the placenta includes congenital malformations, stillbirth, neonatal death, fetal growth retardation of any type, hydrops, meconium in the amniotic fluid, Apgar scores of 0 to 3 at 1 minute or thereafter, any neurologic abnormalities or seizures in the newborn, any evidence of fetal distress during labor and delivery, fetal tachycardia, neonatal respiratory distress or tachypnea, any evidence of infection in the neonate, multiple births, admission to a neonatal intensive care unit, or any clinical abnormalities that keep the neonate in the hospital longer than is usual for normal newborns.

How the Placenta Should Be Fixed

A placenta can be stored for up to 3 days at 4° C without producing artifacts that pose serious problems during microscopic examination. Such artifacts can be completely prevented if placental tissue is fixed within a day of delivery. Permanent sections should not be prepared from tissue that has been frozen without recognizing that freezing and thawing often produce artifacts that can be confused

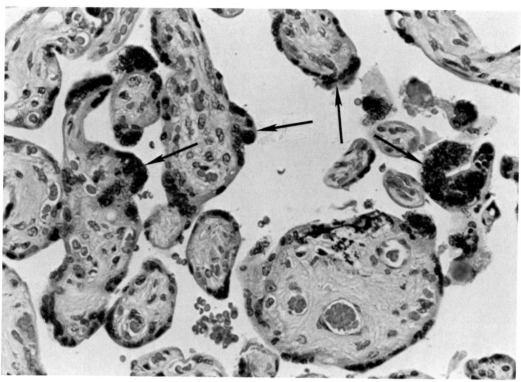

FIG 7–4.
By the 28th week the cytotrophoblast has disappeared and subsequently the nuclei in the syncytiotrophoblast become scarce except at intervals where they proliferate in large numbers to form multinucleated syncytial knots *(arrows)*. HE stain, ×600.

with villous edema. Tissue blocks should be fixed in buffered formalin. Assuming that the formalin is in a concentration of 40% when received from the manufacturer, dissolve 40 g of monosodium phosphate and 65 g of disodium phosphate in 9 L of water. Add the 9 L to 1 L of the 40% formalin to prepare the buffered formalin. For proper fixation to occur, the placenta should be allowed to lie flat, not folded, and be covered with at least three times its own volume of buffered formalin. Consultants receive many requests to review placental tissue that has been poorly fixed. The artifacts produced by this poor fixation are one of the reasons why pathologists sometimes experience difficulties in interpreting microscopic findings in the placenta.

If there is a critical need to evaluate the number, volume, and structure of blood vessels in the villi for research purposes, the placenta should be fixed by perfusion rather than by immersion. Perfusion fixation is also necessary to quantitate the fine structure of the trophoblast. Electron microscopy reveals ischemic changes about 10 minutes after a placenta has been delivered by cesarean section and severe necrosis is evident within an hour.[144] Perfusion with a mixture of glutaraldehyde and formalin should be preceded by perfusion with a heparin–physiologic saline solution. Perfusion pressures should be no higher than 60 mm Hg to avoid artifacts.

Selecting Tissue Blocks for Microscopic Examination

After complete inspection of the two surfaces and the edge of the placenta, cross-section the placenta like a loaf of bread into slices that are 1.5 to 2.0 cm thick. At least three representative blocks of placenta tissue should be removed for microscopic examination. One block should be taken from the periphery, one 3 to 4 cm away from the insertion of the cord, and the third from an area where the fetal plate of the placenta is thinnest. Each block of tissue should be 3 to 4 cm wide and span the entire thickness of the placenta to include both the maternal and the fetal surfaces. Blocks of tissue should also be taken from any grossly visible lesions. Taking additional blocks for microscopic examination will increase the chance of finding villitis and several other disorders. The fetal surface of the placenta should not be wiped by fingers or a towel because such wiping often removes the amnion, particularly when it is edematous. Such edema is often the consequence of a clinically important disorder.

Gross Examination

The extraplacental membranes should be examined for opacity, color, and the point of insertion on the placenta. *Vela-*

mentous insertion of the umbilical cord is diagnosed when the umbilical blood vessels prematurely break out of the umbilical cord and traverse the fetal membranes before they reach the placenta. Small nodular elevations that are several millimeters in diameter and widely distributed over the fetal surface of the placenta are often manifestations of *amnion nodosum*, a consequence of absent amniotic fluid (oligohydramnios) (Fig 7–5). This absence of amniotic fluid prevents exfoliated cells from the fetal skin and the amnion from being washed off the surface of the placenta. These exfoliated cells constitute the small nodules of amnion nodosum. The nodules of amnion nodosum can be distinguished from the nodules of squamous metaplasia by the fact that only the nodules of amnion nodosum can be easily wiped off the surface of the placenta.

The maternal surface of the placenta should be examined for missing tissue that might indicate that fragments of the placenta have been retained in the wall of the uterus as the result of an abnormally deep penetration of the uterine wall by trophoblastic cells *(placenta accreta). Abruption*

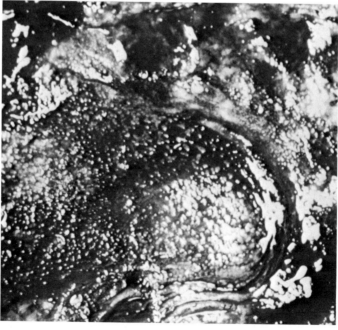

FIG 7–5.
The small opaque nodules of amnion nodosum cover the surface of the placenta.

placentae should be suspected when a blood clot on the maternal surface of the placenta is tightly adherent to the maternal surface or is located in a depression in the substance of the placenta.

DISORDERS OF THE PLACENTA

Placental Weight

Great variations are commonly observed in placental weights. Some of this variation may have a genetic origin, because there are some differences in the genes that regulate fetal and placental growth.[269] Many of the observed variations in placental weights are due to differences in the amounts of umbilical cord, extraplacental membranes, and blood clots that are removed before the organ is weighed, differences in the amount of blood trapped in the intervillous space, and variations in the length of storage before the organ is weighed. Most of these factors need not greatly influence placental weights. The umbilical cord, extraplacental membranes, and attached blood clots should be removed before the organ is weighed. Blood should

be allowed to drain from the umbilical cord and maternal surface for at least 2 hours before the organ is weighed. If the organ is weighed only a few minutes after delivery, as much as 200 g of blood may be retained in the organ.[96] Weights should be measured within a day of delivery. The unfixed placenta will lose about 10% of its weight in 48 hours under refrigeration.[167]

Placental growth percentiles, based on these procedures, are shown in Figure 7–6. We have found that placental weights rarely change more than 7% after fixation in buffered formalin, so the placenta is worth weighing even if it has been fixed.

Small Placentas

An unusually small placenta often has clinical significance. We placed placentas in this category when weights were between the 1st and 10th percentiles for gestational age. Low maternal pregravid body weight, low pregnancy weight gain, and the absence of hand and facial edema in the gravida were all associated with small placentas (Figs 7–7 and 7–8). All of these factors are associated with low maternal gestational blood volume expansion with resulting low blood flow from

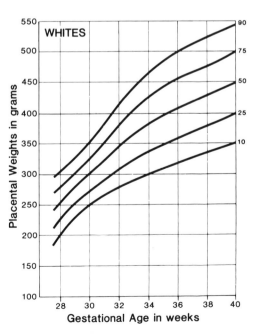
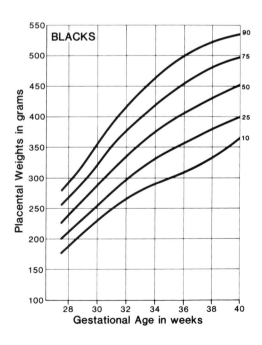

FIG 7–6.
Growth percentiles for normal placental weights.

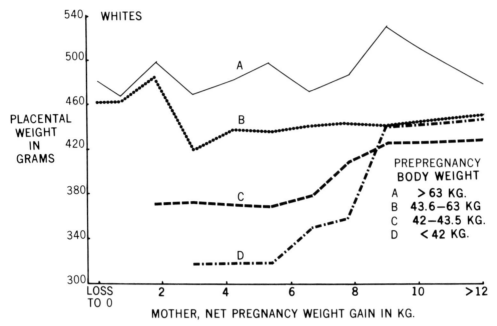

FIG 7–7.
Small placentas were more frequent when women had low pregravid body weights and had small pregnancy weight gains. (From Naeye RL, Tafari N: *Risk Factors in Pregnancy and Diseases of the Fetus and Newborn.* Baltimore, Williams & Wilkins Co, 1983, p 33. Used by permission.)

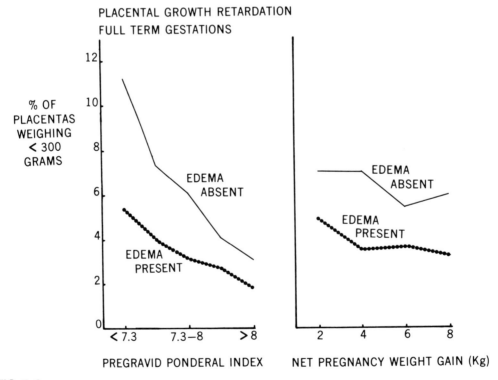

FIG 7–8.
Placental growth retardation was less frequent in full-term gestations when gravidas developed hands and facial edema than when such edema was absent. (From Naeye RL, Tafari N: *Risk Factors in Pregnancy and Diseases of the Fetus and Newborn.* Baltimore, Williams & Wilkins Co, 1983, p 168. Used by permission.)

the uterus to the placenta.[237] Taking these growth factors and the sex of the infant into consideration, we were able to identify several risk factors for placental growth retardation in the Collaborative Perinatal Study (CPS). The most important of these risk factors was fetal growth retardation (Table 7–1). Other factors that were associated with small placental size included accelerated placental maturation and major fetal malformations. Unevenly accelerated placental maturation is the characteristic consequence of preeclampsia and chronic maternal hypertension, which reduce blood flow from the uterus to the placenta (Fig 7–9).[258] This low flow retards placental growth by restricting uterine blood flow into the intervillous space. The retarding effect on placental growth is particularly striking when the low blood flow is present from early gestation. Many of the major autosomal disorders are associated with placental growth retardation. Trisomy 21 is an exception, the fetus often being more growth-retarded than the placenta.

All of these risk factors in combination accounted for 47% of the growth-retarded placentas in the CPS (see Table 7–1). This makes it clear that fetal and placental growth are not always linked. This is not surprising because different genes regulate fetal and placental growth. Paternal antigens are expressed in the placenta and fetal membranes and maternal antigens in the fetus.[140,269] In the CPS a small placenta was associated with an increased frequency of stillbirths and mental retardation at 7 years of age, independent of the size of the fetus, malformations in the child, and the disorders that chronically reduce uteroplacental blood flow (see Table 7–1). The association with stillbirths raises the possibility that small placentas are sometimes functionally inadequate to supply all of the needs of the fetus for oxygen and nutrients.

The microscopic findings in a small placenta often provide clues to the genesis of the placental growth retardation. A frequent example is unevenly accelerated villous maturation and infarcts which are

TABLE 7–1.

Risk Estimates for Antecedents to the Development of an Unusually Small Placenta (Growth Percentiles 1 Through 10)*

Risk Factors	No. of Cases in Which Placenta was Unusually Small per 1,000 Cases With Risk Factor†	Relative Risks (95% Confidence Intervals)	Attributable Risks (95% Confidence Intervals)
All cases	99 (3,315)		
Maternal factors			
Preeclampsia, eclampsia	**126** (906), P < .001	**1.3** (1.1, 1.5)	**.09** (.07, .11)
Fetal factors			
Birth weight, percentiles 1–10	**395** (1,291), P < .001	**8.9** (8.0, 9.9)	**.34** (.32, .37)
Major fetal malformations	**120** (320), P < .001	**1.1** (1.0, 1.3)	**.02** (.00, .05)
Placental factors			
Uniformly accelerated villous maturation	**117** (86), P < .002	**1.6** (1.2, 2.0)	**.02** (.01, .03)
Population attributable risk			**.47** (.43, .53)
Pregnancy outcomes			
Preterm birth	**91** (657), P < .02	**0.9** (0.7, 1.0)	
Stillbirth	**400** (68), P < .001	**4.8** (4.4, 5.3)	
Neonatal death	**80** (85), P < .02	1.4 (0.9, 2.0)	
Neurologic abnormalities at 7 yr	**125** (161), P < .001	**1.2** (1.0, 1.5)	
Mental retardation without motor abnormalities		**1.4** (1.0, 1.9)	

*Significant values are in boldface.
†Numbers of cases are in parentheses.

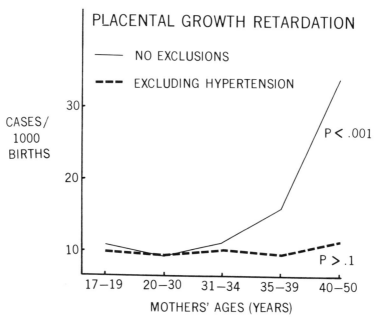

FIG 7–9.
Placental growth retardation became more frequent after age 30 owing to an increasing frequency of chronic hypertension. (From Naeye RL, Tafari N: *Risk Factors in Pregnancy and Diseases of the Fetus and Newborn.* Baltimore, Williams & Wilkins Co, 1983, p 169. Used by permission.)

a characteristic consequence of low blood flow from the uterus to the placenta.[237] Such a low flow markedly restricts the delivery of nutrients to the placenta and is one of the most frequent causes of fetal growth retardation. The low blood flow in such cases is caused by stenotic segments or occlusions in the spiral arteries of the uterus that limit blood flow to the intervillous space of the placenta. If the child is mildly growth-retarded at birth, the prognosis for catch-up growth is good. Only when a child's birth weight is more than 25% below the mean value for its gestational age is some degree of long-term growth retardation likely. With this degree of growth retardation there is also an increased risk of mild mental retardation and learning disorders (see Chapter 11). Maternal cigarette smoking during pregnancy is a well-known cause of fetal growth retardation. It does not cause a parallel retardation of placental growth, so the ratio of fetal to placental weight decreases.

Unusually Large Placentas

Common causes of an unusually large placenta (91st–100th weight percentile) are villous edema, maternal diabetes mellitus, severe maternal anemia, fetal anemia, congenital syphilis, large intervillous thrombi, and a large blood clot beneath the subchorionic (fetal) plate of the placenta. Rare causes of an unusually large placenta include toxoplasmosis, congenital fetal nephrosis, idiopathic fetal hydrops, and multiple placental chorangiomas. Placental enlargement with diabetes mellitus and chronic fetal and maternal anemia are usually related to abnormally large villi for gestational age.

Villous edema is the most frequent cause of a preterm placenta being overweight. This overweight condition is often not recognized because charts of normal placental weights for gestational age are not consulted. Recognizing placental villous edema is important because when it is widespread and severe it makes fetuses hypoxic with resulting low Apgar scores,

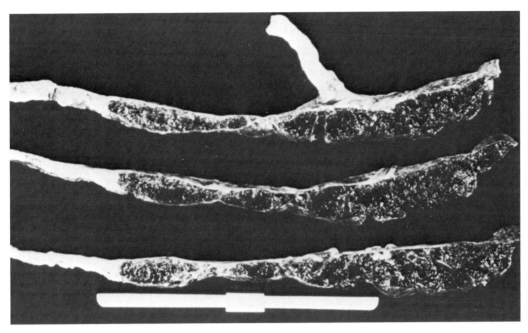

FIG 7–10.
An unusually thin placenta.

difficulty in resuscitation at birth, neonatal respiratory distress, a high neonatal mortality rate, and an increased frequency of long-term neurologic abnormalities.[233] In the CPS, 5% of preterm born infants with normal-weight placentas had one or more neurologic abnormalities at 7 years of age compared with 9% of children of the same gestational age who had overweight placentas.[222] In most of these latter cases the placenta was overweight because it was edematous.

Placental Thickness

Unusually Thin Placentas

Of the full-term placentas in the CPS, 12.1% were classified as thin because they were less than 2 cm in average thickness (Fig 7–10). The antecedents of thin placentas were a placenta that was subnormal in weight, the gravida being short or thin, and major fetal malformations (Table 7–2). Taking all of these risk factors into consideration, an unusually thin placenta increased the risk for both fetal growth retardation and for neonatal death, rais-

ing the possibility that very thin placentas are sometimes functionally insufficient (see Table 7–2). A thin placenta did not increase the risk for long-term neurologic abnormalities.

Thick Placentas

Of the placentas in the CPS, 13.1% were classified as unusually thick because they were 3 cm or greater in average thickness. Only 5% of these unusually thick placentas were explained by risk factors, raising the possibility that they are usually an indication of health rather than of disease (Table 7–3). This possibility is supported by the finding that unusually thick placentas were associated with lower-than-expected frequencies of fetal growth retardation and neonatal death (see Table 7–3).

Bilobed and Trilobed Placentas

Of the placentas in the CPS, 1.7% (791) were bilobed or trilobed (bipartite or tripartite), and 1.5% (738) had an accessory (succenturiate) lobe. To be classified as bipartite or tripartite the two or three

TABLE 7–2.

Risk Estimates for Antecedents to the Development of Unusually Thin Placentas (<2 cm at Full Term)*

Risk Factors	No. of Cases of Unusually Thin Placentas per 1,000 Cases With Risk Factor†	Relative Risks (95% Confidence Intervals)	Attributable Risks (95% Confidence Intervals)
All cases	111 *(4,663)*		
Maternal factors			
Short stature	**161** *(721)*, *P*<.001	**1.5** (1.4, 1.6)	**.05** (.04, .06)
Very thin pregravid	**127** *(1,418)*, *P*<.02	**1.1** (1.0, 1.3)	**.02** (.00, .04)
Fetal factors			
Sex: female	**124** *(2,334)*, *P*<.05	**1.1** (1.0, 1.2)	**.08** (.07, .09)
Major fetal malformations	**132** *(419)*, *P*<.05	**1.1** (1.0, 1.2)	**.01** (.00, .01)
Placental factor			
Low-weight placenta (percentiles 1–10)	**258** *(833)*, *P*<.001	**2.5** (1.7, 3.4)	**.13** (.10, .17)
Population attributable risk			**.29** *(.26, .32)*
Pregnancy outcomes			
Preterm birth (all births in analyses full term)			
Fetal growth retardation	**190** *(659)*, *P*<.001	**1.8** (1.6, 2.0)	
Stillbirth	**240** *(67)*, *P*<.001	1.0 (0.7, 1.4)	
Neonatal death	**173** *(39)*, *P*<.005	**1.5** (1.1, 2.1)	
Neurologic abnormalities at 7 yr	117 *(196)*, *P*>.1	1.0 (0.8, 1.2)	

Significant values are in boldface.
†Numbers of cases are in parentheses.

TABLE 7–3.

Risk Estimates for Antecedents to the Development of an Unusually Thick Placenta (>3 cm at Full Term)*

Risk Factors	No. of Cases of a Thick Placenta per 1,000 Cases With Risk Factor†	Relative Risks (95% Confidence Intervals)	Attributable Risks (95% Confidence Intervals)
All cases	116 *(4,455)*		
Maternal factors			
Obese pregravid	**170** *(485)*, *P*<.001	**1.4** (1.3, 1.5)	**.03** (.02, .04)
Tall (>165 cm)	**144** *(249)*, *P*<.001	**1.1** (1.0, 1.2)	**.01** (.01, .02)
Diabetes mellitus	**188** *(81)*, *P*<.001	**1.4** (1.0, 1.8)	**.01** (.00, .01)
Population attributable risk			**.05** *(.03, .07)*
Pregnancy outcomes			
Preterm birth (all births full term)			
Fetal growth retardation	**106** *(296)*, *P*<.001	**0.7** (**0.6, 0.8**)	
Stillbirth	**189** *(40)*, *P*<.005	1.1 (0.6, 1.8)	
Neonatal death	102 *(19)*, *P*>.1	**0.7** (0.4, 1.0)	
Neurologic abnormalities at 7 yr	137 *(201)*, *P*>.1	1.1 (0.8, 1.6)	

Significant values are in boldface.
†Numbers of cases are in parentheses.

lobes of a placenta should be separated by a membrane and be of equal or near-equal size (Fig 7–11). There is no certain information on how multilobed placentas form. In the CPS a bipartite placenta in one pregnancy was followed by a 2.5-fold greater-than-expected frequency of a bipartite placenta in the next pregnancy. This raises the possibility that some multilobed placentas have a genetic origin.

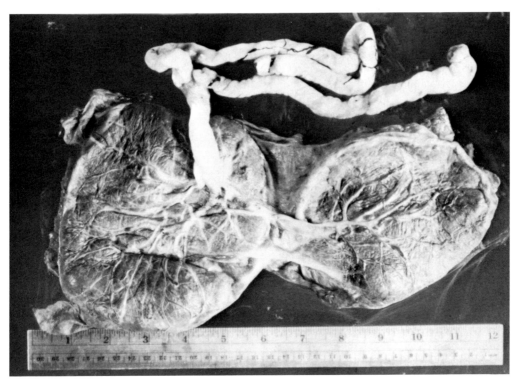

FIG 7–11.
A bilobed (bipartite) placenta.

The umbilical cord most often inserts into the membranes between the two lobes of bipartite placentas but in about a third of the cases it inserts into the larger of the two lobes.

The two clinical manifestations of a bipartite or tripartite placenta most often cited are bleeding in the first trimester of pregnancy, and a failure of one of the lobes to separate at delivery with consequent postpartum hemorrhage.[333] There are also published reports that bilobed placentas increase in frequency with advanced maternal age and with a maternal history of infertility.[24] These associations were not confirmed by our analyses of the CPS findings (Table 7–4). Obvious risks posed by a bilobed placenta, such as thrombosis or hemorrhage from torn vessels in the membranes that connect the two lobes, are rare. Antecedent risk factors for bipartite and tripartite placentas in the CPS were maternal cigarette smoking during pregnancy, mother being over 34 years of age, vomiting excessively during the first

trimester of pregnancy, diabetes mellitus, and one of the parents or a sibling having a chronic seizure disorder (Table 7–4). Combined, these risk factors accounted for 21% of the bipartite and tripartite placentas in the CPS. After taking the aforementioned risk factors into consideration, bipartite and tripartite placentas did not have any unfavorable short-term or long-term pregnancy outcomes (see Table 7–4).

Succenturiate Lobe

A succenturiate (accessory) lobe is a second or third placental lobe that is much smaller than the largest lobe (Fig 7–12). Unlike bipartite lobes, the smaller succenturiate lobe often has areas of infarction or atrophy. In the CPS, risk factors associated with a succenturiate lobe were advanced maternal age, mother a primigravida, proteinuria in the first trimester of pregnancy, and major malformations in the fetus (Table 7–5). In combination these risk factors accounted for 17% of the

TABLE 7–4.

Risk Estimates for Antecedents to the Development of a Bipartite or Tripartite Placenta*

Risk Factors	No. of Cases With a Bipartite or Tripartite Placenta per 1,000 Cases With Risk Factor†	Relative Risks (95% Confidence Intervals)	Attributable Risks (95% Confidence Intervals)
All cases	17 *(791)*		
Maternal factors			
Smoked during pregnancy	**21** *(195)*, *P* < .001	**1.3** (1.1, 1.6)	**.08** *(.06, .09)*
Age ≥ 35 yr	**33** *(93)*, *P* < .001	**2.1** (1.7, 2.7)	**.08** *(.06, .10)*
Excessive vomiting, 1st trimester	**23** *(76)*, *P* < .005	**1.5** (1.1, 1.8)	**.03** *(.02, .04)*
Diabetes mellitus	**35** *(21)*, *P* < .001	**2.0** (1.3, 3.1)	**.01** *(.01, .02)*
Fetal factor			
Seizure disorder, parent or sibling	**22** *(87)*, *P* < .005	**1.3** (1.0, 1.6)	**.02** *(.02, .03)*
Population attributable risk			**.21** *(.19, .23)*
Pregnancy outcomes			
Preterm birth	**13** *(132)*, *P* < .005	0.7 (0.4, 1.2)	
Fetal growth retardation	17 *(66)*, *P* > .1	1.0 (0.3, 1.8)	
Stillbirth	16 *(13)*, *P* > .1	0.9 (0.3, 1.6)	
Neonatal death	13 *(11)*, *P* > .1	0.7 (0.2, 1.4)	
Neurologic abnormalities at 7 yr	**23** *(35)*, *P* < .05	1.1 (1.0, 2.0)	

*Significant values are in boldface.
†Numbers of cases are in parentheses.

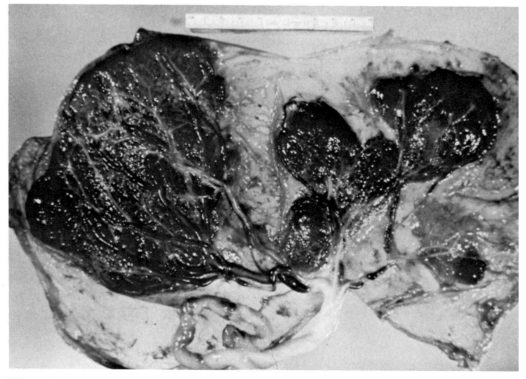

FIG 7–12.
A placenta with several succenturiate (accessory) lobes.

TABLE 7–5.

Risk Estimates for Antecedents to the Development of a Succenturiate Lobe of the Placenta*

Risk Factors	No. of Placentas With Succenturiate Lobes per 1,000 Cases With Risk Factor†	Relative Risks (95% Confidence Intervals)	Attributable Risks (95% Confidence Intervals)
All cases	15 (*738*)		
Maternal factors			
Age ≥35 yr	**30** (*82*), *P* < .001	**2.1** (1.6, 2.2)	**.09** (.07, .10)
Primigravida	**29** (*45*), *P* < .001	**1.8** (1.5, 2.2)	**.03** (.02, .04)
Proteinuria, 1st trimester	**27** (*45*), *P* < .001	**2.0** (1.5, 2.7)	**.03** (.02, .04)
Fetal factor			
Major fetal malformations	**18** (*81*), *P* < .05	**1.2** (1.0, 1.4)	**.02** (.00, .04)
Population attributable risk			***.17*** (*.15, .20*)
Pregnancy outcomes			
Preterm birth	14 (*132*), *P* > .1	0.9 (0.7, 1.2)	
Fetal growth retardation	16 (*64*), *P* > .1	1.0 (0.8, 1.2)	
Stillbirth	11 (*9*), *P* > .1	0.7 (0.4, 1.1)	
Neonatal death	13 (*11*), *P* > .1	0.8 (0.5, 1.2)	
Neurologic abnormalities at 7 yr	19 (*28*), *P* > .1	1.2 (0.9, 1.5)	

Significant values are in boldface.
†Numbers of cases are in parentheses.

succenturiate lobes in the CPS. The membranes between the lobes in such a placenta can be torn during delivery, and the extra lobe can be retained after the rest of the placenta has been delivered, with consequent postpartum bleeding. These complications did not increase the frequency of abnormal short-term or long-term pregnancy outcomes in the CPS (see Table 7–5).

Irregularly Shaped Placentas

An irregularly shaped placenta was present in 0.7% of the pregnancies of the CPS. Most of the antecedents of bilobed placentas and succenturiate lobes were not antecedents of an irregularly shaped placenta (see Tables 7–4 through 7–6). Irregularly shaped placentas were not associated with any increase in unfavorable pregnancy outcomes (Table 7–6).

Placenta Membranacea

Placenta membranacea is a rare disorder in which villi are retained beneath the amnion over all or most of the uterine wall. In some cases the placenta grossly appears to cover most of the uterine wall,

while in other cases there are just a few villi beneath the fetal membranes over much of the uterine wall. In the CPS the most frequent antecedent of placenta membranacea was maternal immunization or infection during the first trimester of pregnancy (Table 7–7). Less important risk factors were maternal obesity, maternal diabetes mellitus, major malformations of the fetus, and a motor disorder in a parent or sibling (Table 7–7). In toto these risk factors accounted for half of the cases of placenta membranacea in the study. Other risk factors mentioned in the literature include previous endometritis, poor development of a decidual blood supply, and atrophy or hypoplasia of the endometrium.[264]

A review of the literature on placenta membranacae up until 1987 revealed only six cases of fetal survival with the disorder.[125] In the CPS there was an increased risk of fetal growth retardation and preterm birth but only 3 of the 19 children associated with placenta membranacea were stillborn or died in the newborn period (see Table 7–7). Since the placenta, or at least some villi, often overlie the cervix in the disorder, there is a high risk of vaginal bleeding as term approaches

TABLE 7–6.

Risk Estimates for Antecedents to the Development of an Irregularly Shaped Placenta*

Risk Factors	No. of Cases of an Irregularly Shaped Placenta per 1,000 Cases With Risk Factor†	Relative Risks (95% Confidence Intervals)	Attributable Risks (95% Confidence Intervals)
All cases	7 (*343*)		
Maternal factors			
Immunization or infection during 1st trimester	**16** (*45*), P < .001	**2.3** (1.7, 3.2)	**.08** (.06, .10)
Smoked during pregnancy	**7** (*259*), P < .02	**1.4** (1.1, 1.8)	**.06** (.05, .07)
Excessive vomiting, 1st trimester	**13** (*44*), P < .001	**1.9** (1.4, 2.7)	**.06** (.04, .07)
Nondiabetic gestational acetonuria	**14** (*35*), P < .001	**2.0** (1.4, 2.9)	**.05** (.04, .06)
Age ≥ 35 yr	**13** (*34*), P < .001	**1.8** (1.4, 2.6)	**.04** (.03, .05)
Preeclampsia, eclampsia	**9** (*76*), P < .001	**1.2** (1.0, 1.4)	**.03** (.01, .05)
Fetal factor			
Motor disorder, siblings	**17** (*10*), P < .05	**1.8** (1.0, 2.9)	**.01** (.00, .02)
Population attributable risk			**.32** (*.29, .35*)
Pregnancy outcomes			
Preterm birth	6 (*60*), P > .1	0.8 (0.4, 1.2)	
Fetal growth retardation	7 (*27*), P > .1	1.0 (0.7, 1.3)	
Stillbirth	11 (*9*), P > .1	1.3 (0.3, 2.4)	
Neonatal death	10 (*9*), P > .1	0.9 (0.4, 1.5)	
Neurologic abnormalities at 7 yr	8 (*12*), P > .1	1.0 (0.8, 1.2)	

*Significant values are in boldface.
†Numbers of cases are in parentheses.

TABLE 7–7.

Risk Estimates for Antecedents to the Development of Placenta Membranacea*

Risk Factors	No. of Cases of Placenta Membranacea per 1,000 Cases With Risk Factor†	Relative Risks (95% Confidence Intervals)	Attributable Risks (95% Confidence Intervals)
All cases	0.4 (*19*)		
Maternal factors			
Immunization or infection during 1st trimester	**1.5** (*4*), P < .05	**4.0** (1.3, 12.1)	**.21** (.10, .32)
Obese pregravid	**1.0** (*4*), P < .02	**2.0** (1.1, 7.9)	**.11** (.02, .21)
Diabetes mellitus	**2.6** (*2*), P < .01	**5.2** (1.3, 9.2)	**.03** (0.1, .05)
Fetal factors			
Major fetal malformations	**8.0** (*2*), P < .05	**4.0** (1.0, 9.6)	**.10** (.00, .28)
Motor disorder, parents or sibling	**5.1** (*3*), P < .001	**11.5** (3.1, 42.1)	**.05** (.00, .12)
Population attributable risk			**.50** (*.46, .54*)
Pregnancy outcomes			
Preterm birth	**0.8** (*8*), P < .02	**2.8** (1.1, 7.0)	
Fetal growth retardation	**1.8** (*7*), P < .001	**6.5** (2.6, 16.0)	
Stillbirth	**1.2** (*1*)		
Neonatal death	**2.3** (*2*), P < .02	0.0	
Neurologic abnormalities at 7 yr	**0.7** (*1*)		

*Significant values are in boldface.
†Numbers of cases are in parentheses.

and the cervix begins to dilate. At times not all of the villi separate at delivery, which results in postpartum bleeding. In the CPS 5 of the 19 gravidas with placenta membranacea bled at delivery and 4 of the 5 also bled earlier in gestation, 3 in both the first and second trimesters and 1 in the second trimester.

Opaque Fetal Surface of Placenta

Membranes were opaque on the fetal surface of 7.7% of the placentas in the CPS. Unusually long umbilical cords (91st through 100th percentiles), excessive fibrin beneath the chorionic (fetal) plate of the placenta, and the other disorders that are associated with vigorous fetal movements were associated with a third of the opaque membranes (Table 7–8). The association of these factors with opaque membranes raises the possibility that the opacity is sometimes the result of trauma to the placental surface by fetal movements. In other cases the fetal membranes were apparently opaque as the result of infection because they were edematous, infiltrated by acute inflammatory cells, and associated with the characteristic findings of acute chorioamnionitis (see Table 7–8 and Fig 7–13). In preterm born infants the frequency of opaque membranes increased progressively from 52/1,000 in placentas without acute chorioamnionitis to 77/1,000 in placentas with mild chorioamnionitis to 139/1,000 in placentas with severe chorioamnionitis ($P < .001$). The comparable frequencies for full-term born infants were 58/1,000, 69/1,000, and 98/1,000 ($P < .001$). When all of the risk factors were taken into account, an opaque surface of the placenta was associated with a frequency of long-term neurologic abnormalities that was 40% greater than expected (see Table 7–8). These neurologic abnormalities fell into two categories: motor disorders accompanied by mental retardation and nonfebrile seizure disorders.

TABLE 7–8.

Risk Estimates for Antecedents to the Development of Opaque Fetal Membranes on the Surface of the Placenta*

Risk Factors	No. of Placentas With Opaque Membranes per 1,000 Cases With Risk Factor†	Relative Risks (95% Confidence Intervals)	Attributable Risks (95% Confidence Intervals)
All cases	77 *(3,764)*		
Fetal factors			
Postterm birth	**102** *(464)*, *P* < .001	**1.4** (1.3, 1.6)	**.04** (.02, .06)
Major fetal malformations	**101** *(299)*, *P* < .001	**1.2** (1.0, 1.4)	**.02** (.01, .04)
Placental factor			
Acute chorioamnionitis	**94** *(85)*, *P* < .001	**1.4** (1.3, 1.5)	**.12** (.11, .13)
Markers for vigorous fetal motor activity			
Diffuse subchorionic fibrin	**107** *(1,418)*, *P* < .001	**1.7** (1.5, 1.8)	**.15** (.14, .16)
Unusually long umbilical cord	**100** *(1,741)*, *P* < .001	**1.6** (1.5, .17)	**.17** (.16, .19)
Other indicators			**.01** (.00, .03)
Population attributable risk			**.50** *(.48, .53)*
Pregnancy outcomes			
Preterm birth	76 *(3,764)*, *P* > .1	1.0 (0.8, 1.1)	
Fetal growth retardation	**85** *(346)*, *P* < .05	1.1 (0.8, 1.2)	
Stillbirth	**266** *(229)*, *P* < .001	**1.2** (1.0, 1.5)	
Neonatal death	**136** *(122)*, *P* < .001	1.0 (0.8, 1.2)	
Neurologic abnormalities at 7 yr	**87** *(137)*, *P* < .05	**1.4** (1.2, 1.6)	
Motor abnormalities + mental retardation		**1.3** (1.0, 1.6)	
Nonfebrile seizure disorder		**1.6** (1.3, 1.9)	

*Significant values are in boldface.
†Numbers of cases are in parentheses.

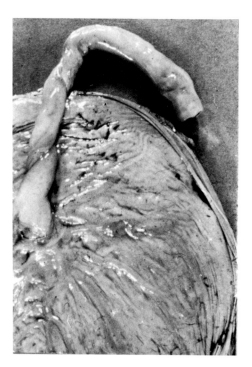

FIG 7–13.
Acute chorioamnionitis has made the surface of the placenta opaque. The chorionic vessels are barely visible through the cloudy amnion. (From Blanc WA: Pathology of the placenta, membranes, and umbilical cord in bacterial, fungal and viral infections in man, in Naeye R, Kissane J, Kauffman N: *Perinatal Diseases.* Baltimore, Williams & Wilkins Co, 1981. Used by permission.)

Disorders of Placental Maturation

Villi go through a sequence of structural changes as they mature. In early gestation a double layer of epithelial cells, the inner cytotrophoblast and the outer syncytiotrophoblast, cover the villi. The inner cytotrophoblastic layer disappears as gestation progresses and persists only as isolated cells in the third trimester. During this period syncytiotrophoblastic nuclei divide without the cell dividing, so multinucleated cells (syncytial knots) progressively increase in number and size. The relative number and size of these syncytial knots are important aids in evaluating villous maturation. Villous size is another guide to maturity. After about 25 weeks of gestation the size of terminal villi progressively decreases until term and beyond.

Accelerated Maturation

In making the diagnosis one must be certain that the gestational age is accurate. Relying solely on a gestational age calculated from the start of the last menstrual period is unwise because some women bleed at the end of their first month of pregnancy, which can make their newborns a month older than their menstrual history would indicate. Accelerated maturation is identified by finding abnormally small villi, an abnormally thin syncytiotrophoblastic cell layer covering the villi, and both larger and more numerous syncytial knots than are normal for gestational age (Fig 7–14).[81] These findings are so frequent in preterm placentas that they are not always recognized as abnormal. This high frequency of accelerated maturation in preterm placentas has convinced many that the microscopic appearance of the placenta is an unreliable guide to gestational age. This is an error. It is a useful guide when some areas of normal maturation can be found among the areas of hypermaturity. When the entire placenta appears hypermature for gestational age, other means must be employed to evaluate gestational age.

When present, accelerated maturation can be relatively uniform throughout the placenta, or it can be interspersed with areas that appear normally mature for gestational age. The two patterns of evenly

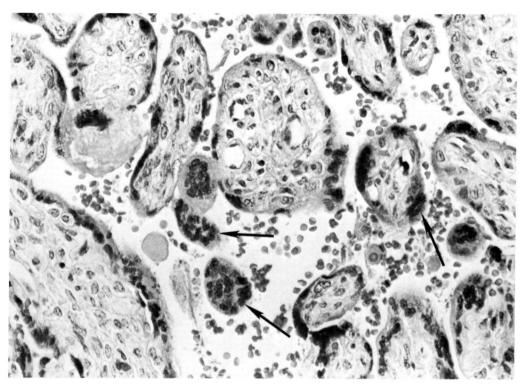

FIG 7–14.
Villous maturation is markedly accelerated in this 11-week-gestational-age placenta. The cytotrophoblast has already disappeared and large numbers of multinucleated syncytial knots *(arrows)* have developed. HE stain, ×600.

and unevenly accelerated maturation have different origins and clinical outcomes.

Uniformly Accelerated Maturation. — Uniformly accelerated maturation is present when the entire placenta appears hypermature for gestational age. Such maturation was observed in 3.5% (925) of the placentas in the CPS. The antecedents were being black, an absence of maternal third-trimester peripheral edema, low maternal net pregnancy weight gain, and low maternal pregravid body weight for height (Table 7–9). Maternal net pregnancy weight gain was a mother's total pregnancy weight gain minus the weight of her newborn infant and the weight of the placenta. It mainly reflects maternal gestational increases in blood volume, other extracellular fluids, breast changes, and fat stores.[237] Both low maternal net pregnancy weight gain and the absence of

maternal peripheral edema are usually manifestations of a low maternal gestational blood volume increase, which in turn commonly leads to low blood flow from the uterus to the placenta.[128] Being thin pregravid is also associated with a relatively low uteroplacental blood flow.[128] A low maternal gestational blood volume increase, manifested by a failure of maternal hemoglobin values to decrease between early and midgestation, explained more than half of the uniformly accelerated placental maturation that we observed in the CPS.

A lower maternal blood volume could be the reason why blacks had more uniformly hypermature placentas than whites at each gestational age in the CPS (see Table 7–9). It could also explain why whites grow faster than blacks in late gestation. This growth difference is not genetic in origin because until the last 6

TABLE 7–9.

Risk Estimates for Antecedents to Uniformly Accelerated Placental Maturation in the Absence of Infarcts Before 38 Weeks of Gestation or Infarcts >3 cm in Diameter After 38 Weeks of Gestation*

Risk Factors	No. of Cases of Accelerated Placental Maturation per 1,000 Cases With Risk Factor†	Relative Risks (95% Confidence Intervals)	Attributable Risks (95% Confidence Intervals)
All cases	57 *(2,996)*		
Maternal factors			
No hands or ankle edema	**71** *(2,095)*, *P* < .001	**1.4** (1.3, 1.5)	**.14** (.12, .15)
Net pregnancy weight gain < 4 kg	**80** *(1,335)*, *P* < .001	**1.5** (1.4, 1.6)	**.10** (.09, .11)
Very thin pregravid	**61** *(551)*, *P* < .05	**1.1** (1.0, 1.2)	**.01** (.00, .02)
Fetal factor			
Race: black	**79** *(1,959)*, *P* < .001	**2.0** (1.9, 2.1)	**.21** (.20, .23)
Population attributable risk			**.45** (.42, .49)
Pregnancy outcomes			
Fetal growth retardation	**58** *(108)*, *P* > .1	1.1 (0.8, 1.4)	
Stillbirth	**89** *(88)*, *P* < .001	1.2 (1.0, 1.4)	
Neonatal death	**24** *(47)*, *P* < .001	1.0 (0.5, 1.9)	
Neurologic abnormalities at 7 yr	**66** *(100)*, *P* > .1	1.1 (0.9, 1.4)	

Significant values are in boldface.
†Numbers of cases are in parentheses.

weeks of gestation blacks grew as fast as whites in the CPS, while after birth blacks grew faster than whites.[217,237] When children with uniformly hypermature placentas were excluded from the analysis, blacks grew as fast as whites until the 38th week of gestation. This is just what would be expected if low uteroplacental blood flow was responsible for the slower growth of blacks than of whites, because low uteroplacental blood flow exerts its largest influence on fetal growth late in gestation.[237]

The clinical consequences of uniformly accelerated placental maturation were small in the CPS. When race and other antecedent factors were taken into consideration, the only unfavorable pregnancy outcome was a relative risk of 1.2 for stillbirths (see Table 7–9). Fetal growth retardation had a low frequency when the various antecedents of accelerated maturation were taken into consideration.

Unevenly Accelerated Maturation. – An uneven acceleration of placental maturation is widely recognized as a manifestation of stenoses and occlusions in the uterine spiral arteries that unevenly re-

duce blood flow to the intervillous space in the placenta. This uneven blood flow, when present for several weeks or longer, accelerates villous maturation in those areas of the placenta where blood flow into the intervillous space is low, while acceleration is absent in the areas where blood flow into the intervillous space is normal. The result is a mosaic in which irregularly sized areas of accelerated villous maturation alternate with areas in which villi are normally mature. The acceleration is identified by the presence of abnormally small villi, a thinning of the syncytiotrophoblastic cell layer that covers the villi, trophoblastic basement membrane thickening, and syncytial knots that are larger in size and have more nuclei than would be expected for gestational age (see Fig 7–14).[81] Affected placentas are often growth-retarded as the consequence of the chronic low uteroplacental blood flow.[258]

The cause of the uneven blood flow is presumed to be a combination of fluctuating vasoconstriction and longstanding stenotic lesions in the spiral arteries.[149,181] The vasoconstriction is a plausible explanation for the fibrinoid necrosis and acute atherosis that are sometimes

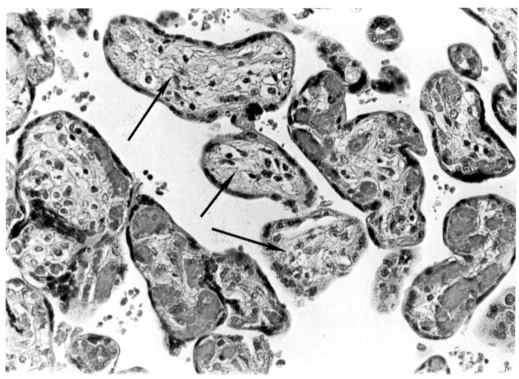

FIG 7–15.
Alternating zones of normal and fibrotic villi in the placenta of a gravida who had severe preeclampsia. The fibrotic villi are marked by *arrows*. This fibrosis is presumably the result of low blood flow through stenotic arteries like those seen in Figure 7–16. HE stain, ×600.

seen in decidual arteries. Placental infarcts are a common associated finding. These infarcts develop when obstructive lesions in one or more spiral arteries reduce blood flow into the intervillous space to a level too low to keep villi alive. The thinning of the syncytiotrophoblastic layer that covers the villi is presumably an adaptation to low blood flow in the intervillous space (Figs 7–14 and 7–15).

At the ultrastructural level placentas subjected to uneven low uteroplacental blood flow show both a loss and a distortion of syncytial microvilli, a dilatation of syncytial rough endoplasmic reticulum, a decrease in the number of syncytial pinocytotic vesicles, an increase in stromal fibrosis, and an obliterative enlargement of endothelial cells in some villous capillaries.[82] As previously mentioned, the low uteroplacental blood flow that causes these abnormalities is due to stenotic areas in uterine spiral arteries that origi-

nate from a failure of trophoblastic cells to completely remodel these arteries and to vasoconstriction (Fig 7–16).[149,276] Doppler measurements often show an increased resistance to blood flow in uterine vessels that are presumed to be the spiral arteries.[337] The placental lesions of uneven placental maturation can occur without maternal hypertension and with increased circulating levels of maternal serum lupus anticoagulant.[61,62,112,116]

Immunoglobulins, including antinuclear antibodies and complement, are sometimes deposited along villi, the trophoblast, the amnion, and in decidual vessels in cases of preeclampsia, diabetes mellitus, and lupus erythematosus.[112] It is unlikely that these deposited immunoglobulins cause the various placental abnormalities that are characteristic of chronic low uteroplacental blood flow. Most speculation has centered on the possibility that the immunoglobulins are involved in the

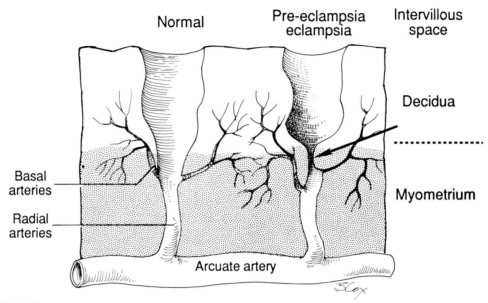

FIG 7–16.
The *arrow* points to an area in a spiral artery that is stenotic because it has not been remodeled by trophoblastic cells early in gestation.

genesis of the fibrinoid necrosis and atherosis that are often present in decidual blood vessels in cases of preeclampsia, diabetes mellitus, and lupus erythematosus.[319] There is also a possibility that the immunoglobulin deposition may be the consequence of the fibrinoid necrosis and atherosis.[152] Atherosis refers to an invasion of blood vessel walls by foamy macrophages.

The other cause of the uneven low blood flow into the intervillous space is vasoconstriction. Blood levels of the vasoconstrictor angiotensin II are not increased with preeclampsia, but the uterine vascular responsiveness to angiotensin II is greatly increased as early as the second trimester in gravidas who subsequently develop preeclampsia.[91] This change in the pressor response to angiotensin II is related to a change in the number and avidity of vascular receptors.[327] The placental production of thromboxane, a potent vasoconstrictor, is increased severalfold in preeclampsia.[348] Prostacyclin, which relaxes blood vessels, is produced by the endothelial cells of uterine blood vessels, umbilical arteries, and placental veins.[51] In both preeclampsia and in normotensive

gestations complicated by fetal growth retardation, the production of prostacyclin is reduced in all of these vessels.[39,135,321] As a result, the vasoconstrictor effects of angiotensin II, thromboxane, and catecholamines are not efficiently opposed, leading to maternal and often fetal and placental hypertension, fetal growth retardation, stillbirth, and neonatal death.[27,74,338,348]

Various authors have reported that an obliterative thickening of arterial walls and a reduced number of small arteries in the villi explain the increase in placental vascular resistance in preeclampsia and eclampsia (Fig 7–17).[78,99,190] Some of these arterial lesions may be the result of vasoconstriction induced by a reduction of unopposed thromboxane and angiotensin II. Reduced oxygen tension in the maternal blood supplied to the intervillous space may also play a role. This latter role is based on the observation that oxygen deprivation can initiate vasoconstriction in the placental cotyledons.[123] This would appear to reflect the activity of a local homeostatic mechanism that normally matches the blood flow to individual cotyledons with the available oxygen in the

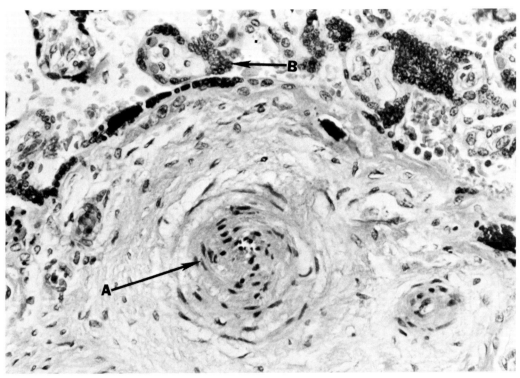

FIG 7–17.
In this case of severe preeclampsia a proliferative process has markedly reduced the luminal size of an artery in a stem villus *(A).* The peripheral villi are abnormally small and some of the syncytial knots are abnormally large *(B)* for the gestational age of 30 weeks. HE stain, ×600.

intervillous blood. In this regard it resembles the circulation in the lung where a drop in alveolar oxygen levels causes the local arteries to constrict, thereby shunting blood to better-ventilated areas of the lung. Rodgers et al.[278] and Rappaport et al.[266] have demonstrated antibodies to human umbilical vein endothelial cells in gravidas with preeclampsia.

The percentage of placental arteries affected by the aforementioned lesions reportedly correlates with vascular resistance in the placenta.[78] The terminal villi served by arteries with these lesions often have a marked increase in stroma and few or no blood vessels (see Fig 7–15). A correlation has also been reported between the extent of these arterial lesions and hypoxic changes in the villi, namely fibrinoid necrosis, infarcts, thickening of the trophoblastic basement membrane, and a reduced capillary bed.[23] Teasdale has reported a low ratio of peripheral villi

to stem villi owing to a relatively low number of peripheral villi in disorders that produce chronic low uteroplacental blood flow.[330]

To recognize and properly interpret the microscopic findings that are characteristic of low uteroplacental blood flow, tissue from grossly normal as well as from grossly abnormal areas of the placenta should be examined. Findings at the edge of the placenta and just below the fetal plate should not be used to assess the state of placental maturation because blood flow is normally lower at these sites than in more central areas of the placenta, so that findings at the periphery often give an unrepresentative impression of chronic low blood flow.

Some pathologists think that because the placenta rapidly matures after fetal death, that abnormally small villi and large numbers of syncytial knots are a normal finding with stillbirth. The placentas of some stillborn children show a mosaic of varying maturity with some areas normally mature and other areas hypermature. Such a finding in the absence of another explanation for stillbirth is often an indication that chronically low uteroplacental blood flow was the likely cause of the death. It is therefore important to distinguish between a uniformly hypermature and a unevenly hypermature placenta in stillborn infants.

The placental findings associated with maternal hypertension and proteinuria during pregnancy appear to be strongly influenced by the time of onset and the duration of the low uteroplacental blood flow that may have accompanied the hypertension. Both the fetus and the placenta are often growth-retarded when gravidas are hypertensive before midgestation, presumably because low blood flow into the intervillous space started early in gestation. Accelerated villous maturation and often placental infarcts are usually prominent in such cases. Low uteroplacental blood flow from early gestation greatly increases the risk of spontaneous abortion, abruptio placentae, fetal death, spontaneous preterm labor, and preterm delivery.[225,237] It is important to know that all of these outcomes can be present without hypertension with placental findings being the only clue that low uteroplacental blood flow was responsible for the outcome.[225] Such cases pose a particularly high risk for a repeat of the disorder with preterm delivery in the next pregnancy.[225] In the CPS more than half of the next pregnancies ended preterm with the same placental findings. This repeating disorder is probably not a prehypertensive manifestation of preeclampsia because preeclampsia is characteristically not a repeating disorder. Circulating lupus anticoagulants and anticardiolipin antibodies are probably the explanation for some of these cases.[336] Details of these latter conditions are found later in this chapter.

Metabolic abnormalities in the placenta may potentiate the effects of low uteroplacental blood flow. Low oxygen consump-tion, poor glucose utilization, and impairments in glycolytic pathways have been reported in placentas from eclamptic and preeclamptic pregnancies.[30,326,335] This may reflect impaired nutrient synthesis that could add to the fetal growth retardation that is often associated with preeclampsia and eclampsia.

Risk factors were identified for 81% of the unevenly accelerated placental maturation in the CPS (Table 7–10). As would be expected, preeclampsia and eclampsia were the dominating factors. Other antecedent risk factors included being white, a primigravida, low maternal pregnancy weight gain, and a mother being overweight for height before pregnancy (see Table 7–10). A low net pregnancy weight gain is often associated with a low maternal gestational blood volume expansion.[128] Preeclampsia and eclampsia are mainly disorders of primigravidas.

Stillbirth and neonatal death rates were increased in the CPS when placentas had the findings of unevenly accelerated maturation, even after the identified risk factors that predispose to these placental findings had been taken into consideration (see Table 7–10). The risk of long-term mental retardation, learning disorders, and a flat, passive personality also increased with the presence of unevenly accelerated placental maturation (see Chapter 11).

There appear to be major differences in the frequencies and character of hypertensive disorders in different populations. In the CPS unevenly accelerated placental maturation was more frequent in whites than in blacks whereas evenly accelerated maturation was much more frequent in blacks than in whites (see Tables 7–9 and 7–10). Among Asians preeclampsia with proteinuria is reportedly most frequent in China and least frequent in Vietnam.[106] A high frequency would be expected in China where most pregnancies are in primigravidas. In the United States preeclampsia is most frequent in primigravidas and in multigravidas who are having a child with a different man than fathered their previous children. In some

TABLE 7–10.

Risk Estimates for Antecedents to Placental Findings With Unevenly Accelerated Maturation, With or Without Accompanying Placental Infarcts*

Risk Factors	No. of Cases of Uneven Accelerated Placental Maturation per 1,000 Cases With Risk Factor†	Relative Risks (95% Confidence Intervals)	Attributable Risks (95% Confidence Intervals)
All cases	28 *(1,425)*		
Maternal factors			
Net pregnancy weight gain < 4 kg	**34** *(391)*, *P* < .001	**1.2** (1.0, 1.4)	**.04** (.02, .06)
Primigravida	**38** *(490)*, *P* < .001	**1.4** (1.3, 1.5)	**.07** (.06, .08)
Preeclampsia, eclampsia	**106** *(1,034)*, *P* < .001	**3.6** (3.3, 4.0)	**.54** (.52, .56)
Overweight pregravid	**40** *(131)*, *P* < .001	**1.2** (1.1, 1.3)	**.01** (.01, .02)
Fetal factor			
Race: white	**38** *(998)*, *P* < .001	**1.4** (1.3, 1.6)	**.17** (.15, 1.8)
Population attributable risk			**.81** *(.78, .85)*
Pregnancy outcomes			
Preterm birth	**58** *(663)*, *P* < .02	**3.6** (3.4, 3.9)	
Fetal growth retardation	**38** *(145)*, *P* < .001	**1.4** (1.3, 1.6)	
Stillbirth	**38** *(36)*, *P* < .05	**1.6** (1.3, 1.9)	
Neonatal death	**39** *(72)*, *P* < .001	**1.3** (1.0, 1.6)	
Neurologic abnormalities at 7 yr	**38** *(55)*, *P* < .001	**1.4** (1.2, 1.7)	

Significant values are in boldface.
†Numbers of cases are in parentheses.*

African populations the disorder repeats without changing the father of the children. The explanation for these population differences appears to include differing levels of maternal pregravid fatness, differing diets during pregnancy, and perhaps immunologic mechanisms.[137,225,227]

Placental Infarction

A *placental infarct* is defined as an area of ischemic villous necrosis. Infarcts are usually the result of the occlusion of one or more spiral arteries in the uterine wall. Such occlusions are common with disorders that unevenly reduce uteroplacental blood flow. The most common of these disorders are preeclampsia, eclampsia, and chronic maternal hypertension. On a cut surface a fresh infarct is dark red and moderately soft. It subsequently becomes brown, then yellow, and eventually white and firm (Fig 7–18). The first evidence of an infarct is the marked narrowing or disappearance of the intervillous space so that villi touch each other. Soon after, syncytiotrophoblastic nuclei shrink and become pyknotic. Thereafter, necrosis develops, and eventually all that remains are ghostlike outlines of former villi and other structures (Figs 7–19 and 7–20).

One or two small infarcts (<2 cm in diameter), and even larger infarcts that are at the margin of the placenta, are not usually associated with unfavorable pregnancy outcomes in full-term gestations.[212,237,352] As the number and size of infarcts increase, so do the frequencies of stillbirth and neonatal death. Overall the perinatal mortality rate associated with placental infarction increases with the size of the infarct, with preterm delivery, and with the presence of disorders that reduce placental function such as preeclampsia, eclampsia, chronic maternal hypertension, and lupus erythematosus. In preterm placentas an infarct of any size is usually associated with unevenly accelerated maturation. Infarcts greater than 3 cm in diameter are associated with an increase in abnormal pregnancy outcomes at every gestational age.[212,237] Of the placentas in the CPS, 2.5% (781) had four or more grossly visible infarcts and

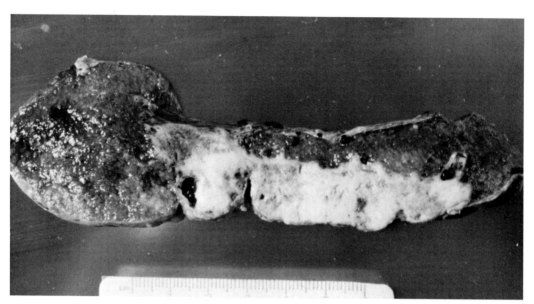

FIG 7–18.
This old placental infarct is white, firm, and shrunken.

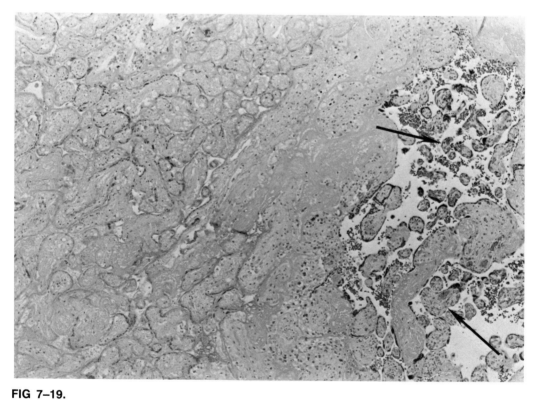

FIG 7–19.
In this old placental infarct all that remains of the original placental tissue are ghostlike outlines of former villi and other structures. A few semi-intact fibrotic villi are present on the right *(arrows)*. HE stain, ×4.

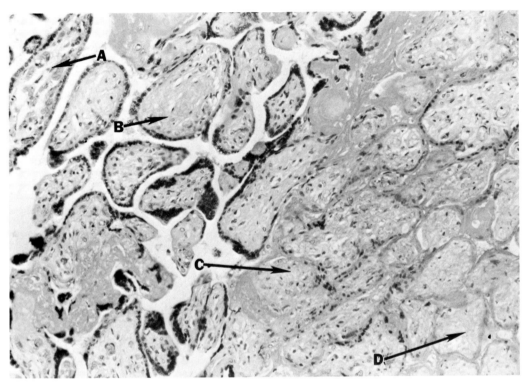

FIG 7–20.
This higher-power view of a placental infarct shows the transition from a normal villus *(A)* to fibrotic villi *(B)*, to fibrotic villi surrounded by fibrin *(C)*, to old "ghost" villi *(D)*. HE, ×300.

2.9% (1,663) had infarcts greater than 3 cm in diameter (Tables 7–11 and 7–12). The most frequent antecedents of such infarcts were preeclampsia, eclampsia, being a primigravida, and being white (see Tables 7–11 and 7–12 and Fig 7–21). Being a primigravida was presumably a risk factor because the spiral arteries are sometimes incompletely remodeled in first pregnancies, which leads to stenotic zones which in turn restrict blood flow to the placenta. Being white may be a risk for infarcts because the renin-angiotensin system is more active in whites than in blacks.[237] As previously mentioned, unevenly accelerated placental maturation is more frequent in whites and evenly accelerated maturation more frequent in blacks.

The frequency of maternal gestational hypertension, a major antecedent of placental infarcts, changed with the season of

the year in the CPS and there were parallel changes in the frequency of large placental infarcts (Fig 7–22). There are various speculations about the reason for these seasonal changes. They could be related to the pressor effects of cold outdoor temperatures, or they could be due to uteroplacental blood flow that increased with the feasting of the holiday season and decreased after New Year's Day as the result of fasting (see Chapter 3).

After taking all the identified risk factors for placental infarcts into consideration, one to four grossly visible infarcts and infarcts greater than 3 cm in diameter were associated with increased risks for fetal growth retardation (see Tables 7–11, 7–12). The risk for long-term neurologic abnormalities increased with four or more grossly visible infarcts (see Table 7–11). The increased risk was mainly in the category of mild mental retardation. The

TABLE 7–11.

Risk Estimates for Antecedents to the Development of Four or More Grossly Visible Placental Infarcts*

Risk Factors	No. of Placentas With Four or More Infarcts per 1,000 Cases With Risk Factor†	Relative Risks (95% Confidence Intervals)	Attributable Risks (95% Confidence Intervals)
All cases	25 (*1,281*)		
Maternal factors			
Race: white	**34** (*559*), *P* < .001	**2.3** (2.0, .27)	**.27** (.25, .28)
Preeclampsia, eclampsia	**63** (*385*), *P* < .001	**4.2** (3.6, 4.8)	**.25** (.23, .27)
Primigravida	**36** (*304*), *P* < .001	**1.7** (1.4, 1.9)	**.10** (.09, .12)
Population attributable risk			**.61** (*.58, .63*)
Pregnancy outcomes			
Preterm birth (only full-term births included in analyses)			
Fetal growth retardation	**49** (*130*), *P* < .001	**1.9** (1.6, 2.3)	
Stillbirth	**78** (*16*), *P* < .001	0.7 (0.3, 1.4)	
Neonatal death	23 (*4*), *P* > .1	0.9 (0.4, 1.5)	
Neurologic abnormalities at 7 yr	**34** (*46*), *P* < .05	**1.3** (1.0, 1.7)	

*Significant values are in boldface.
†Numbers of cases are in parentheses.

TABLE 7–12.

Risk Estimates for Antecedents to the Development of Large Placental Infarcts (>3 cm in Diameter)*

Risk Factors	No. of Placentas With Large Placental Infarcts per 1,000 Cases With Risk Factor†	Relative Risks (95% Confidence Intervals)	Attributable Risks (95% Confidence Intervals)
All cases	29 (*1,663*)		
Maternal factors			
Preeclampsia, eclampsia	**105** (*335*), *P* < .001	**3.5** (3.1, 4.0)	**.19** (.17, .21)
Race: white	**37** (*913*), *P* < .001	**2.0** (1.8, 2.3)	**.17** (.15, .19)
Primigravida	**32** (*390*), *P* < .02	**1.1** (1.0, 1.3)	**.03** (.02, .04)
Population attributable risk			**.39** (*.36, .41*)
Pregnancy outcomes			
Preterm birth	27 (*238*), *P* > .1	0.9 (0.7, 1.3)	
Fetal growth retardation	**45** (*172*), *P* < .001	**1.2** (1.0, 1.4)	
Stillbirth	**73** (*24*), *P* < .001	1.0 (0.8, 1.3)	
Neonatal death	35 (*9*), *P* > .1	1.1 (0.6, 1.4)	
Neurologic abnormalities at 7 yr	**40** (*73*), *P* < .01	1.1 (0.5, 1.9)	

*Significant values are in boldface.
†Numbers of cases are in parentheses.

risk for preterm birth increased markedly when ten or more grossly visible infarcts were present.

Lupus Erythematosus

Women who have lupus erythematosus have a higher-than-expected rate of spontaneous abortions, stillbirths, placental abruptions, preterm births, and growth-retarded neonates.[75,179,180,289] Clues to these outcomes can be found in a number of findings in the placenta and decidua. Many of the placentas are growth-retarded and have both an unevenly accelerated villous maturation and infarcts, which suggests that blood flow into the intervillous space is low with the disorder (Fig 7–23). Such placentas cannot be easily distinguished from the placentas of

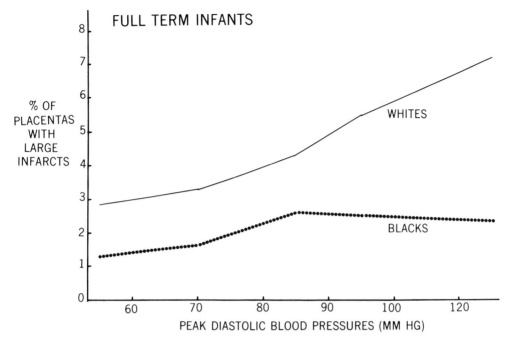

FIG 7–21.
The frequency of large placental infarcts increases more rapidly with increasing maternal blood pressure in whites than in blacks.

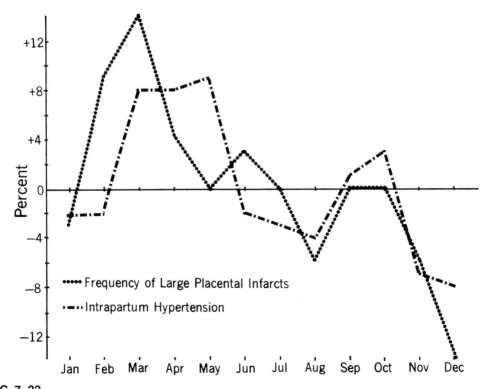

FIG 7–22.
The frequency of maternal gestational hypertension and large placental infarcts changed with the season, reaching their low point in the Thanksgiving–New Year's Day period and their high point after New Year's Day.

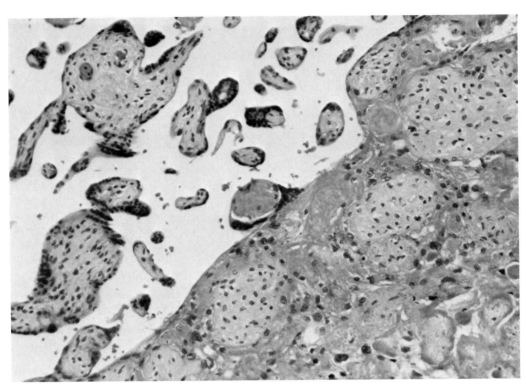

FIG 7–23.
An infarct is present on the right in this 33-week-gestational-age placenta from a gravida with lupus erythematosus.
HE stain, ×300.

gravidas who had gestational preeclampsia or eclampsia. Vascular lesions in the decidua appear to be responsible for the low blood flow into the intervillous space. Blood vessels in the decidua reportedly have large infiltrates of plasma cells and lymphocytes, fibrinoid necrosis, and are sometimes thrombosed.[1,24] Benirschke and Kaufmann note that the decidual vascular lesions are most easily seen in retroplacental curettings and in the decidua capsularis.[24] Deposits of IgM and C3 have been identified on the walls of these blood vessels and on the basement membranes of villi.[110] It is not known if these deposits have any role in the genesis of the decidual and placental lesions in lupus erythematosus.

Lupus Anticoagulants

A group of immunoglobulins, misnamed *lupus anticoagulants*, have been described in some women with lupus erythematosus and in a number of women with other disorders.[336] Lupus anticoagulants and anticardiolipin antibodies are antiphospholipids that paradoxically promote thrombosis via a myriad of prothrombotic mechanisms.[75,175] Their presence is sometimes associated with bleeding because of the presence of thrombocytopenia or a qualitative platelet defect.[75] Some of the affected women have a history of repeat abortions, repeat fetal losses, a false-positive serological test for syphilis, or unexplained thrombosis. Poor pregnancy outcomes reportedly correlate better with circulating levels of lupus anticoagulants and anticardiolipin antibodies than with the clinical severity of lupus erythematosus when it is present.[176] As many as three-fourths of pregnancies in which lupus anticoagulants are present and untreated have complications with the pregnancy, the fetus, or both.[175,180] Lupus anticoagulants and anticardiolipin antibodies are reportedly present in about

20% of women with lupus erythematosus.[14] When they are present, a previous pregnancy loss more than doubles the risk for a loss in the current pregnancy.[175] Suppressing these anticoagulants and antibodies by glucocorticoids or by prophylactically administered heparin, warfarin, aspirin, or IgG reportedly reduces the frequencies of placental infarction, fetal growth retardation, and perinatal death.[75,180,289,300]

Damage in the spiral arteries, intervillous thrombi, and immune-mediated trophoblast damage are the mechanisms that are postulated to be responsible for the poor pregnancy outcomes with high circulating levels of antiphospholipid antibodies.[62,174,180] Many of the placentas are growth-retarded and have both an unevenly accelerated villous maturation and infarcts which are characteristic consequences of chronic low blood flow into the intervillous space. Such placentas cannot be distinguished from the placentas of gravidas who had preeclampsia or eclampsia. However, there are clinical differences. The antiphospholipid antibody disorders often develop before midgestation, whereas preeclampsia and eclampsia usually make their clinical appearance later in gestation.

The presence of circulating autoantibodies, unrelated to lupus erythematosus or to another recognized autoimmune disorder, appear to have little or no effect on pregnancy outcome.[72] The production of such autoantibodies normally increases at term, probably because fetal antigens on trophoblastic cells often enter the maternal circulation at that time.

Cocaine (Benzoylmethylecgonine) Use

The possibility of cocaine use arises when a placenta has alternating zones of normal and hypermature villi in the absence of a maternal history of gestational hypertension.[225,249] Episodes of vasoconstriction may be the cause of damage in the walls of stem villus arteries in the placentas of some cocaine users (Fig 7–24). This arterial damage is a likely explanation for the uneven peripheral villous fibrosis that is present in the placentas of some cocaine users (Fig 7–25). Such findings are not surprising since cocaine in its various forms produces severe hypertension and vasoconstriction in the placenta.[355] One of the major complications of preeclampsia and eclampsia is abruptio placentae, so it is not surprising that abruptio placentae is increased in frequency in cocaine users.[195,237,249]

The fetal growth retardation reported in the offspring of cocaine users could be due to periods of hypertension-related low uteroplacental blood flow that are induced by cocaine. Poor maternal nutrition could be another cause of the fetal growth retardation.[42,83] Cocaine users often smoke cigarettes, use alcohol, amphetamines, marijuana, and opiates during pregnancy, all of which are risk factors for fetal growth retardation.[83,219] Many cocaine users are teenagers, who sometimes produce growth-retarded neonates because their own growth needs compete with the needs of their fetuses for available nutrients.[218] All of these are possible reasons, apart from the use of cocaine, why cocaine users sometimes produce growth-retarded neonates.

Maternal Floor Infarction

Maternal floor infarction is a frequently misdiagnosed and poorly understood disorder of the placenta. It is initiated by a heavy deposition of fibrin in the decidua beneath the placenta and adjacent villi, which then extends to engulf more and more villi, making them atrophic (Figs 7–26 and 7–27). Grossly, the maternal surface of the placenta is yellow or white, stiff, and has a reflective surface. This process can be uniform over the entire surface of the placenta or spotty in its distribution (Fig 7–28). On cross section the process can also be massive and diffuse or irregular in its distribution (Fig 7–29). Quite often so many villi are destroyed that placental insufficiency develops and the fetus dies.

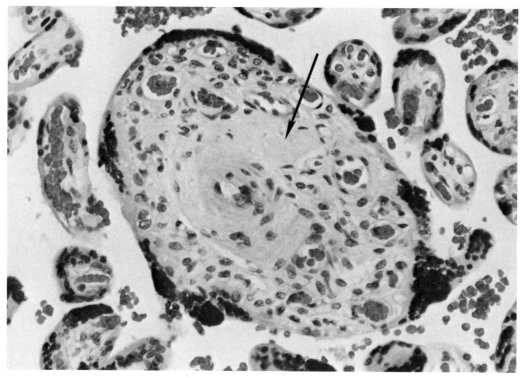

FIG 7–24.
The wall of this artery in a stem villus has some fibrinoid necrosis and it is partially hyalinized *(arrow)*. The gravida used cocaine throughout the pregnancy. HE stain, ×600.

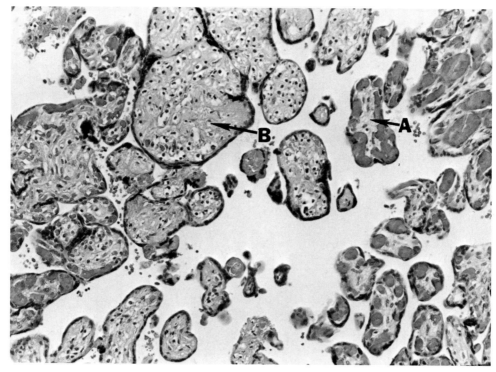

FIG 7–25.
Alternating areas of normal *(arrow A)* and fibrotic *(arrow B)* villi in the placenta of a cocaine addict. HE stain, ×300.

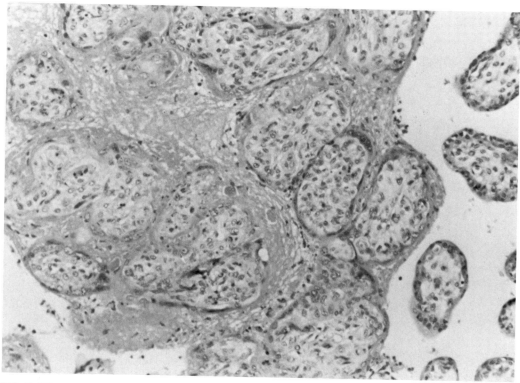

FIG 7–26.
Villi are being progressively surrounded by fibrin in this maternal floor infarct. Note that villi immediately adjacent to the affected areas have no ischemic changes. This helps distinguish floor infarcts from true infarcts where villi adjacent to the infarcted area almost always have ischemic changes. HE stain, ×600.

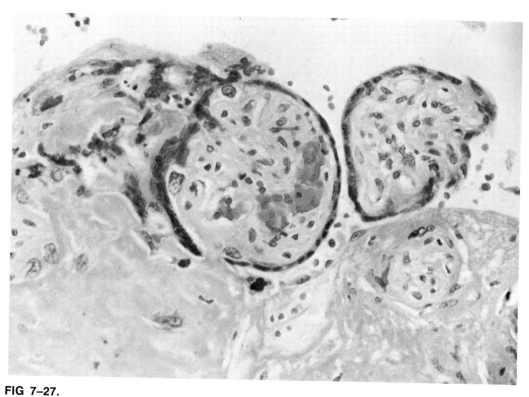

FIG 7–27.
A higher-power view of villi being engulfed and destroyed by fibrin in a maternal floor infarct. The villus at the center is partially surrounded and is undergoing early degenerative changes while the villus to the right is still intact. HE stain, ×600.

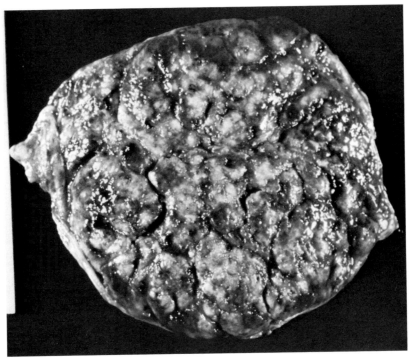

FIG 7–28.
The pale yellow, firm, highly reflective maternal surface of a placenta with maternal floor infarction. In this case not all of the maternal surface is affected. In many cases the entire maternal surface is pale and shiny.

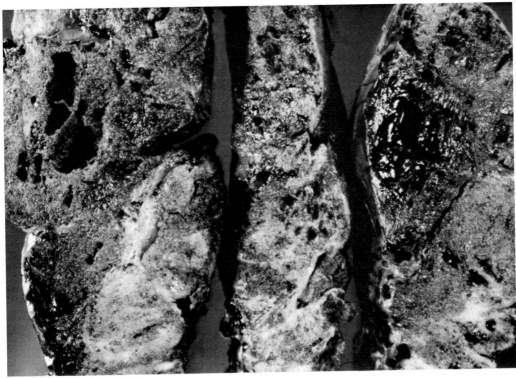

FIG 7–29.
Cross sections of the placenta in Figure 7–28 show that the floor infarction is irregular in its distribution.

Since ischemic necrosis is not a feature of the disorder, it is not an infarct and hence is misnamed. It can be easily distinguished from a true infarct by the fact that villi immediately adjacent to the affected areas show no ischemic changes. Specifically, these nearby villi are not subnormal in size, are not fibrotic, and do not have syncytial knots that are excessive in number or size (see Figs 7–19, 7–20, 7–26, and 7–27). The disorder is often not recognized and thus it is not widely known that it may be present in as many as 1 in every 845 placentas (Table 7–13).[220] Fetal mortality was high with the disorder in the CPS. The risk of stillbirth was 26 times that of the study population as a whole (see Table 7–13). The most important antecedents were major malformations in the fetus, an unusually long umbilical cord (91st–100th percentiles) and diffuse fibrin beneath the chorionic (fetal) plate of the placenta (see Table 7–13). Taken together these risk factors accounted for 31% of the maternal floor infarcts in the CPS. The association of unusually long cords with maternal floor infarcts raises the possibility that trauma to the placenta by fetal movements initiated some of the floor

infarcts. This reasoning is based on the fact that long umbilical cords often appear to be the result of vigorous fetal movements putting traction on the cord (see Chapter 6). If trauma to the placenta by fetal movements is the cause of some maternal floor infarcts, it has much in common with intervillous thrombi, which in many respects it resembles.

Maternal floor infarcts often recur in successive pregnancies, so recognizing the disorder is an indication that the next pregnancy should be carefully monitored to identify the disorder before it kills another fetus.[46,142,245] Clewell and Manchester observed a maternal floor infarct in progress and obtained a living baby by promptly delivering the child by cesarean section.[46] Maternal floor infarction may sometimes cause an elevation in the level of alpha-fetoprotein in maternal serum.[142]

After all of the risk factors for maternal floor infarcts had been taken into account, the surviving CPS children had an increased risk of neurologic abnormalities at 7 years of age. All of this increased risk was in the category of mental retardation with accompanying motor abnormalities

TABLE 7–13.
Risk Estimates for Antecedents to the Development of Maternal Placental Floor Infarction*

Risk Factors	No. of Placentas With Floor Infarcts per 1,000 Cases With Risk Factor†	Relative Risks (95% Confidence Intervals)	Attributable Risks (95% Confidence Intervals)
All cases	1 *(52)*		
Fetal factor			
Major fetal malformations	**7** *(7)*, P<.05	**1.7** (1.2, 2.3)	**.05** (.03, .07)
Markers for vigorous fetal motor activity			
Unusually long umbilical cord	**5** *(64)*, P<.001	**2.5** (1.1, 5.9)	**.18** (.13, .22)
Diffuse subchorionic fibrin	**4** *(45)*, P<.001	**2.1** (1.0, .49)	**.07** (.04, .11)
Other indicators			**.01** (.00, .02)
Population attributable risk			**.31** *(.28, .38)*
Pregnancy outcomes			
Preterm birth	2 *(18)*, P>.1	1.1 (0.6, 1.7)	
Fetal growth retardation	3 *(7)*, P>.1	1.3 (0.3, 1.7)	
Stillbirth	**30** *(18)*, P<.001	**26.2 (8.2, 97.4)**	
Neonatal death	3 *(3)*, P>.1	1.0 (0.2, 2.3)	
Neurologic abnormalities at 7 yr	**5** *(10)*, P<.05	**1.6 (1.0, 23.3)**	
Motor abnormalities + mental retardation		**2.7 (1.0, 4.6)**	

*Significant values are in boldface.
†Numbers of cases are in parentheses.

(see Table 7–13). Many fetuses survived maternal floor infarcts in the CPS. This is strong evidence against the view of Fox that maternal floor infarction is a change that follows stillbirth.[79]

Delayed Maturation of the Placenta

Delayed maturation of the placenta is identified by finding villi that are larger than normal, a syncytiotrophoblastic cell layer thicker than normal covering the villi, smaller and less numerous syncytial knots than are normal for gestational age, increased villous stromal density, and sometimes cytotrophoblastic cells retained beyond the gestational age when they usually disappear. Delayed placental maturation is less frequent than is accelerated maturation. The frequency of delayed maturation was 7.5% in full-term placentas in the CPS (Table 7–14). Antecedents or risk factors were identified for only 6% of these delays. These antecedents were maternal cigarette smoking during pregnancy, maternal diabetes mellitus, major fetal malformations, and erythroblastosis fetalis (see Table 7–14). After

taking these four risk factors into consideration, delayed placental maturation was associated with an increased risk of stillbirth, neonatal death, and mental retardation accompanied by neurologic abnormalities at 7 years of age (see Table 7–14). Delayed maturation has sometimes been claimed to be present in congenital syphilis, but it has not been present in the many syphilitic placentas that I have examined in Africa.[81]

Prolonged (Postterm) Gestation

About 1 pregnancy in 10 extends beyond 42 weeks and is thereby considered to be postterm. Perinatal mortality rates have long been known to increase progressively each week after the 42nd week of gestation. In the CPS the perinatal mortality rate was 21/1,000 births for postterm gestations vs. 12/1,000 for gestations that ended between 38 and 42 weeks of gestation ($P < .001$). Part of this mortality increase postterm was related to an increase in lethal fetal malformations.[213,237] Placental weights increase very slowly after 40 weeks and this has

TABLE 7–14.

Risk Estimates for Antecedents to Slow Maturation of the Placenta*

Risk Factors	No. of Cases of Slow Placental Maturation per 1,000 Cases With Risk Factor†	Relative Risks (95% Confidence Intervals)	Attributable Risks (95% Confidence Intervals)
All cases	75 (*3,305*)		
Maternal factors			
Smoked during pregnancy	**85** (*402*), *P* < .05	**1.1** (1.1, 1.2)	**.02** (.00, .03)
Diabetes mellitus	**97** (*22*), *P* > .1	**1.2** (1.0, 1.6)	**.01** (.00, .01)
Hemoglobin value < 9 g/dL			
Fetal factors			
Major malformations	**92** (*191*), *P* < .001	**1.3** (1.1, 1.5)	**.02** (.01, .03)
Rh disease	**147** (*26*), *P* < .001	**2.1** (1.7, 2.6)	**.01** (.00, .01)
Population attributable risk			**.06** (*.04, .08*)
Pregnancy outcomes			
Preterm birth (analyses included only full-term births)			
Fetal growth retardation	**111** (*242*), *P* < .001	**1.6** (1.4, 1.9)	
Stillbirth	**253** (*42*), *P* < .001	**4.1** (2.8, 5.8)	
Neonatal death	**200** (*23*), *P* < .001	**2.8** (1.8, 4.5)	
Neurologic abnormalities at 7 yr	**98** (*68*), *P* < .01	**1.5** (1.1, 1.9)	
Motor abnormalities + mental retardation		**1.5** (1.1, 2.0)	

Significant values are in boldface. All cases analyses are in birth weight and birth length percentiles > 30.
†Numbers of cases are in parentheses.

been postulated to place the postterm fetus at an increased risk of stress or death by creating a relative mismatch between the increasing needs of the growing fetus for oxygen and nutrients and the amount of oxygen and nutrients that the placenta can transfer.

Several types of evidence support the likelihood that many fetuses experience increasing stress postterm.[213,237] In the CPS, hemoglobin values were more often greater than 20 g/dL in neonates born postterm than at term, suggesting that a larger proportion of the postterm neonates had experienced antenatal hypoxemia.[237] In this same study much of the increase in perinatal mortality postterm was due to an increased case fatality rate for a wide variety of seemingly unrelated disorders.[213,237] These case fatality rate increases could be due to progressively insufficient blood flow from the uterus to the placenta, or to an aging of the placenta that leads to progressively decreasing function, or to the ever increased needs of the fetus for nutrients and oxygen. Neither of the first two explanations will explain the increase in perinatal mortality that occurs postterm. Most postterm placentas do not show gross or microscopic evidences of either low uteroplacental blood flow or of degenerative changes that might reduce placental function. Placental vascular resistance is reported to be normal postterm and when fetal acidosis develops postterm, it is usually not associated with an increase in cord blood carbon dioxide levels.[111,309]

Taken together, the aforementioned findings suggest that it is mainly the increasing needs of the fetus, rather than an insufficiency of placental function, that is responsible for the increasing frequency of fetal stress and death after 42 weeks of gestation. This possibility is also supported by the fact that fetal growth normally slows in the third trimester of pregnancy and then accelerates after birth. This is an indication that the placenta normally supplies less nutrients than the fetus needs to achieve its full growth potential in late gestation.

The only placental disorder whose frequency increased postterm in the CPS was acute chorioamnionitis.[213,237] At first glance this increase might be considered no more than a continuation of the progressive increase in the frequency of acute chorioamnionitis that starts in early gestation and continues to term. However, the increase greatly accelerates postterm, so explanations linked to specific postterm circumstances must be considered. One such a circumstance is the loss of the cervical mucous plug which often occurs around term, particularly in multigravidas. Its loss gives bacteria and mycoplasmas in the cervix direct access to the fetal membranes where they can initiate acute chorioamnionitis.

Developmental Disorders

Placenta Accreta, Increta, and Percreta

Placenta accreta is a disorder in which all or part of the placental villi are in direct contact with the myometrium and are anchored to muscle fibers rather than to decidual cells (Fig 7–30). It is usually attributed to a lack of decidua beneath the placenta, which allows placental villi to invade the uterine wall.[66] Reported risk factors include old cesarean section scars, fibroids, a prior myomectomy, and uterine malformations.[81] Clinically, placenta accreta presents as a failure of the placenta to separate spontaneously from the uterus after the birth of the child. There were four such cases in the CPS. This is presumably an underestimate because placenta accreta is quite frequent with placenta previa.[26] The true frequency of placenta accreta is difficult to establish because the diagnosis is usually based on clinical findings, and when microscopic criteria are used, appropriate sections of the uterine wall are often not available.

The frequency of placenta accreta was 1/10,000 in the CPS, which is close to some published estimates.[255] Three of the four gravidas who developed placenta accreta in the CPS had either a uterine leiomyoma or a history of prior uterine

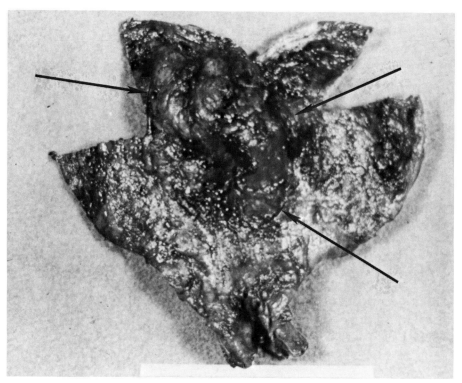

FIG 7–30.
Placenta accreta. The *arrows* point to parts of a retained placenta that required a hysterectomy.

surgery (Table 7–15). Two of the four cases terminated with placenta previa and vaginal bleeding and one of the infants was stillborn.

Some recent findings suggest that placenta accreta sometimes has a more complex origin.[151] To interpret these findings it must be remembered that there are two successive invasions of the uterine wall by trophoblastic cells during the course of normal implantation. In the first invasion trophoblastic cells infiltrate the inner myometrium for several millimeters. In the second invasion trophoblastic cells invade and remodel the spiral arteries, which permits these vessels to expand to accommodate a large blood flow to the intervillous space of the placenta. In placenta accreta both trophoblastic invasions may be abnormal.[151] Trophoblastic giant cells that are normally plentiful in the interstitium of the inner myometrium are reported to be rare or absent in cases of placenta accreta, and the trophoblastic cells that normally remodel the spiral

arteries invade far beyond their usual stopping point in the spiral arteries to infiltrate the walls of the radial and arcuate arteries.[151] An interstitial infiltrate of chronic mononuclear cells reportedly often accompanies these findings, and a hyalinization of the myometrium is often present at those sites where the villi implanted. Khong and Robertson suggest that these findings are the result of a defective interaction between the maternal decidua and the two trophoblastic invasions of the uterine wall.[151] This is not an explanation for all cases of placenta accreta which also occurs with tubal pregnancies, abdominal pregnancies, and implantation in the cervical canal.[24]

In *placenta increta* placental villi invade the myometrium. In *placenta percreta* trophoblastic cells penetrate the entire thickness of the uterine wall and the uterus ruptures (Fig 7–31). Such ruptures are associated with about a 10% maternal mortality. Up until 1988, 76 cases of placenta percreta were reported in the

TABLE 7–15.

Risk Estimates for Antecedents to the Development of Placenta Accreta*

Risk Factors	No. of Cases of Placenta Accreta per 1,000 Cases With Risk Factor†	Relative Risks (95% Confidence Intervals)	Attributable Risks (95% Confidence Intervals)
All cases	0.1 *(4)*		
Maternal factor			
Uterine leiomyoma or prior uterine surgery	**0.5** *(3)*, $P<.02$	**234** (192, 291)	**.77** *(.01, .99)*
Placental factor			
Placenta previa	**9.8** *(2)*, $P<.001$	**86** (32, 233)	**.11** *(.00, .41)*
Population attributable risk			**.88** *(.55, .99)*
Pregnancy outcomes			
Preterm birth	250 *(1)*		
Fetal growth retardation	0 *(0)*		
Stillbirth	250 *(1)*		
Neonatal death	0 *(0)*		
Neurologic abnormalities at 7 yr	0 *(0)*		

*Significant values are in boldface.
†Numbers of cases are in parentheses.

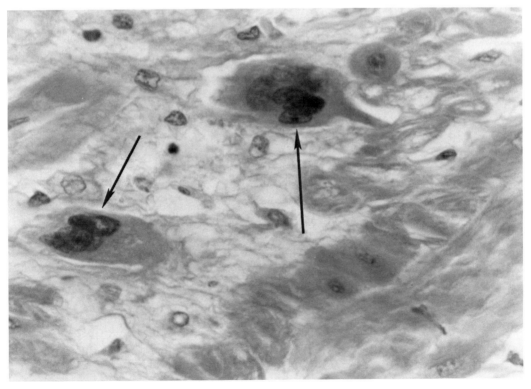

FIG 7–31.
Placenta percreta. Trophoblastic cells are invading an area of the myometrium just beneath the serosal surface of the uterus in a case in which trophoblastic elements penetrated the entire thickness of the uterine wall. HE stain, ×1,200.

literature with an overall fetal-neonatal mortality rate of 96% (73/76). Placenta accreta is usually recognized after delivery because the placenta fails to separate completely, whereas placenta increta and placenta percreta usually manifest during pregnancy with bleeding.

Placenta accreta is a major cause of maternal morbidity and mortality in some Third World populations, where its frequency may be 20 times that in the industrial nations.[18,322] Reported predisposing factors include a previously untreated retained placenta, suppurative postpartum endometritis, and incomplete and missed abortions.[18] Such disorders are postulated to predispose to placenta accreta by causing necrosis with consequent fibrosis in the uterine wall.[18]

The low frequency of placenta accreta in the industrial nations does not mean that it has little clinical significance in these societies. In these societies it is one of the most frequent reasons for emergency hysterectomy undertaken to control severe obstetric hemorrhage or uterine atony.[44] It is reportedly responsible for up to a third of hysterectomies undertaken to stop uncontrolled bleeding at delivery. Placenta accreta is also a frequent complication of the Asherman syndrome, a disorder in which replacement of most of the functioning endometrium by scar tissue is followed by endometrial failure.[85]

Extrachorial Placentas

Extrachorial placentas are placentas in which the chorion leave inserts at some distance inside of the rim of the placenta instead of at the rim. This includes circummarginate and circumvallate placentas. The term *extrachorial* derives from the fact that the edge of the placenta is uncovered except for fibrin and sometimes old clotted blood. It is from this site that vaginal bleeding occasionally originates.[299] When the membrane that normally covers the surface of the placenta is folded back over itself (plicated) inside the edge of the placenta, the condition is designated *circumvallate*. When it is not plicated it is termed *circummarginate*.

Both presumably originate from an early separation of the membranes from the edge of the placenta. This origin was demonstrated by Scott et al. who showed that many fetal chorionic vessels pursue a straight course through and beyond the points where the membranes are inserted into the placental surface.[299] The bleeding that presumably initiates the separation of the membranes from the edge of the placenta can clinically mimic a placental abruption and either exsanguinate a fetus or produce an infant that is anemic at birth.[24,200]

Circummarginate Placenta.—Of the placentas in the CPS, 4% (2,367) received this diagnosis. Some of the risk for a circummarginate placenta may be due directly or indirectly to low uteroplacental blood flow to the edge of the placenta (Table 7–16). White race was the most important risk factor. It may be a risk factor because uneven maturation of the placenta, a manifestation of low uteroplacental blood flow, is more frequent in whites than in blacks. Other risk factors that may be markers for low blood flow to the periphery of the placenta include maternal cigarette smoking during pregnancy, preeclampsia, eclampsia, decidual necrosis at the margin of the placenta, and major malformations in the fetus (see Table 7–16). Taken together these risk factors accounted for 28% of the circummarginate placentas in the study. The finding that cigarette smoking was a risk factor raises the possibility of a blood flow abnormality because maternal blood pressure drops for 5 to 15 minutes after smoking a cigarette and this drop likely affects uterine blood flow to the edge of the placenta more than to more central areas. This is evident because in the CPS decidual necrosis at the edge of the placenta was much more frequent in cigarette smokers than in nonsmokers. Decidual necrosis at the edge of the placenta was also nearly twice as frequent when major fetal malformations were present as when they were absent.[237] It has long been known that placental villous maturation is

TABLE 7–16.

Risk Estimates for Antecedents to the Development of Circummarginate Placenta*

Risk Factors	No. of Cases of Circummarginate Placenta per 1,000 Cases With Risk Factor†	Relative Risks (95% Confidence Intervals)	Attributable Risks (95% Confidence Intervals)
All cases	40 (*2,367*)		
Maternal factors			
Race: white	**44** (*1,394*), *P* < .001	**1.5** (1.4, 1.6)	**.17** (.16, .19)
Smoked during pregnancy	**49** (*557*), *P* < .001	**1.3** (1.1, 1.4)	**.04** (.03, .05)
Parity ≥ 5	**45** (*407*), *P* < .005	**1.2** (1.1, 1.3)	**.02** (.01, .03)
Preeclampsia, eclampsia	**52** (*154*), *P* < .001	**1.2** (1.0, 1.4)	**.01** (.00, .02)
Fetal factor			
Major fetal malformations	**55** (*280*), *P* < .001	**1.4** (1.2, 1.6)	**.03** (.02, .04)
Placental factor			
Decidual necrosis, edge of placenta	**49** (*260*), *P* < .01	**1.3** (1.1, 1.5)	**.03** (.01, .05)
Population attributable risk			**.28** (.26, .31)
Pregnancy outcomes			
Preterm birth	40 (*483*), *P* > .1	1.0 (0.9, 1.2)	
Fetal growth retardation	40 (*179*), *P* > .1	1.0 (0.8, 1.3)	
Stillbirth	15 (*32*), *P* < .001	0.9 (0.7, 1.1)	
Neonatal death	38 (*41*), *P* > .1	1.0 (0.6, 1.9)	
Neurologic abnormalities at 7 yr	*36* (*61*), *P* > .1	0.9 (0.6, 1.4)	

*Significant values are in boldface.
†Numbers of cases are in parentheses.

usually much more advanced at the edge than in other areas of the placenta. All of this raises the possibility that low maternal blood flow to the edge of the placenta during early gestation is the factor responsible for many extrachorial placentas. Having a circummarginate placenta did not increase the risk of stillbirth or any other unfavorable pregnancy outcome in the CPS when antecedent risk factors were taken into consideration (see Table 7–16).

Circumvallate Placenta.—As previously mentioned, when the fetal surface has a raised ring of fused, folded membrane at some distance inside of the placental margin, the condition is termed a *circumvallate placenta* (Figs 7–32 and 7–33). Six percent (3,687) of the placentas in the CPS received this designation. This included placentas in which a ring of folded membranes was present around the entire circumference of the placenta as well as cases in which only part of the circumference was affected. The raised folded membrane contains chorion and often amnion, decidual tissue, blood clot, and villi in varying stages of degeneration (Fig 7–34). As would be expected, the risk factors for circumvallate placenta were the same as those for circummarginate placentas, another evidence of the common genesis of the two disorders (Tables 7–16 and 7–17). Taking all of the risk factors into consideration the presence of a circumvallate placenta slightly increased the risk for fetal growth retardation but not for other unfavorable pregnancy outcomes (see Table 7–17). Previous investigators have reported that circumvallate placentas are associated with increased frequencies of abortion, antepartum hemorrhage, and preterm birth.[81] These associations were not present in the CPS when antecedent risk factors for circumvallate placentas were taken into consideration.

Cysts

Cysts are relatively frequent in the placenta, particularly just beneath the

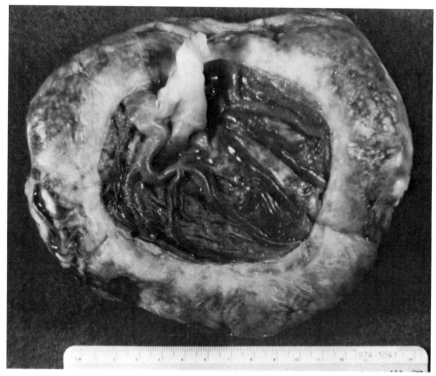

FIG 7–32.
Typical circumvallate placenta at 38 weeks of gestation.

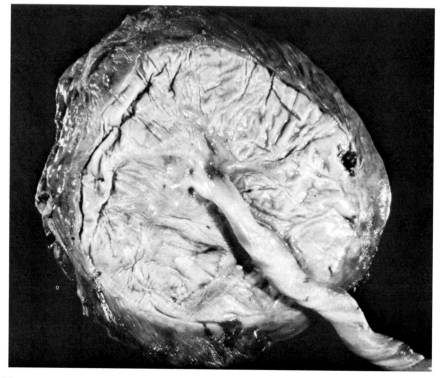

FIG 7–33.
There is a lesser degree of circumvallation than in Figure 7–32.

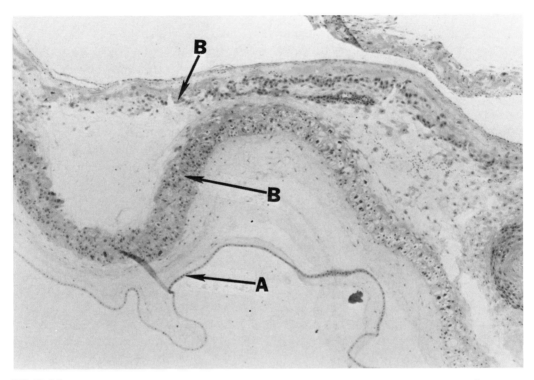

FIG 7–34.
This section is taken from the overhanging margin of membranes in a circumvallate placenta. Note that the amnion *(A)* has not infolded with the chorion *(B)* in this case. HE stain, ×120.

TABLE 7–17.
Risk Estimates for Antecedents to the Development of Circumvallate Placenta*

Risk Factors	No. of Cases of Circumvallate Placenta per 1,000 Cases With Risk Factor†	Relative Risks (95% Confidence Intervals)	Attributable Risks (95% Confidence Intervals)
All cases	62 *(3,687)*		
Maternal factors			
Race: white	**77** *(2,464)*, P < .02	**2.1** (1.9, 2.2)	**.26** (.25, .28)
Smoked during pregnancy	**92** *(1,004)*, P < .001	**1.5** (1.4, 1.6)	**.08** (.07, .09)
Parity ≥5	**72** *(654)*, P < .001	**1.3** (1.1, 1.4)	**.03** (.02, .04)
Preeclampsia, eclampsia	**78** *(932)*, P < .001	**1.2** (1.1, 1.3)	**.03** (.02, .04)
Fetal factor			
Major fetal malformations	**71** *(366)*, P < .005	**1.1** (1.0, 1.3)	**.01** (.00, .02)
Placental factor			
Decidual necrosis, edge of placenta	**86** *(440)*, P < .001	**1.4** (1.2, 1.6)	**.04** (.02, .06)
Population attributable risk			**.43** *(.40, .45)*
Pregnancy outcomes			
Preterm birth	**60** *(737)*, P < .005	1.0 (0.8, 1.2)	
Fetal growth retardation	**80** *(361)*, P < .001	1.2 (1.1, 1.3)	
Stillbirth	**27** *(59)*, P < .001	0.6 (0.1, 1.1)	
Neonatal death	**80** *(85)*, P < .02	1.0 (0.8, 1.2)	
Neurologic abnormalities at 7 yr	64 *(120)*, P > .1	1.0 (0.8, 1.2)	

*Significant values are in boldface.
†Numbers of cases are in parentheses.

amnion where they are often the remnants of chorionic cells that have liquefied (Fig 7–35). Large cysts at this site are sometimes the result of large subchorionic blood clots that have contracted.[24] Cysts are also common in cell islands and in placental septa. Cysts in villi are often an exaggerated form of villous edema, and placentas that have such villous cysts often have multiple areas where the villi are edematous. A small proportion of placental cysts are chorangiomas or the remnant of an atrophied member of a twin pair. Septal cysts are frequent if placentas are cross-sectioned at close intervals.[24]

Three or more cysts were recognized during the gross examination in 0.4% (230) of the placentas in the CPS. Antecedents were identified for 9% of these placentas. The only identified risk factor was white race (Table 7–18). Taking this risk factor into consideration, placental cysts were associated with lower-than-expected risks for both preterm birth and stillbirth (Table 7–18). Bret et al. have published the most detailed review of the literature on placental cysts.[34]

Chorangioma (Hemangioma)

Chorangioma, often called *chorioangioma, hemangioma, fibroma,* and a number of other names in the literature, had a frequency of 0.4% (228) in the placentas of the CPS. It is the only common nontrophoblastic tumor of the placenta and it can be classified as a hamartoma because it is comprised of elements derived from primitive chorionic mesenchyme.[263] It is a benign neoplasm that does not metastasize. Most chorangiomas are single, small, red, and they can be present in any part of the placenta but are most often nearer the fetal than the maternal surface. On microscopic examination they are comprised of blood vessels, loose stroma, and areas of degeneration. The relative mixture of these three tissue types varies from chorangioma to chorioangioma and within chorangiomas, which has confused many observers. The angiomatous areas are

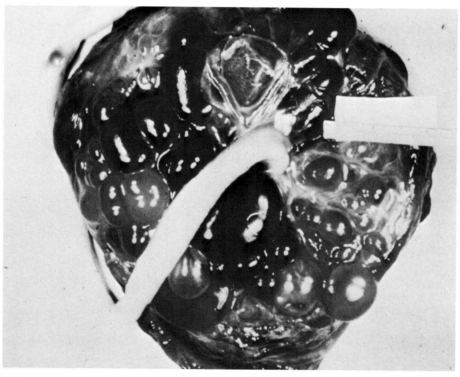

FIG 7–35.
Subamniotic cysts in a placenta. Many of these cysts were lined by squamous epithelium.

easiest to recognize with their many thin-walled blood vessels crowded together between a stroma of loose connective tissue (Fig 7–36). Most of the vessels are capillary-sized, but larger, cavernous-sized vessels are often present. Stromal areas of the neoplasm are usually comprised of loose, spindle-shaped cells with a few poorly formed vessels. The degenerate areas of chorangiomas often show admixtures of myxoid stroma, calcification, hyalinized connective tissue, and necrosis.

TABLE 7–18.

Risk Estimates for Antecedents to the Development of Three or More Cysts in the Placenta*

Risk Factors	No. of Placentas With Three or More Cysts per 1,000 Cases With Risk Factor†	Relative Risks (95% Confidence Intervals)	Attributable Risks (95% Confidence Intervals)
All cases	4 (*230*)		
Maternal factor			
Race: white	**5** (*130*), *P* < .01	**1.3** (1.1, 1.5)	**.09** (.07, .11)
Population attributable risk			**.09** (.07, .11)
Pregnancy outcomes			
Preterm birth	**2** (*30*), *P* < .002	**0.6** (0.3, 1.0)	
Fetal growth retardation	3 (*13*), *P* > .1	0.8 (0.5, 1.2)	
Stillbirth	**1** (*3*), *P* < .05	**0.4** (0.1, 0.9)	
Neonatal death	1 (*1*), *P* > .1		
Neurologic abnormalities at 7 yr	1 (*12*), *P* > .1	0.4 (0.0, 1.7)	

*Significant values are in boldface.
†Numbers of cases are in parentheses.

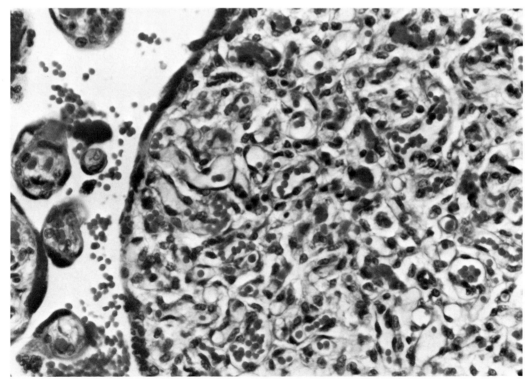

FIG 7–36.
Chorangioma with a mainly capillary appearance. HE stain, ×600.

Quite a number of very large chorangiomas have been reported in the literature.[24] They are often encapsulated, red-purple in color, and sometimes can be identified by ultrasound. Occasionally, more than one large chorangioma is present. A few large chorangiomas have been associated with polyhydramnios, fetal cardiomegaly, and fetal hydrops due to high output fetal heart failure.[325] Some chorangiomas have red cells and platelets trapped in their vascular channels with a resultant consumptive coagulopathy and microangiopathic hemolytic anemia. Rarely, chorangiomas have such a large blood flow through them that they act as arteriovenous shunts that reduce blood flow through the rest of the placenta, thereby depriving the fetus of needed nutrients. This has occasionally produced fetal growth retardation, fetal distress, and intrauterine death.[20,126,255,270] Hydramnios is the most frequently reported clinical complication of a chorangioma and it would seem likely that it is the result of fetal heart failure.[20,32,255,347] There is a case report in which fetal heart failure and hydramnios disappeared after a chorangioma underwent necrosis.[70]

In the CPS only a few antecedent risk factors for chorangiomas were identified. These included unevenly accelerated placental maturation, minor malformations in the fetus, and the fetus being male (Table 7–19). Several authors have previously reported an association between chorangiomas and preeclampsia or eclampsia which produced an uneven acceleration of placental maturation.[120] It is difficult to imagine what the mechanism might be, but perhaps the abnormal blood flow through the placenta that is associated with large chorangiomas might somehow initiate preeclampsia or eclampsia. It is well known that the low blood flow into the placental intravillous space often initiates a vasoconstrictive response in the placental circulation, but is the reverse sequence possible? Can low intravillous blood flow in those parts of the placenta that are away from the chorangioma initiate a vasoconstrictive response in the uterus and other maternal vascular beds?[78] After taking all of the identified risk factors for chorangiomas into consideration, there were no residual unfavorable pregnancy outcomes associated with chorangiomas in the CPS (see Table 7–19).

Several other types of neoplasms have been reported in the placenta.[182] These include partial hydatidiform moles, which

TABLE 7–19.

Risk Estimates for Antecedents to the Development of Multiple Chorangiomas*

Risk Factors	No. of Placentas With Multiple Placental Chorangiomas per 1,000 Cases With Risk Factor†	Relative Risks (95% Confidence Intervals)	Attributable Risks (95% Confidence Intervals)
All cases	4 *(228)*		
Maternal factor			
Preeclampsia, eclampsia	**5** *(928)*, *P* < .001	**1.3** (1.1, 1.5)	**.05** *(.03, .07)*
Fetal factors			
Minor malformations	**65** *(19)*, *P* < .05	**1.7** (1.1, 2.8)	**.04** *(.02, .05)*
Sex: male	**5** *(126)*, *P* < .05	**1.1** (1.0, 1.3)	**.05** *(.03, .07)*
Population attributable risk			**.14** *(.11, .17)*
Pregnancy outcomes			
Preterm birth	4 *(52)*, *P* > .1	1.0 (0.8, 1.2)	
Fetal growth retardation	4 *(20)*, *P* > .1	1.2 (0.8, 1.5)	
Stillbirth	5 *(11)*, *P* > .1	1.2 (0.3, 2.2)	
Neonatal death	**9** *(10)*, *P* < .001	1.4 (0.8, 2.1)	
Neurologic abnormalities at 7 yr	4 *(11)*, *P* > .1	1.0 (0.5, 1.8)	

*Significant values are in boldface.
†Numbers of cases are in parentheses.

are not true tumors; rare teratomas, which may be the remnants of twins; and heterotopic tissues representing other organs such as the adrenal.[24]

Chorangiosis

This is a condition in which there is a marked increase in the number of capillaries inside villi in a circumscribed area of the placenta. Chorangiosis has been reported sporadically in the past and has been of particular interest to Altshuler.[6] He has made the diagnosis when microscopic inspection with a ×10 objective showed ten villi, each with ten or more vascular channels in ten or more noninfarcted and nonischemic zones of at least three different areas of the placenta (Fig 7–37). He has graded the lesion and found it to be strongly associated with perinatal death and with fetal malformations.[6,131]

Thrombi in the Surface Vessels of the Placenta

Such thrombi were observed in 0.3% (159) of the placentas of the CPS (Fig 7–38). When the thrombosis is in a large artery on the fetal surface of the placenta, it produces a well-demarcated triangular pale zone of parenchyma that otherwise is normal in appearance and consistency. Villi in the affected zone are hypovascular or avascular, are devoid of blood, and display both villous stromal fibrosis and increased numbers of syncytial knots. In the CPS the principal risk factor for such thrombi was a very long (91st–100th percentile) umbilical cord and other indicators of vigorous fetal motor activity (Table 7–20). As is explained later in this chapter, unusually long cords are the characteristic consequence of traction applied to the cord by vigorous fetal movements. Children with these long umbilical cords have a greater-than-expected frequency of hyperactive behavior both as neonates and as older children. From these associations we postulate that trauma to the placental surface by fetal movements is the likely explanation for many thrombi that develop in the surface vessels of the placenta.

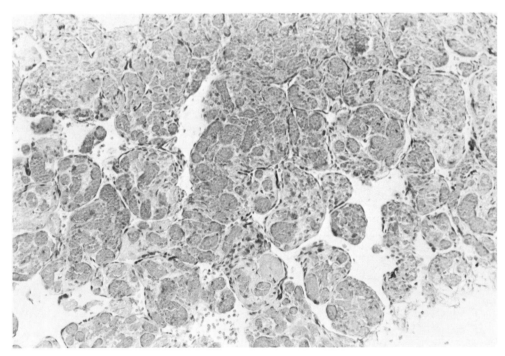

FIG 7–37.
Chorangiosis. HE stain, ×300.

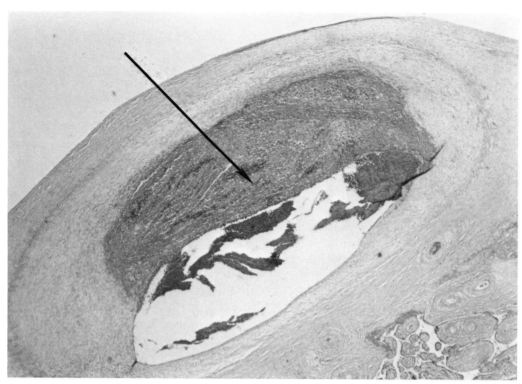

FIG 7–38.
A thrombus partially occludes a vessel just beneath the fetal surface of the placenta. HE stain, ×120.

TABLE 7–20.

Risk Estimates for Antecedents to the Development of Thrombi in Vessels on the Surface of the Placenta*

Risk Factors	No. of Placentas With Vascular Thrombi per 1,000 Cases With Risk Factor†	Relative Risks (95% Confidence Intervals)	Attributable Risks (95% Confidence Intervals)
All cases	3 (*159*)		
Maternal factor			
Preeclampsia, eclampsia	**4** (*34*), P < .05	**1.4** (1.1, 1.7)	**.08** (.05, .11)
Placental factors			
Acute chorioamnionitis	5 (*78*), P > .1	**1.4** (1.0, 2.0)	**.05** (.04, .07)
Markers for vigorous fetal motor activity			
Unusually long umbilical cord	**4** (*78*), P < .005	**2.0** (1.4, 2.9)	**.26** (.21, .30)
Other indicators			**.17** (.14, .20)
Population attributable risk			**.55** (*.50, .61*)
Pregnancy outcomes			
Preterm birth	**5** (*49*), P < .005	**1.6** (**1.0, 2.3**)	
Fetal grwoth retardation	2 (*9*), P > .1	0.7 (0.3, 1.1)	
Stillbirth	**35** (*31*), P < .001	**21.4** (15.9, 39.1)	
Neonatal death	**7** (*6*), P < .02	1.0 (0.2, 2.6)	
Neurologic abnormalities at 7 yr	4 (*6*), P > .1	1.0 (0.6, 1.6)	

Significant values are in boldface.
†*Numbers of cases are in parentheses.*

In the CPS other antecedents of thrombi in placental surface vessels were acute chorioamnionitis, preeclampsia, and eclampsia (see Table 7–20). Preeclampsia and eclampsia produce low uteroplacental blood flow (see Table 7–20). Invasion of the vessel walls by bacteria, mycoplasmas, or the associated products of the infection is presumably the reason why acute chorioamnionitis was a risk factor for thrombi in surface vessels of the placenta. The association of preeclampsia and eclampsia with such thrombi may be due to the vasoconstriction and vascular damage that such low blood flow initiates in the placental circulation.[78] After taking all of the identified risk factors into consideration, placental surface vessel thrombosis was associated with a high risk for stillbirth and a somewhat smaller increased risk for preterm birth (see Table 7–20). There were no other unfavorable pregnancy outcomes.

Grossly Visible Calcium Deposits

Grossly visible calcium deposits are common in the basal plate and in the septa of the placenta in late gestation (Figs 7–39 and 7–40). Jeacock et al. found that the amount did not increase very much postterm, so its quantity is not a reliable indicator of postmaturity.[134] Grading the amount of calcium in the placenta by ultrasonography has not proved to be a reliable indicator of fetal lung maturity.[117] Grossly visible calcium deposits do not increase with placental infarcts or with most other placental disorders, and they reportedly decrease as parity increases.[88] All of these findings suggest that calcium in the basal plate and septa of the placenta is more likely a physiologic than a pathologic finding. On gross examination this calcium at first has a dirty brown color and subsequently it has a bluish tinge.

Such calcifications were identified by gross examination in 9.5% (5,659) of the

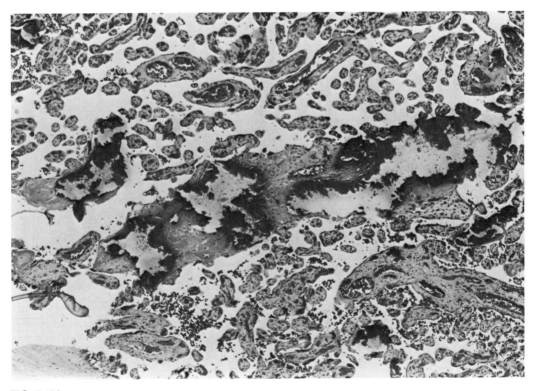

FIG 7–39.
Black calcium deposits in the septa of a term placenta. The section was not decalcified so the calcium deposits have torn the septa. HE stain, ×120.

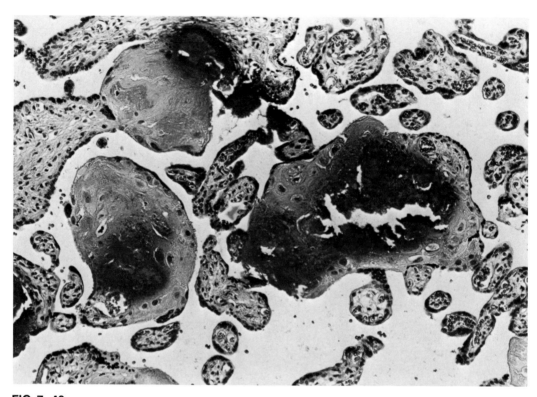

FIG 7–40.
Black calcium deposits in nests of decidual cells at the point where villi attach to the decidua. This placenta was from a full-term, normal pregnancy. HE stain, ×300.

TABLE 7–21.

Risk Estimates for Antecedents to the Development of Gross, Diffuse Calcification of the Placenta*

Risk Factors	No. of Cases With Diffuse Placental Calcification per 1,000 Cases With Risk Factor†	Relative Risks (95% Confidence Intervals)	Attributable Risks (95% Confidence Intervals)
All cases	95 (5,659)		
Maternal factor			
Race: white	**117** (3,728), P < .001	**1.7** (1.6, 1.8)	**.23** (.21, .24)
Fetal factors			
Full-term birth	**109** (4,717), P < .001	**1.8** (1.7, 1.9)	**.32** (.31, .34)
Major fetal malformations	**113** (359), P < .001	**1.2** (1.0, 1.5)	**.02** (.00, .04)
Placental factors			
Unevenly accelerated maturation	**102** (382), P < .05	**1.2** (1.0, 1.5)	**.01** (.00, .02)
Uniformly accelerated maturation	**115** (122), P < .02	**1.3** (1.0, 1.7)	**.01** (.00, .02)
Population attributable risk			**.58** (.56, .62)
Pregnancy outcomes			
Fetal growth retardation	94 (426), P > .1	0.7 (0.4, 1.1)	
Stillbirth	**25** (54), P < .001	**0.3** (0.1, 0.6)	
Neonatal death	**48** (51), P < .001	**0.6** (0.4, 0.8)	
Neurologic abnormalities at 7 yr	99 (280), P > .1	0.8 (0.5, 1.1)	

*Significant values are in boldface.
†Numbers of cases are in parentheses.

placentas of the CPS. The two major antecedents were full-term birth and being white (Table 7–21). Additional antecedents were major fetal malformations and, microscopically, an acceleration of villous maturation. Taking these antecedent factors into consideration, gross calcium in the basal plate and septa of the placenta was associated with a lower risk for stillbirth and neonatal death than was the case for the CPS as a whole (see Table 7–21).

Disorders of the Villi

Calcium Localized in the Terminal Villi

Calcium localized in the terminal villi of the placenta had a 0.7% (401) frequency in the CPS. Its identified antecedent risk factors were being black, acute chorioamnionitis, preeclampsia and eclampsia (Table 7–22). After taking these risk factors into consideration, such calcification was not associated with any unfavorable pregnancy outcome (see Table 7–22). Calcium often deposits in villi that have undergone degeneration (Fig 7–41). Calcium also commonly deposits in terminal villi after fetal death.

Chronic Villitis

Chronic villitis is defined as chronic inflammation in one in more placental villi. Various studies have reported it to be present in from 1% to 34% of placentas, depending upon the number of microscopic sections examined, the stringency of the diagnostic criteria, and the population group examined.[32,153,160,162,205] In about 85% of the affected villi, only chronic inflammatory cells are present, usually lymphocytes and less often plasma cells (Fig 7–42). Sometimes villi are completely destroyed leaving only fibrotic remnants of their original structure and a few lymphocytes still visible (Fig 7–43). Necrosis is sometimes a feature of villitis. In some instances villitis has a granulomatous character with giant cells (Fig 7–44). In more than 95% of the cases of chronic villitis no etiologic agent can be identified and the neonate shows no signs of infection. In one study 90% of the cord bloods from placentas with villitis had IgM levels that were within normal levels, which is strong evidence that most of the villitis in that study was not caused by infection.[205]

Specific viruses have been isolated from 1% to 2% of placentas with villitis, usu-

TABLE 7–22.

Risk Estimates for Antecedents to the Development of Widespread Calcification of Terminal Villi in the Placenta*

Risk Factors	No. of Cases of Calcification of Placenta Villi per 1,000 Cases With Risk Factor†	Relative Risks (95% Confidence Intervals)	Attributable Risks (95% Confidence Intervals)
All cases	7 (401)		
Maternal factor			
Preeclampsia, eclampsia	**10** (122), P<001	**1.6** (1.3, 2.0)	**.09** (.07, .11)
Placental factor			
Acute chorioamnionitis	**9** (139), P<.001	**1.4** (1.3, 1.6)	**.18** (.14, .22)
Fetal factor			
Race: black	**9** (205), P<.001	**1.3** (1.1, 1.6)	**.39** (.35, .44)
Population attributable risk			**.65** (.61, .70)
Pregnancy outcomes			
Preterm birth	8 (92), P>.1	1.0 (0.7, 1.3)	
Fetal growth retardation	11 (33), P>.1	1.7 (0.8, 2.7)	
Stillbirth	**12** (26), P<.01	1.0 (0.7, 1.3)	
Neonatal death	**16** (17), P<.001	0.9 (0.6, 1.3)	
Neurologic abnormalities at 7 yr	10 (10), P>.1	1.3 (0.5, 2.3)	

*Significant values are in boldface.
†Numbers of cases are in parentheses.

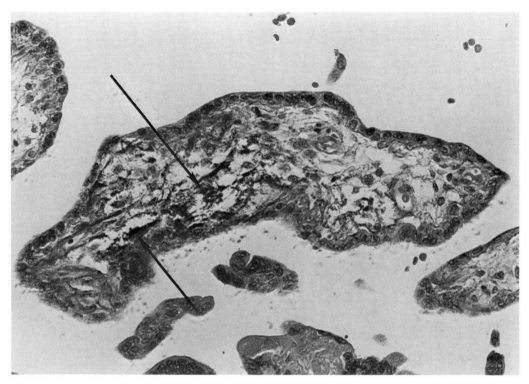

FIG 7–41.
Black-stained calcium deposits in a degenerating villus. HE stain, ×600.

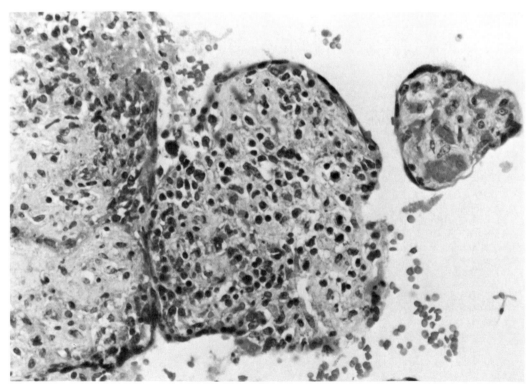

FIG 7–42.
Chronic villitis of unknown etiology in a 37-week gestation. There is intensive infiltration by lymphocytes, plasma cells, and histiocytes. HE stain, ×300.

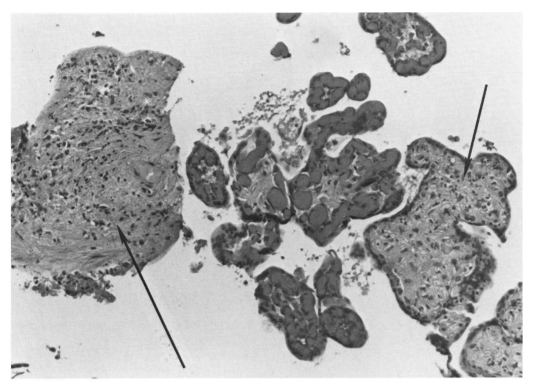

FIG 7–43.
A widespread, destructive chronic villitis of unknown etiology in a stillborn fetus. The mother had two previous stillbirths with this same placental disorder. HE stain, ×120.

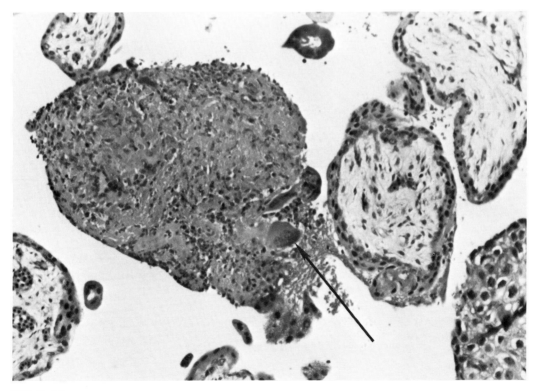

FIG 7–44.
Chronic granulomatous villitis of unknown etiology in a 13-week gestation. The villus has been destroyed and is infiltrated by lymphocytes and several giant cells. One of the giant cells is marked by an *arrow*. HE stain, ×120.

ally cytomegalovirus, rubella, or herpes-virus.[25] Vaccinia, varicella, hepatitis virus, enterovirus, polio virus, *Toxoplasma gondii*, and trypanosomes have been isolated from a few placentas with villitis. With all of these agents the fetus is usually infected when the placenta is infected. The only bacterium that commonly causes villitis is *Listeria monocytogenes*. Villitis caused by this agent is usually different from that produced by viruses, in that listerial infections often produce microabscesses that affect one part of a villus more than another, producing a characteristic asymmetric or eccentrically located lesion.[232] The antecedent infection in the gravida characteristically manifests as a flulike illness.

Chronic villitis had a 0.6% (314) frequency in the CPS, which is a lower figure than has been reported by many other investigators (Table 7–23). There are several reasons for this low figure in the CPS. First, in determining this frequency we excluded from the analysis placentas with acute chorioamnionitis or with the findings that are produced by low uteroplacental blood flow. Placentas with the findings of low uteroplacental blood flow

were excluded because low uteroplacental blood flow sometimes produces lesions that superficially resemble chronic villitis in ischemic areas. If an infarct is just out of the plane of section, the degenerative process at the edge of the infarct can be mistaken for villitis (Figs 7–45 and 7–46).[87,160] Benirschke and Kaufmann have termed these lesions *subinfarctive villous degenerations*.[24] We did not want to confuse these lesions with chronic villitis, particularly because chronic low uteroplacental blood flow is a common cause of fetal growth retardation, stillbirth, and neonatal death.[29,225,237] Acute bacterial chorioamnionitis, a common disorder caused by a wide variety of bacteria and mycoplasmas, on rare occasions causes acute villitis and we did not want to include cases with acute villitis in our analyses.

After making these exclusions, we found antecedents or risk factors for 13% of the chronic villitis in the CPS (see Table 7–23). All of these antecedents were nonspecific except for maternal immunization and clinically diagnosed maternal infection during the first trimester of pregnancy (see Table 7–23). After taking these

TABLE 7–23.

Risk Estimates for Antecedents to the Development of Chronic Placental Villitis*

Risk Factors	No. of Placentas With Chronic Villitis per 1,000 Cases With Risk Factor†	Relative Risks (95% Confidence Intervals)	Attributable Risks (95% Confidence Intervals)
All cases	6 (*314*)		
Maternal factors			
Very thin pregravid	**8** (*110*), P < .05	**1.3** (1.1, 1.6)	**.06** (.05, .08)
Race: black	**8** (*159*), P < .01	**1.2** (1.0, 1.4)	**.05** (.03, .07)
1st trimester immunization or infection	**9** (*25*), P < .001	**2.4** (1.1, 2.1)	**.02** (.00, .03)
Fetal factor			
Twins	**41** (*20*), P < .002	**2.0** (1.3, 3.2)	**.02** (.01, .04)
Population attributable risk			**.13** (*.11, .14*)
Pregnancy outcomes			
Preterm birth	8 (*77*), P > .1	1.2 (0.8, 1.5)	
Fetal growth retardation	**13** (*13*), P < .02	**1.6** (1.1, 2.3)	
Stillbirth	4 (*8*), P > .1	0.7 (0.2, 1.4)	
Neonatal death	7 (*6*), P > .1	0.6 (0.2, 1.1)	
Neurologic abnormalities at 7 yr	10 (*11*), P > .1	1.5 (0.7, 2.4)	

*Significant values are in boldface.
†Numbers of cases are in parentheses.

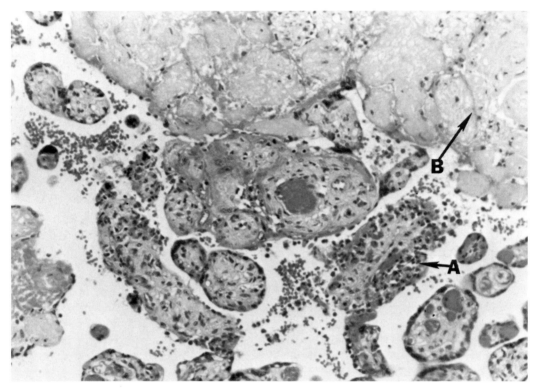

FIG 7–45.
False villitis *(A)*. Ischemic changes in villi that are near an infarct *(B)* sometimes resemble chronic villitis. Benirschke and Kaufmann have termed this inflammatory process *subinfarctive villous degeneration.*[24] *HE stain,* ×120.

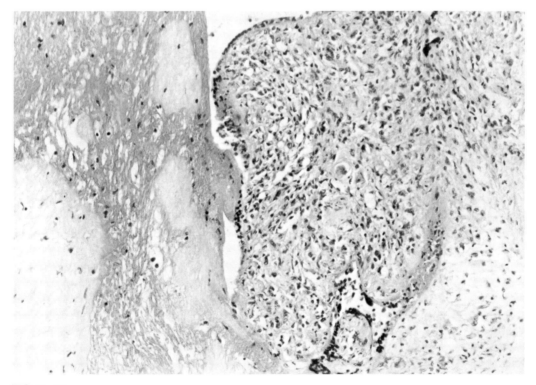

FIG 7–46.
In rare instances the false villitis that is caused by ischemia is florid. In this case the true infarct on the left is adjacent to the false villitis on the right. HE stain, ×120.

identified risk factors into consideration, chronic villitis had almost no clinical significance. The only unfavorable pregnancy outcome was a small increase in the risk for fetal growth retardation (see Table 7–23). This growth retardation was no longer present at 7 years of age, so its clinical significance appears to be negligible. There are some who strongly suspect that chronic villitis is an infectious process or an immunologic disorder akin to an organ rejection phenomenon.[24] It would be surprising if either of these possibilities were true because the clinical consequences of chronic villitis are usually benign.

Our findings are at odds with most published studies of chronic villitis, which have reported it to be associated with increased frequencies of fetal growth retardation and fetal and neonatal death.[24,291] Very high figures for these poor outcomes have been reported when chronic villitis had been present in successive pregnancies.[4,268] Several such cases have been sent to me for consultation (see Fig 7–43). We looked for these repeating unfavorable outcomes associated with chronic villitis in the CPS. They were absent when disorders that accelerate placental maturation and cause placental infarcts were excluded from the analyses. This raises the possibility that some of the poor outcomes associated with recurrent villitis in previous studies may have been due to low uteroplacental blood flow disorders. When hypertension is absent, apparent low uteroplacental blood flow disorders characteristically repeat in successive pregnancies and cause fetal growth retardation, preterm birth, and increased frequencies of both stillbirth and neonatal death.[225] It has been postulated that immunoglobulins, including antinuclear antibodies deposited on villi, may be responsible for some chronic villitis.[161] This too could be a manifestation of chronic low uteroplacental blood flow because other immunoglobulins, once thought to cause the fibrinoid necrosis and artherosis in decidual vessels in cases of preeclampsia and eclampsia, now seem more likely to be secondary to vascular damage.[152]

There may be still another reason why chronic villitis lacked clinical significance in the CPS. The CPS findings were derived from a prospectively selected segment of the general population, while most earlier studies have included at least some placentas that were sent for consultation because of a poor pregnancy outcome. In several consultation cases referred to me, chronic villitis was widespread and destroyed a large proportion of the villi in a placenta. In two of these cases the villitis had repeated in successive pregnancies and by widely destroying villi had led to repeat stillbirths. All of this indicates that case selection is probably a major factor in the widely divergent views expressed about the clinical significance of chronic villitis.

Placental Villous Edema

In recent years placental villous edema has been the most frequent cause of stillbirth, neonatal death, and neonatal morbidity in children born at our institution before 28 weeks of gestation.[233] The edema develops inside of intravillous cells and does not appear as dilated lymphatics because there are no lymphatics in the villi (Figs 7–47 and 7–48). When the edema is both diffuse and severe, it makes fetuses hypoxic by compressing blood vessels inside of the villi. All that is known about the genesis of this edema is that it is initiated by fetal stress.[233] The most frequent causes of this stress are acute chorioamnionitis, major fetal malformations, and abruptio placentae (Table 7–24). Whatever its cause, the edema is initiated by the fetus. This is known because the edema is usually present on only one side of twin placentas that do not have transplacental shunts, while twin placentas with such shunts usually have a similar degree of edema on both sides of the placenta.[233] In the first instance the two twins have separate placental circulations, while in the second the same blood circulates through both fetuses. The edema is most frequent and severe in

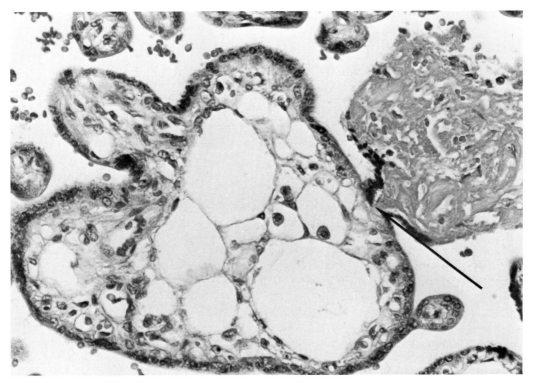

FIG 7–47.
Severe edema in a villus. At the point of the *arrow* the trophoblast covering the edematous villus is disrupted and an intervillous thrombus has formed. A syncytiotrophoblastic cell has begun to grow out from the villus to cover this intervillous thrombus. HE stain, ×600.

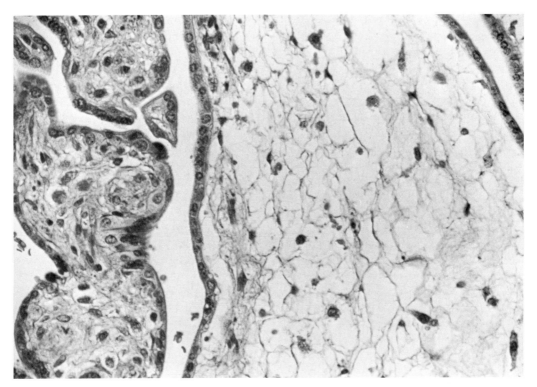

FIG 7–48.
An edematous villus on the right is adjacent to nonedematous villi. HE stain, ×600.

TABLE 7–24.

Risk Estimates for Antecedents to the Development of Edema in the Placental Villi*

Risk Factors	No. of Placentas With Villous Edema per 1,000 Cases With Risk Factor†	Relative Risks (95% Confidence Intervals)	Attributable Risks (95% Confidence Intervals)
All cases	29 (*1461*)		
Fetal factor			
Major fetal malformations	**42** (*198*), P < .001	**1.5** (1.3, 1.7)	**.04** (.02, .06)
Placental factors			
Acute chorioamnionitis	**63** (*991*), P < .01	**1.9** (1.6, 2.0)	**.36** (.32, .42)
Diffuse subchorionic fibrin	**31** (*1862*), P < .001	**1.1** (1.0, 1.2)	**.06** (.04, .08)
Abruptio placentae	**57** (*54*), P < .001	**1.8** (1.2, 2.6)	**.01** (.01, .02)
Population attributable risk			**.46** (.43, .51)
Pregnancy outcomes			
Preterm birth	**61** (*808*), P < .005	**4.2** (3.9, 4.7)	
Fetal growth retardation	26 (*119*), P > .1	0.9 (0.4, 1.4)	
Stillbirth	**72** (*71*), P < .001	**3.1** (2.1, 4.6)	
Neonatal death	**88** (*96*), P < .001	**5.3** (4.1, 7.1)	
Neurologic abnormalities at 7 yr	**44** (*112*), P < .02	**1.3** (1.0, 1.7)	
Motor abnormalities + severe mental retardation		**1.7** (1.1, 2.6)	

Significant values are in boldface.
†Numbers of cases are in parentheses.

placentas delivered before 28 weeks of gestation after which both its frequency and its severity decrease. The risk of developing severe villous edema relates much more to the microscopic maturity of the placenta than to its gestational age. The more advanced the maturity, the less frequently severe edema occurs. Thus fetal stress produces no edema or only mild edema in placentas that are histologically mature whether they are full term or preterm in actual gestational age. Quite often edema is severe in normally mature areas of a preterm placenta and absent or only mild in areas of the same placenta where villous maturation is more advanced.

When it develops, placental villous edema usually reaches its peak shortly after fetal stress begins and then it slowly recedes, even though the fetal stress continues. Thus, edema that is only mild at delivery may have been severe some days earlier when it first developed. This is sometimes reflected by poor renal function in the first 1 to 3 days of life which then rapidly improves. This sequence re-

flects the repair phase in the early neonatal period of a hypoxic renal injury that took place some days before birth. When hypoxia severely damages the kidneys during labor and delivery, renal function does not usually improve until 5 to 7 days after birth.

Villous edema appears to be the most frequent cause of severe fetal hypoxia in infants born before 30 weeks of gestation. In such children the extent and severity of the edema correlates inversely with umbilical arterial blood oxygen levels and pH values.[233] Severe, diffuse villous edema is almost always associated with the need to resuscitate vigorously at birth, persistently low Apgar scores, and the need for prolonged mechanical ventilation of a neonate (Table 7–25). The fetal hypoxia caused by severe villous edema often damages the type II pneumocytes in the lungs. The resulting deficiency of surfactant predisposes to the development of hyaline membrane disease and the neonatal respiratory distress syndrome (see Table 7–25).[233,237] The neonatal respiratory distress syndrome often continues and

TABLE 7–25.

Placental Villous Edema: Neonatal Morbidity and Mortality

Gestation: 27–31 wk	Severity of Placental Villous Edema*		
	Mild	Moderate	Severe
Apgar score <6 at 1 min	0	63% (5)	95% (19)
Neonatal resuscitation, none	60% (3)	0	0
Intubation required	0	50% (4)	85% (17)
Neonatal respiratory distress syndrome	20% (1)	13% (1)	90% (18)
Neonatal deaths	0	24% (2)	55% (11)

Numbers of cases are in parentheses.

potentiates the hypoxia and acidosis started by the villous edema.[178] The hypoxia and acidosis in turn often lead to a breakdown in the autoregulation of the cerebral circulation. Vasoparalysis appears to be a major cause of this loss of autoregulation.[169] Fluctuations in blood pressures and blood flow then lead to bleeding from capillaries in the subependymal germinal matrix, germinal matrix destruction, subsequent rupture of the blood into a lateral ventricle, periventricular hemorrhagic infarction, which is termed *periventricular leukomalacia,* and at times posthemorrhagic hydrocephalus (see Table 7–24; Fig 7–49).[170,177,346]

There are several reasons why this sequence of events does not occur at term. The germinal matrix capillary bed is immature before 30 weeks of gestation when intraventricular hemorrhages usually take place. The germinal matrix capillary bed

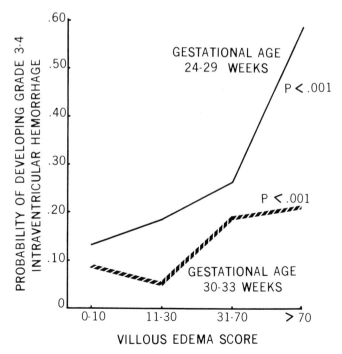

FIG 7–49.
The frequency of combined grades 3 and 4 intraventricular cerebral hemorrhage increased in preterm born infants with the extent and severity of placental villous edema. An edema score of 0–10 represents absent, or very mild, focal villous edema. A score above 70 represents severe diffuse edema.

regresses by term. By this time placental villi have matured and resist becoming edematous and autoregulation of the cerebral circulation is less easily disturbed than earlier in gestation.[233,345] In an ultrasound study only leukomalacia was found during the first 7 days that followed the first identification of periventricular leukomalacia.[59] The first cysts appeared between 10 days and 9 weeks after the leukomalacia was identified. Thereafter, cysts, old glial scars, and delayed myelination were present.[59,279,340] The long-term consequences of leukomalacia are serious and can include cerebral palsy, blindness, cognitive impairments, a seizure disorder, and hearing loss. In some studies as many as a third of very low-birth-weight infants born before 28 weeks of gestation have one or more of these impairments.

The frequency of intraventricular hemorrhages has declined in recent years, presumably because means have been discovered to reduce fluctuations in cerebral blood pressure and flow in preterm born neonates.[256,257] However, intraventricular hemorrhages, white matter necrosis, and consequent quadriplegic and diplegic cerebral palsy will probably not be completely prevented in preterm born children until ways are found to prevent placental villous edema.

In evaluating the role of placental villous edema in a newborn's clinical course the extent and severity of any edema that is present should be assessed from representative areas of the placenta. Observing the placenta through a low-power (4 mm or 2 mm) microscope objective is the simplest way to make this assessment. By using one of these low-power objectives the observer will not easily see villous edema which is too mild to have clinical significance, whereas moderate and severe villous edema that is capable of producing clinically significant fetal hypoxia is readily apparent. If more than half of a placenta appears moderately or severely edematous under this magnification, the associated newborn will usually have clinical evidence of antenatal hypoxia. If the edema involves most of the placenta and is severe, the infant will be stillborn or severely acidotic with a low level of oxygen in its umbilical cord arterial blood (see Tables 7–24, 7–25).[233]

In 1989 Shen-Schwarz et al. reported no correlation between villous edema, Apgar scores, and neonatal death.[304] They found a 10% frequency of villous edema in full-term placentas and a 38% frequency of such edema in full-term placentas with villous fibrosis. These percentages are at least 40-fold greater than we have observed in full-term placentas, so it is likely the authors scored a far milder process as villous edema than is our practice or else the placentas were too long in the refrigerator, incompletely fixed, or they used an improperly prepared fixative. Poorly fixed and partially autolyzed villi have artifacts that mimic villous edema.

Villous edema is so frequent in placentas delivered before 25 to 26 weeks of gestation that many have assumed it is a normal finding.[304] This can easily be disproved when comparisons are made between the extent and severity of the edema and umbilical cord arterial blood pH, Po_2, and base excess values. When the edema is severe and generalized, these cord blood values invariably reflect severe fetal acidosis and hypoxia. When edema is absent, these cord blood values will usually be normal, even when the infant is born before 25 weeks of gestation. Benirschke and Kaufmann suggest that the villous edema we observe is often not edema but rather normal stromal channels in immature intermediate villi.[24] We originally viewed mild villous edema as normal stromal channels. What changed our interpretation was the observation that such "normal stromal channels" were occasionally not present under low-power magnification in the placentas of neonates born between 23 and 25 weeks of gestation. When we visited these infants in the newborn nursery we found that their Apgar scores had been normal or near normal, they had not needed resuscitation, and were experiencing no respiratory distress the day after delivery. By contrast, neonates of the same gestational age who had diffuse, severe placental villous edema by our criteria always had a history of low Apgar scores, had been difficult to resuscitate, and had severe respiratory distress that usually required mechanically assisted ventilation the day after delivery. The group without severe placental villous edema had normal umbilical arterial blood pH values, and the group with the severe edema had low pH values.

Widespread Fibrosis of the Terminal Villi

A few villi are fibrotic in most placentas. Widespread fibrosis of terminal villi is abnormal (Fig 7–50). It had a frequency of 2.1% (1,223 cases) in the CPS (Table 7–26). In the literature it is usually attributed to one or more of three causes: (1) ischemia in an area adjacent to an infarct, (2) inflammation, usually viral in origin, and (3) a dead fetus. In the CPS identified risk factors for widespread villous fibrosis fell into four categories: (1) disorders and conditions that predispose to low uteroplacental blood flow, (2) fetal malformations, (3) chronic villitis, (4) fetal death (see Table 7–26). The low uteroplacental blood flow category includes the mother being thin pregravid which predisposes to low uteroplacental blood flow by limiting maternal gestational blood volume expansion.[127,128] It also includes disorders in which uteroplacental blood flow is characteristically low, namely preeclampsia, eclampsia, and chronic maternal hypertension. Overall, 17% of the diffuse villous fibrosis in the CPS could be attributed to one of these disorders (see Table 7–26). After taking these antecedent risk factors into consideration, widespread villous fibrosis was associated with increased risks for preterm birth and neonatal death (see Table 7–26). Children whose placentas had such villous fibrosis did not

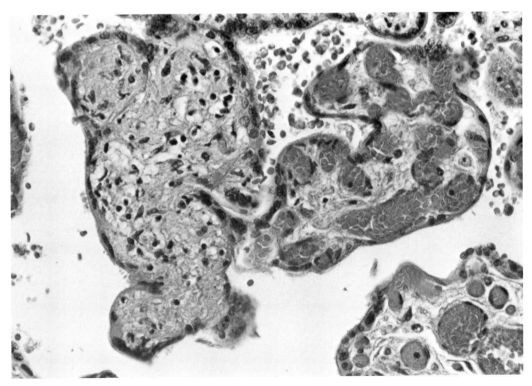

FIG 7–50.
A fibrotic villus on the left is adjacent to two normal villi. HE stain, ×600.

TABLE 7–26.

Risk Estimates for Antecedents to the Development of Widespread Fibrosis of Terminal Villi in the Placenta*

Risk Factors	No. of Cases of Fibrosis of Terminal Villi per 1,000 Cases With Risk Factor†	Relative Risks (95% Confidence Intervals)	Attributable Risks (95% Confidence Intervals)
All cases	21 (1,223)		
Maternal factors			
Thin pregravid	**25** (422), P < .001	**1.4** (1.2, 1.5)	**.09** (.08, .10)
Preeclampsia, eclampsia, chronic hypertension	**27** (321), P < .001	**1.5** (1.3, 1.7)	**.08** (.07, .09)
Fetal factors			
Stillbirth	**181** (137), P < .001	**9.3** (8.6, 10.1)	**.10** (.08, .13)
Major fetal malformations	**29** (148), P < .001	**1.3** (1.1, 1.6)	**.03** (.02, .04)
Minor fetal malformations	**30** (90), P < .001	**1.3** (1.7, 1.7)	**.01** (.01, .02)
Placental factor			
Chronic villitis	**74** (72), P < .001	**3.4** (2.9, 4.0)	**.04** (.02, .06)
Population attributable risk			**.34** (.31, .38)
Pregnancy outcomes			
Preterm birth	**29** (351), P < .001	**1.4** (1.3, 1.7)	
Fetal growth retardation	**26** (117), P < .01	1.2 (0.9, 1.6)	
Neonatal death	**35** (38), P < .01	**1.9** (1.5, 2.4)	
Neurologic abnormalities at 7 yr	21 (422), P > .1	1.0 (0.6, 1.5)	

*Significant values are in boldface.
†Numbers of cases are in parentheses.

have an increase of long-term neurologic abnormalities.

A careful inspection should always be made of the placentas of stillborn infants to try to distinguish between villous fibrosis of antemortem and postmortem origins. If the fibrosis appears much older in some than in other areas and spares still other areas, it could have antedated death rather than been its consequence.

Intervillous Thrombi

Intervillous thrombi are blood clots that usually start where the trophoblast covering a villus or the underside of the chorionic plate of the placenta has been disrupted (see Fig 7–47). These thrombi then frequently spread to reach and partially cover adjacent villi. They are termed *intervillous thrombi* because they commonly fill the space between villi (Fig 7–51). They are very frequent under the microscope and a few sometimes reach a size at which they are grossly visible. They are present in almost every placenta and are more frequent at term than preterm. The more

such thrombi are grossly visible, the greater the likelihood that they will have clinical significance, either as markers of vigorous fetal movements that have traumatized the placenta or as a disorder that impairs placental function by cutting off blood flow around large number of villi and leading to their atrophy.

Intervillous thrombi that reach several centimeters in diameter sometimes displace as well as surround villi. These large intervillous thrombi are usually round or oval in gross appearance, and are more frequent at the edge than in other areas of the placenta. Initially they are red in color and firm. When they are somewhat older and when they have formed in a moving flow of blood they are multilayered. As they age they turn brown, yellow, and eventually become white and hard. Initially they are comprised of red cells with intermixed fibrin. As time passes the red cells lyse and fibrin dominates. Villi atrophy after the blood clot forms around them. Hemosiderin is often visible at the periphery of a large intervillous thrombus

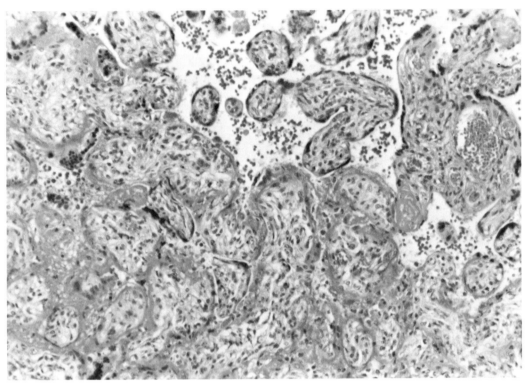

FIG 7–51.
Intervillous thrombi in the lower part of the photo surround many villi and cut off the flow of maternal blood around them. As a result they are becoming atrophic. HE stain, × 120.

if the thrombus has been present for many days or weeks.

The formation of intervillous thrombi has often been interpreted as a normal, clinically benign process caused by turbulence in the blood flowing through the intervillous space.[32] Experimental studies have shown that agents or conditions that damage the syncytiotrophoblast can lead to intervillous thrombi.[24] We found by examining serial sections that the intervillous clots are anchored at one or more sites where the trophoblastic covering of the villi has been disrupted (see Fig 7–47). Often the trophoblastic cells adjacent to this site make abortive attempts to cover the thrombus (see Fig 7–47).

In the CPS the most important antecedents of multiple, grossly visible intervillous thrombi were a long umbilical cord and the other markers for vigorous fetal motor activity, including the fetus being male (Table 7–27). As explained later in this chapter, unusually long umbilical cords are frequently the consequence of tension greater than normal applied to the cord by vigorous fetal movements. Since there is a strong association between long cords and intervillous thrombi, traumatic breaks in the trophoblastic covering of the villi, caused by these vigorous fetal movements, is the likely explanation for many intervillous thrombi. The increasing strength of fetal movements with advancing gestational age is a likely reason why intervillous thrombi increase in frequency as term approaches. Less important risk factors for intervillous thrombi in the CPS were fetal malformations and maternal immunization or infection during the first trimester of pregnancy (see Table 7–27). After taking all of these risk factors into consideration, multiple intervillous thrombi that were grossly visible posed no risk for any unfavorable pregnancy outcome (see Table 7–27).

It has sometimes been suggested that intervillous thrombi are the consequence

TABLE 7–27.

Risk Estimates for Antecedents to the Development of Five or More Grossly Visible Intervillous Thrombi in the Placenta*

Risk Factors	No. of Placentas With Five or More Intervillous Thrombi per 1,000 Cases With Risk Factor†	Relative Risks (95% Confidence Intervals)	Attributable Risks (95% Confidence Intervals)
All cases	6 *(302)*		
Maternal factor			
Immunization or infection during 1st trimester	**7** *(50)*, *P* < .05	**1.2** (1.0, 1.5)	**.01** (.00, .02)
Fetal factors			
Major fetal malformations	**8** *(27)*, *P* < .05	**1.3** (1.0, 1.7)	**.02** (.00, .04)
Sex: male	**7** *(156)*, *P* < .005	**1.3** (1.0, 1.7)	**.14** (.11, .16)
Markers for vigorous fetal motor activity			
Unusually long umbilical cord	**8** *(104)*, *P* < .001	**1.6** (1.3, 2.1)	**.19** (.16, .22)
Other indicators			**.46** (.41, .52)
Population attributable risk			**.81** *(.76, .88)*
Pregnancy outcomes			
Preterm birth	**4** *(38)*, *P* < .01	**0.7** (0.4, 1.0)	
Fetal growth retardation	6 *(13)*, *P* > .1	1.1 (0.6, 1.6)	
Stillbirth	**29** *(22)*, *P* < .001	1.0 (0.4, 1.9)	
Neonatal death	10 *(8)*, *P* > .1	1.5 (0.7, 2.4)	
Neurologic abnormalities at 7 yr	8 *(9)*, *P* > .1	1.3 (0.7, 1.9)	

*Significant values are in boldface.
†Numbers of cases are in parentheses.

of fetal blood leaking into the intervillous space and mixing with Rh- and ABO-incompatible maternal blood.[19,80] If this occurs, intervillous thrombi should be more frequent when Rh and ABO blood group incompatibility exists between mother and fetus than when it is absent.[81] In the CPS the frequency of multiple intervillous thrombi was the same (6/1,000) whether mother and baby had the same or different Rh and ABO blood types. In a few cases intervillous thrombi have been reported in the placentas of gravidas who have lupus erythematosus with high circulating levels of antiphospholipid antibodies.[180]

Effects of High Altitude

Placentas are often abnormally large at high altitude. Normally the thickness of the syncytiotrophoblastic layer that covers the villi decreases progressively as gestation advances. This presumably facilitates the passage of gases and nutrients across the trophoblast into the fetal circulation. At high altitude the syncytiotrophoblastic layer reportedly varies more in thickness and intravillous capillaries are closer to the trophoblastic membrane than is the case in placentas delivered at low altitudes.[130] These adaptations at high altitude presumably facilitate oxygen transport from the intervillous space into the fetal blood.

Hemorrhagic Endovasculitis

Hemorrhagic endovasculitis is a fetal blood vessel disorder of uncertain etiology and poor prognosis.[298] Its characteristic features are endothelial cell degeneration, vessel thrombosis, and the escape of red cells into the vessel wall and surrounding tissue of a stem or terminal villus (Fig 7–52).[303] Occasionally the lesions are partially calcified, suggesting that the process was in progress for some time before delivery.

Sander et al. originally described the lesion in 19.5% of placentas referred to a placental registry.[298] The lesions were associated with fetal growth retardation, a high perinatal mortality rate, and subse-

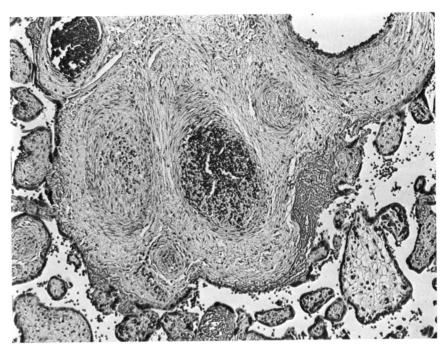

FIG 7–52.
Hemorrhagic endovasculitis. HE stain, ×60.

quent developmental delays. In a subsequent study Shen-Schwarz et al. found the lesion in 13 of 1,938 (0.6%) placentas.[303] This last figure is probably too low because Shen-Schwarz et al. reviewed only two pieces of tissue from each placenta and apparently excluded many placentas from analysis that were associated with poor pregnancy outcomes. The lesions of hemorrhagic endovasculitis are most frequent in the placentas of macerated stillborns and many view the lesion in this situation as a postmortem phenomenon.[24] A somewhat similar lesion has been produced in placental tissue culture under hypoxic conditions.[308] In my view hemorrhagic endovasculitis does exist as an antemortem lesion but its pathogenesis is as yet undetermined.

Bacterial and Mycoplasmal Infections

Acute Chorioamnionitis

Acute chorioamnionitis develops when bacteria or mycoplasms gain access to the extraplacental membranes and spread along the surface of the chorion. There are several routes by which these bacteria reach the membranes, but most often it is through the cervix. Usually the bacteria or mycoplasmas pass from the membranes into the amniotic fluid, overcome its antimicrobial systems, and then grow freely. This disorder is the most frequent cause of preterm labor wherever it has been studied and it was responsible for more than a third of the preterm births in the CPS.[235,237] Since these infections develop outside of the control of the health care system and the resulting labor cannot be stopped, they remain a major public health problem. This is one of the main reasons why the frequency of preterm births has hardly changed in the United States during the last three decades.[147] Acute chorioamnionitis is particularly important as a cause of poor pregnancy outcome in women of low socioeconomic status. Populations that have impaired antimicrobial systems in their amniotic fluid also have high frequencies of acute chorioamnionitis and its consequences.[11,328]

Identifying the Disorder and Its Causes.—Acute chorioamnionitis manifests as an acute, sometimes diffuse inflammatory process in the extraplacental membranes, the chorionic plate of the placenta, and the umbilical cord (Fig 7–53).[235,237] It can be severe in some areas of the umbilical cord and extraplacental membranes and absent in other areas, so the diagnosis cannot be excluded if no inflammation is found in one or two tissue samples from these sites. When present, acute chorioamnionitis very early affects the chorionic (fetal) plate of the placenta and it is at this site that the diagnosis is most reliably made (Fig 7–54).

There is considerable evidence that nonmicrobial substances that appear in the amniotic fluid do not cause acute chorioamnionitis. Lauweryns et al. produced all of the histologic features of acute chorioamnionitis by introducing various bacterial species into the amniotic fluid of experimental animals, but not by intro-

ducing various mixtures of meconium, gastric juice, and amniotic fluid debris into the amniotic fluid.[163] There is good evidence that viral infections do not cause acute chorioamnionitis. In the CPS there was no correlation between the presence of acute chorioamnionitis and increasing maternal gestational antibody titers to the ten viruses that most often infect the placenta.[237]

Many have doubted that infectious agents are responsible for acute chorioamnionitis because older studies failed to culture bacteria from half or more of the placentas in which the inflammatory process was present. In recent years improved culture techniques have permitted the recovery of bacteria and mycoplasmas from up to 80% of placentas with acute chorioamnionitis, which is strong evidence that acute chorioamnionitis is an infectious process.[63,121] The mycoplasmas include *Mycoplasma hominis* and *Unreaplasma urealyticum*.[97,265] The bacteria and mycoplasmas recovered from cases of

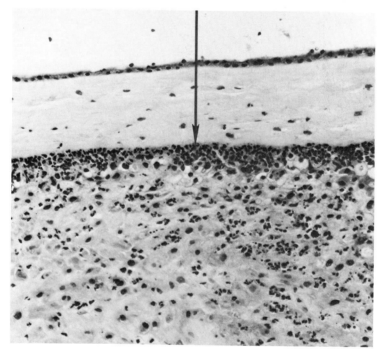

FIG 7–53.
A large number of polymorphonuclear leukocytes are infiltrating along the chorion of the extraplacental fetal membranes in a case of acute chorioamnionitis. HE stain, ×225.

acute chorioamnionitis are the organisms that are normally present in the vagina and cervix during pregnancy. About two-thirds of the cultures yield a single organism, nearly half of which are anaerobic bacteria. Some of these anaerobic bacteria take many days to isolate because they have fastidious growth characteristics. Older studies did not have the technology to isolate and identify many of these organisms and none of the older studies cultured for mycoplasmas. Bacteria and mycoplasmas are less frequently recovered from the amniotic fluid than from the fetal membranes, perhaps because the antibacterial systems in amniotic fluid are often strongly antimicrobial, particularly late in gestation.[287] Endotoxin has been demonstrated in some amniotic fluids in which bacteria are present.[287] The finding of leukoattractants in the amniotic fluid is currently the most sensitive laboratory

method available for identifying the presence of acute chorioamnionitis.[250]

Several organisms that are well-known pathogens in the uterus and fallopian tubes rarely if ever cross intact fetal membranes to cause acute chorioamnionitis. These include *Neisseria gonorrhoeae*, *Chlamydia trachomatis*, and group B streptococci.[183,312] In one study 64% of the newborns infected with group B streptococcus had acute chorioamnionitis, but in every case the membranes were ruptured before delivery.[246] In our laboratory fetal membranes with chorioamnionitis have repeatedly been culture-negative for chlamydia when these membranes were intact at the onset of labor. Many but not all investigators have reported that premature membrane rupture and preterm delivery are more frequent when the cervix is colonized by *C. trachomatis*.[76,109,187,260,293,324] In one study, gravi-

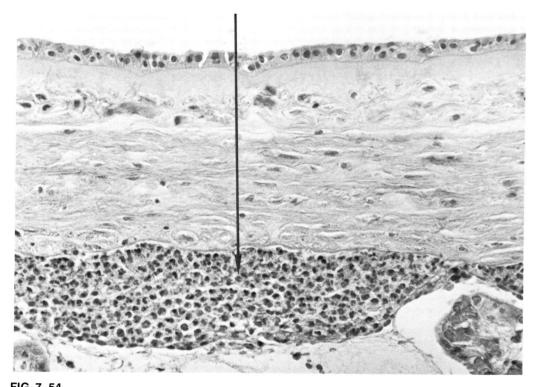

FIG 7–54.
Large numbers of polymorphonuclear leukocytes have accumulated beneath the chorionic (fetal) plate of the placenta in response to leukoattractants that have diffused through the chorionic plate from infected amniotic fluid. HE stain, ×120.

das whose cervical cultures were positive for chlamydia had fewer premature membrane ruptures when they received antibiotics.[293] This suggests that chlamydia may sometimes be a marker for factors or conditions that predispose to acute chorioamnionitis. The gonococcus is an even less frequent cause of acute chorioamnionitis. Only one case has been reported in which the gonococcus was grown from the placenta when the fetal membranes were intact at the onset of labor.[68,312]

Bacterial vaginosis reportedly increases the risks for developing acute chorioamnionitis and for preterm delivery.[109,192,307] Bacterial vaginosis is diagnosed when Gram's stain of vaginal smears shows few lactobacilli and many *Gardnerella vaginalis* and some *Mobiluncus* species.[307] As in the case of chlamydial colonization, one can speculate that the presence of bacterial vaginosis is a marker for other factors that predispose to acute chorioamnionitis.

Positive cultures from placentas without chorioamnionitis often yield organisms that are characteristic contaminants acquired from the cervix or vagina during delivery.[12] Such contamination has usually taken place when *Propionibacterium acnes*, coagulase-negative staphylococci, or lactobacillis are recovered from a placenta or the extraplacental fetal membranes. Such contamination is least frequent when cultures are taken between the amnion and the chorion of the extraplacental membranes. This is the best site for taking cultures because the surface of the chorion within the extraplacental membranes is the primary route by which bacteria and mycoplasmas invade to cause acute chorioamnionitis.

Special stains are only occasionally useful in the diagnostic or treatment of acute chorioamnionitis. Very few of the bacteria that cause acute chorioamnionitis are visible by the use of Gram's stain unless they are present in very large numbers.[281] None of the mycoplasmas that cause acute chorioamnionitis are stained by Gram's stain. Acridine orange stains mycoplasmas but not most of the bacteria that cause acute chorioamnionitis.[282] Both the Brown-Hopps and the Warthin-Starry stains can demonstrate some organisms not made visible by Gram's or acridine orange stains.[8] If acute chorioamnionitis is severe, the diagnosis can sometimes be made at birth by making a smear of an infant's gastric contents (Fig 7–55).

Measurements of maternal serum C-reactive protein and the products of infection in the amniotic fluid have been used to try to diagnose acute chorioamnionitis before delivery. All of these tests are expensive and time-consuming; most lack sensitivity, and some also lack specificity.[286] The leukocyte esterase assay is a simple bedside test that rapidly identifies the presence of neutrophil activity in the amniotic fluid.[69] It is highly specific, but its sensitivity is too low to recognize most cases of acute chorioamnionitis before delivery. This points up the need to develop an inexpensive, sensitive, selective noninvasive test that women can use in their own homes to detect acute chorioamnionitis during its earliest stages. If such a test can be developed, it might be possible to treat acute chorioamnionitis at a very early stage and thereby prevent some preterm deliveries.

Routes of Infection. – The cervical os is the usual route through which bacteria and mycoplasmas reach the extraplacental membranes to initiate acute chorioamnionitis (Fig 7–56). The infection usually starts in the membranes adjacent to the cervical os.[235–237] Inflammation is almost always present at this site and is often more advanced than inflammation at other sites in the membranes, the placenta, or the umbilical cord.[22] In vaginally delivered twins, acute chorioamnionitis usually involves the first-born when only one member of a pair is affected. This would be expected if the infection usually originates in membranes near the cervical os, because the membranes of the first-born are adjacent to the cervical os just

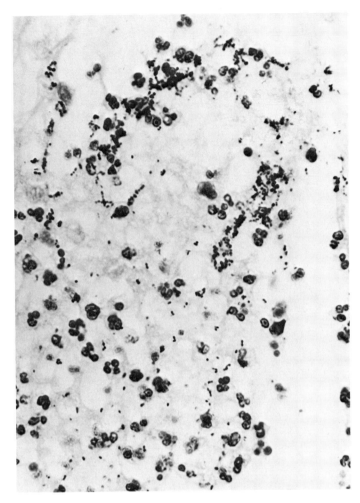

FIG 7–55.
This smear of a newborn infant's gastric contents shows numerous maternal polymorphonuclear leukocytes and chains of streptococci that had been aspirated from infected amniotic fluid. HE stains, ×900. (From Blanc WA: Pathology of the placenta, membranes, and umbilical cord in bacterial, fungal and viral infections in man, in Naeye R, Kissane J, Kauffman N: *Perinatal Diseases.* Baltimore, Williams & Wilkins Co, 1981, p 81. Used by permission.)

prior to delivery. The bacteria that reach the fetal membranes must first pass through the mucous plug in the cervix, which normally resists bacterial penetration.[48] In rare instances diagnostic amniocentesis, fetoscopy, villous sampling, intrauterine transfusion, and a medically induced abortion introduce the bacteria or mycoplasmas into the amniotic fluid which then cause acute chorioamnionitis (Fig 7–56).[272]

When the organisms that cause acute chorioamnionitis have low virulence, the fetal membranes often remain intact until the start of labor. In such cases the infecting organisms spread along the surface of the chorionic cell layer in the extraplacental membranes within 12 to 24 hours after the infection has started.[236]

Bacteria appear often to enter the amniotic fluid during this early phase of the infection. Fetal bacteremia or septicemia is presumed to be the result of the fetus inhaling bacteria that have entered the amniotic fluid, but there is speculation that bacteria may occasionally reach the fetus through placental villi after they have been shed into the intervillous blood from infected decidua (Fig 7–57).[49]

It has long been known that gravidas with asymptomic bacteriuria have an increased frequency of spontaneous preterm labors and deliveries. Treating the bacteriuria with antibiotics appears to reduce this risk.[285] This may not be related to the prevention of pyelonephritis because pyelonephritis is reportedly not associated with preterm birth.[101] Romero

ROUTES OF FETAL INFECTION

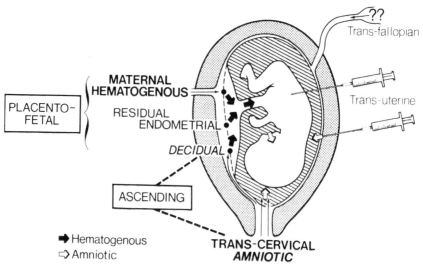

FIG 7–56.
Routes of bacterial entry that produce acute chorioamnionitis. (From Blanc WA: Pathology of the placenta, membranes, and umbilical cord in bacterial, fungal and viral infections in man, in Naeye R, Kissane J, Kauffman N: *Perinatal Diseases.* Baltimore, Williams & Wilkins Co, 1981, p 67. Used by permission.)

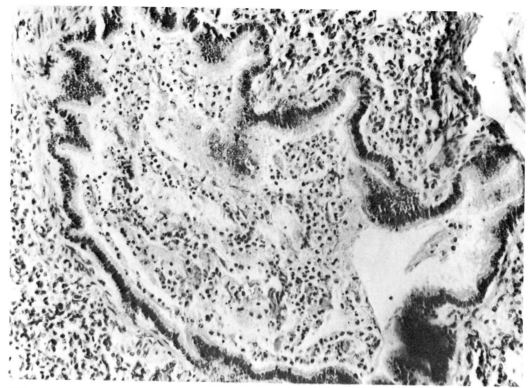

FIG 7–57.
Large numbers of polymorphonuclear leukocytes, most derived from the mother, have been aspirated from infected amniotic fluid into the airway of a stillborn infant, HE stain, ×225.

et al. have suggested that the elimination of an abnormal cervicovaginal flora might be the mechanism by which the antibiotics given for bacteriuria prevent preterm births.[287] As previously noted, there is considerable evidence that an abnormal flora predisposes to acute chorioamnionitis. In the CPS maternal urinary tract infections during pregnancy were associated with an increased risk for spontaneous preterm delivery (relative risk 1.2; 95th percentile, 1.1, 1.4). Part of this increase was associated with the presence of acute chorioamnionitis, so there is still a possibility that urinary tract infections on rare occasions predispose to acute chorioamnionitis. Whether this predisposition is related to the hematogenous spread of bacteria or to an abnormal cervical bacterial flora has not been determined.

Course of the Infection.—Fetal neutrophils in the umbilical vessels are often attracted by chemotactic substances in the amniotic fluid to migrate out of the umbilical vessels toward the amniotic cavity. Less often, neutrophils in the amniotic fluid migrate into the umbilical cord. These processes are termed *funisitis* (see Chapter 6). In the course of the infection acute inflammatory cells first migrate out of the umbilical vein, and only later out of the umbilical arteries. Even when acute chorioamnionitis is severe, some segments of the umbilical cord may be unaffected, so the absence of funisitis in several sections of an umbilical cord does not exclude the presence of acute chorioamnionitis. Neutrophils can also be absent in several sections of the extraplacental membranes when acute chorioamnionitis is present. A systematic effort should be made to look for neutrophils in the extraplacental membranes when these membranes are edematous. The finding of just a few neutrophils between the amnion and chorion in edematous membranes is a strong clue that acute chorioamnionitis will be present when the chorionic (fetal) plate of the placenta is examined. Perinatal mortality was higher in the CPS in cases of acute chorioamnionitis when the extraplacental membranes were edematous than when they were not edematous.

The definitive criterion for making the diagnosis of acute chorioamnionitis is the presence of maternal neutrophils in the blood clot beneath the chorionic (fetal) plate of the placenta (see Figs 7–54, 7–58, and 7–59). Maternal neutrophils in the intervillous blood are attracted to infiltrate this blood clot, attach to the chorionic plate, and then migrate through it. There is some relationship between the length of time the infection has been in progress and the stage of the chorioamnionitis at the time of delivery. This information on timing was derived in the CPS from an analysis of the stage of acute chorioamnionitis at progressively greater time intervals after fetal membrane rupture. Initially, the neutrophils stick to the underside of the chorionic plate of the placenta (stage I, Figs 7–54 and 7–60).[235,236] Next, they migrate into the plate (stage II). When they reach the basement membrane just beneath the amnion, the process is classified as stage III (see Figs 7–58, 7–59). Neutrophils do not usually pass this basement membrane because they do not possess a collagenase that will cleave the type V collagen that is a major constituent of this membrane.[16] This process of neutrophils passing through the chorionic plate of the placenta is rapid when the inflammatory process is severe. When severe, the inflammatory process usually reaches stage III within 24 hours of membrane rupture (see Figs 7–58, 7–59). When the inflammation is mild it is almost always at stage I for the first 3 days after membrane rupture. Between 3 and 4 days many such cases reach stage II and by 7 days half of the mild inflammatory processes are at stage II and a few at stage III. Thus, only when the inflammatory process is mild can any conclusion be drawn about its duration.

In making the diagnosis of acute chorioamnionitis, the examiner should rely primarily on the presence of acute inflammatory cells in an area of the chorionic plate of the placenta that is very thin. One

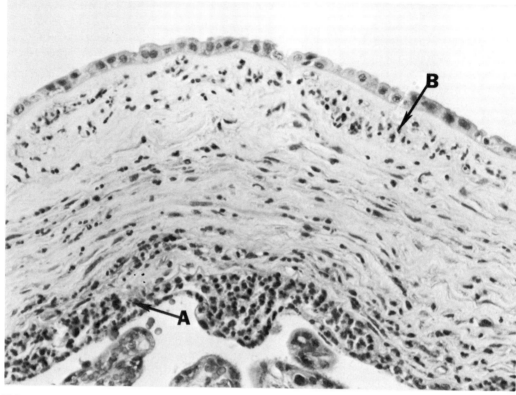

FIG 7–58.
Maternal polymorphonuclear leukocytes have gathered beneath the chorionic plate of the placenta *(A)* and have migrated through the chorionic plate to reach the amnion *(B)*. This is stage III acute chorioamnionitis. HE stain, ×600.

can never be sure that chorioamnionitis is absent unless a thin area of the plate has been examined (Fig 7–61). The failure to examine a thin area of the fetal plate is responsible for missing many diagnoses of acute chorioamnionitis.

Cooperstock et al.[50] have provided strong evidence that acute chorioamnionitis initiates labor through mechanisms that are different from those that start normal labor. Normal labor starts most frequently in the hours between midnight and morning. Cooperstock et al. found that this circadian peak was absent when chorioamnionitis was present.[50] Acute chorioamnionitis appears to start labor when neutrophils and bacteria release an intermediate that initiates the prostaglandin cascade.[21,28] One of the intermediates may be interleukin-1.[280] Another possibility is that leukotriene B and tumor necrosis factor, derived from the inflammatory process, stimulate macrophages in the decidua and uterine wall to release prostaglandins.[283,284] With either mechanism the resulting prostaglandin cascade causes the cervix to dilate through the release of prostaglandin E_2 and the uterus to contract through the action of prostaglandin $F_{2\alpha}$.

Morbidity and Mortality.—Many observers have doubted the clinical importance of acute chorioamnionitis because so many of the affected neonates appear healthy at birth and remain well. Furthermore, only about 10% of the associated mothers have clinical evidence of infection. The reason for the absence of clinical evidence of infection is that the responsible bacteria and mycoplasmas usually have low virulence and the infections reach their peak frequency at term when most fetuses can effectively defend them-

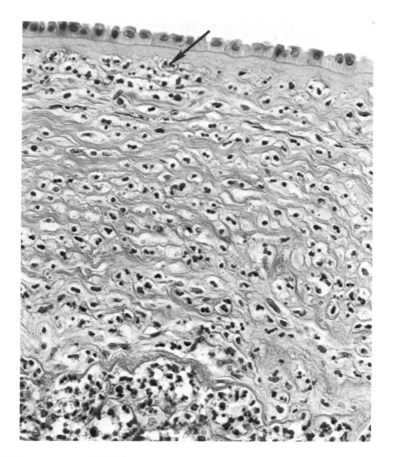

FIG 7–59.
This is severe stage III acute chorioamnionitis. Polymorphonuclear leukocytes have migrated to a position just beneath the amnion *(arrow)*. HE stain, ×600.

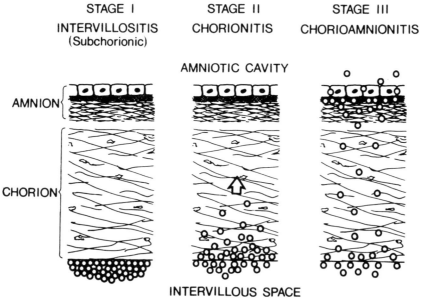

FIG 7–60.
The stages of inflammation of acute chorioamnionitis. (From Blanc WA: Pathology of the placenta, membranes, and umbilical cord in bacterial, fungal and viral infections in man, in Naeye R, Kissane J, Kauffman N: *Perinatal Diseases*. Baltimore, Williams & Wilkins Co, 1981, p 109. Used by permission.)

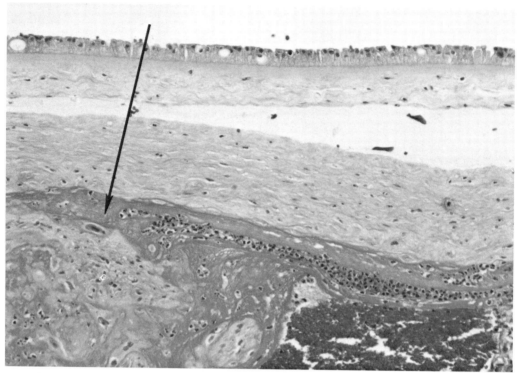

FIG 7–61.

Note the point *(arrow)* at which maternal polymorphonuclear leukocytes no longer collected beneath the chorionic plate of the placenta. Beyond this point the chorionic plate and its underlying tissue became too thick for leukoattractants to diffuse through it and attract maternal leukocytes to stick to the underside of the chorionic plate. HE stain, ×300.

selves against the effects of the infections. We have recovered bacteria or mycoplasmas from nearly 80% of the placentas with chorioamnionitis in our medical center and about 10% of these bacteria are virulent strains. Invariably it is these virulent strains that are recovered when gravidas have clinical evidence of infection.[356] In the CPS most of the chorioamnionitis that was present at term had no unfavorable consequences for mother or infant. However, there were some exceptions. Fetal and neonatal deaths increased 2.6-fold with mild chorioamnionitis and 4.1-fold with moderate or severe chorioamnionitis (Table 7–28). Most of these deaths were related to sepsis, so at no stage of pregnancy is acute chorioamnionitis completely benign. The fetus is reported to stop breathing movements often, and other body movements decrease in frequency when acute chorioamnionitis is present.[107]

Salafia et al. have recently dealt with the issue of acute chorioamnionitis in a community hospital.[296] They found that acute chorioamnionitis was infrequent (4%) in the placentas of uncomplicated term pregnancies. Evidence was found that membrane weakening by acute chorioamnionitis was likely responsible for many premature membrane ruptures. The extraplacental membranes were acutely inflamed twice as often (54%) at the site of membrane rupture with normal vaginal delivery as when delivery was by cesarean section without prior labor. Inflammation was nearly twice as frequent in the extraplacental membranes when labor preceded cesarean section as when there was no labor before cesarean section.

Acute chorioamnionitis has important consequences in addition to the direct effects of infection, namely fetal hypoxia and preterm birth. In the CPS more than a third of all preterm births could be

TABLE 7–28.

Infections of the Placenta*

Acute Chorioamnionitis	Frequency of Abnormalities	Perinatal Mortality Rate	Fetal Growth Retardation	Neurologic Abnormalities at 7 yr	
Preterm births					
Acute chorioamnionitis absent		82 (450)	54 (297)	37 (369)	
Acute chorioamnionitis present					
Mild chorioamnionitis	111 (731)	155 (113), $P<.001$	81 (59), $P<.001$	31 (23)	
Relative risks		2.0, $P<.001$	1.5, $P<.01$	0.9	
Moderate or severe	60 (400)	323 (129), $P<.001$	60 (24)	48 (19)	
Relative risks		5.2, $P<.001$	0.9	1.2	
Funisitis, vein	133 (879)	179 (157), $P<.001$	73 (64), $P<.02$	44 (39)	
Relative risks		2.1, $P<.001$	1.3, $P<.05$	1.2	
Funisitis, artery	79 (523)	256 (134), $P<.001$	94 (49), $P<.001$	42 (22)	
Relative risks		3.5, $P<.001$	1.8, $P<.001$	1.1	
Full-term births					
Acute chorioamnionitis absent		*9 (223)*	91 (2,054)	29 (658)	
Acute chorioamnionitis present					
Mild chorioamnionitis	87 (2,213)	25 (55), $P<.001$	92 (203)	24 (54)	
Relative risks		2.6, $P<.001$	1.0	0.8	
Moderate or severe	24 (595)	40 (24), $P<.001$	108 (64)	20 (12)	
Relative risks		4.1, $P<.001$	1.2	0.7	
Funisitis, vein	122 (3085)	186 (55), $P<.001$	84 (260)	30 (91)	
Relative risks		1.6, $P<.01$	0.9	1.0	
Funisitis, artery	32 (815)	42 (34), $P<.001$	144 (117), $P<.001$	23 (19)	
Relative risks		4.0, $P<.001$	1.7, $P<.001$	0.8	
Fungal infections					
All cases (controls)		*41 (2,281)*	81 (4,528)	30 (1,684)	161 (8,976)
Candida albicans	0.2 (12)	167 (2)	0 (0)	0 (0)	583 (7)
Relative risks		0.9			1.5

*Frequencies per 1,000. Numbers of cases are in parentheses. Relative risk values have been calculated to take major congenital malformations and disorders of low uteroplacental blood flow into consideration. P values compared with chorioamnionitis and funisitis absent.

attributed to labor initiated by acute chorioamnionitis.[236,237] Since perinatal mortality was much higher for preterm than for full-term births, acute, chorioamnionitis was the most frequent cause of stillbirth and neonatal death in the study (see Table 7–28).

Immaturity is not the only reason why infants who are born preterm as the result of acute chorioamnionitis are often ill as neonates. Often they are ill because placental edema made them hypoxic before birth. This hypoxia presents with low 5- and 10-minute Apgar scores, the need to resuscitate vigorously at birth, the neonatal respiratory distress syndrome, and recurrent apneic episodes.[233,235,237] These findings correlate much more strongly with the severity and the extent of placental villous edema than with the severity and stage of the chorioamnionitis.[233] The edema is postulated to impede the movement of oxygen and nutrients from the intervillous space into the fetal circulation by compressing capillaries and veins inside of the placental villi. The severe respiratory distress experienced by many of these neonates is due to the combined effects of lung immaturity and hypoxic damage to the lungs before birth.[233,237]

Funisitis often develops in the course of acute chorioamnionitis, and in the CPS perinatal mortality was higher when funisitis was present than when it was absent. In the course of funisitis inflammatory cells invade the walls of the umbilical vein, and at a later time the walls of the umbilical arteries (see Chapter 6). Stillbirth, neonatal morbidity, and mortality were higher when the arteries were inflamed than when the inflammation was limited to the wall of the umbilical vein (see Table 7–28).

Many fetuses that are exposed to amniotic fluid bacterial infections aspirate some of the infected fluid (see Fig 7–57). Overall, only a small proportion of the neonates have signs and symptoms of infection. The most frequent of these clinical findings is pneumonia. In the CPS this aspiration pneumonia was both less frequent and less often lethal when it arose near term than when it developed preterm, presumably because antibacterial defense mechanisms were more mature and thus more effective at term than preterm. Neonatal pneumonia increased progressively in frequency from 14/1,000 in preterm born neonates without chorioamnionitis to 36/1,000 in those with mild chorioamnionitis to 61/1,000 in those with severe chorioamnionitis ($P < .001$). The comparable rates in full-term neonates were 3/1,000, 6/1,000 and 9/1,000 ($P < .02$).

A small proportion of the fetuses that aspirate infected amniotic fluid develop bacteremia or septicemia. In the CPS the frequency of neonatal septicemia increased progressively with the severity of acute chorioamnionitis from a frequency of 3/1,000 in preterm born children without chorioamnionitis to 5/1,000 in those with mild chorioamnionitis to 9/1,000 in those with moderate or severe chorioamnionitis ($P < .001$). The comparable figures in full-term born children were 0.3/1,000, 0.5/1,000 and 0.8/1,000 ($P < .001$). Septicemia was usually accompanied by pneumonia, so most of the bacteria probably entered the circulation as the result of the fetus aspirating infected amniotic fluid. As might be expected, perinatal mortality rates were severalfold higher when pneumonia or septicemia accompanied acute chorioamnionitis than when neither was present. Fetal tachycardia, a reduction in fetal breathing movements, neonatal neutropenia, and thrombocytopenia are the most frequent manifestations of the bacteremia or septicemia that is associated with acute chorioamnionitis.[114,344]

Severe acute chorioamnionitis can also lead to manifestations of fetal distress that resemble those of hypoxia, namely fetal bradycardia, and variable and late fetal heart rate decelerations.[295] Since this occurs in full-term fetuses, it is presumably a consequence of the infection rather than a reflection of hypoxia caused by infection-induced placental villous edema.[233]

Acute chorioamnionitis often repeated in successive pregnancies in the CPS. When it was responsible for preterm birth in one pregnancy, it repeated preterm in 46% of the mothers' next pregnancies.[225] This is one of several reasons why all preterm delivered placentas should have a microscopic examination.

Excessive perinatal mortality was not the only adverse outcome of acute chorioamnionitis in the CPS. Acute chorioamnionitis was followed by a 20% greater-than-expected frequency of neurologic abnormalities at 7 years of age. This was almost entirely related to the many pre-term births initiated by the chorioamnion-itis. The neurologic abnormalities in those born preterm were usually the conse-quence of placental villous edema. The fetal hypoxia produced by the villous edema damages fetal lungs, which leads to the neonatal respiratory distress syn-drome (RDS). RDS in turn predisposes to brain damage by impairing the autoregu-lation of the cerebral circulation.[177] Ninety-four percent (16/17) of the preterm born children in the CPS who had acute chorioamnionitis followed by severe neo-natal respiratory distress had neurologic abnormalities at 7 years of age vs. 5% (34/668) of gestational age-matched neo-nates who had chorioamnionitis without neonatal RDS (*P* < .001). Other studies have also found evidence that the devel-opmental abnormalities that follow acute chorioamnionitis are mainly related to

neonatal RDS and the severity of cerebral intraventricular hemorrhage.[202]

In the CPS neonatal serum bilirubin levels were significantly higher at every gestational age when chorioamnionitis was present. The frequency of a bilirubin value greater than 18 mg/dL in preterm born children increased progressively from 44/1,000 in neonates without cho-rioamnionitis to 67/1,000 in those with mild chorioamnionitis to 92/1,000 in those who had moderately severe or severe chorioamnionitis (*P* < .001). The compa-rable values in full-term born children were 11/1,000, 13/1,000 and 17/1,000 (*P* < .01). Chorioamnionitis was followed by long-term neurologic abnormalities at serum bilirubin levels far lower than those that usually damage neonates' brains (Fig 7–62).[237]

There are other less frequent conse-quences of acute chorioamnionitis. The

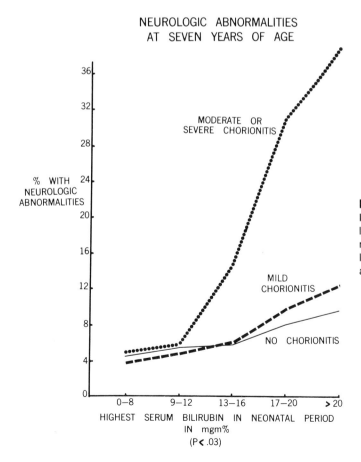

NEUROLOGIC ABNORMALITIES
AT SEVEN YEARS OF AGE

FIG 7–62.
In the CPS chorioamnionitis was fol-lowed by long-term neurologic abnor-malities at neonatal serum bilirubin levels far lower than those that usu-ally damage neonates' brains.

infection sometimes invades the decidua basalis where it can damage blood vessels, lead to hemorrhage, and thereby initiate a placental abruption.[216,237] A very small proportion of the neonates exposed to acute chorioamnionitis develop otitis media, meningitis, septic arthritis, or other evidences of disseminated infection. The site of bacterial entry for meningitis may often be the middle ear because middle ear infections are usually present when meningitis follows chorioamnionitis.

There is indirect evidence that acute chorioamnionitis may sometimes have a role in the genesis of the Wilson-Mikity syndrome. In a study from Japan 30 of 35 children (86%) with the syndrome had been exposed to moderate or severe acute chorioamnionitis.[89] Only 2 of 12 children (17%) with bronchopulmonary dysplasia and 29 of 43 children (67%) with unexplained chronic lung disease had been exposed to acute chorioamnionitis. Neonatal serum levels of IgM were sevenfold higher in children who developed the Wilson-Mikity syndrome than in children who did not develop a chronic pulmonary disorder. Pulmonary emphysema is the underlying disorder in the Wilson-Mikity syndrome and it develops during the first weeks of life. Children with the Wilson-Mikity syndrome have reportedly had large numbers of neutrophils in their amniotic fluid and significant levels of neutrophil elastase in their tracheal aspirates soon after birth.[89] Fujimura et al. postulate that this infection-generated elastase overwhelmed the antiproteinase activity in the affected children's lungs, leading to emphysema by a rapid destruction of the elastic tissue in alveolar walls.[89]

In the CPS fetal growth retardation (1st–10th birth weight percentiles) was about 15% more frequent when chorioamnionitis was present than when it was absent, both in preterm and in full-term born children (see Table 7–28). This raises the possibility that the factors that predispose to growth retardation may also predispose to acute chorioamnionitis.

The presence of acute chorioamnionitis can affect the course of labor and delivery.

It has long been known that women who develop acute bacterial chorioamnionitis have a higher frequency of slow cervical dilatation and ineffective uterine contractions than uninfected gravidas.[86] These effects on labor are most frequent and severe when the bacteria responsible for chorioamnionitis have a high level of virulence. Virulence is the key factor because less virulent bacteria in the amniotic fluid do not appear to affect the rate of cervical dilatation, the level of uterine contractions, the total duration of labor, or the dose of oxytocin that is required to accelerate labor.[310] In the CPS both uterine dysfunction and a failure of the uterus to respond to oxytocin stimulation increased in frequency with the presence and severity of acute chorioamnionitis. In full-term gestations the frequency of uterine dysfunction during labor increased from 66/1,000 when acute chorioamnionitis was absent to 122/1,000 when it was mild and to 183/1,000 when it was moderately severe or severe ($P < .001$). This is not surprising because in more than two-thirds of the cases of chorioamnionitis the infection extends into the myometrium, sometimes reaching the serosal surface of the uterus.[17] There is a strong, positive correlation between the virulence of the organism causing acute chorioamnionitis and the severity of the inflammatory process.

Factors Predisposing to Acute Chorioamnionitis.—It is not known why the frequency of acute chorioamnionitis differs so much from one population to another. Possibilities include differing levels of antimicrobial activity in the amniotic fluid, differences in the character of cervical mucous plugs, and differing bacterial flora in the cervix and vagina.[236,237] Normally, antimicrobial activity first appears in the amniotic fluid in the second trimester of pregnancy, progressively increases in titer to term, and is active against a wide spectrum of aerobic and anaerobic bacteria. When this antibacterial activity is absent or weak, almost any among the great variety of bacteria that are normally present in the vagina and cervix can readily propagate in the amniotic fluid and lead to acute chorioamnionitis. The high frequencies in amniotic fluid of inhibitory activities against *C. trachomatis, M. hominis,* and *U. urealyticum* may explain why these organisms are rarely isolated from placentas and extraplacental membranes with acute chorioamnionitis when the fetal membranes were intact at the onset of labor.[183,332] In one study amniotic fluids collected during preterm labors that could not be stopped by tocolytic agents rarely inhibited the growth of *Escherichia coli, Staphylococcus aureus,* and *Bacteroides fragilis.*[240] Fluids taken during labors that were successfully inhibited by tocolytic agents more often inhibited the growth of these bacteria. In a small study conducted at term we found that about 5% of both US whites and blacks had abnormally low levels of antimicrobial activity in their amniotic fluid, whereas over 90% of the malnourished mothers in some Third World populations we have studied have lacked this antimicrobial activity.[11,235,237] There are factors that likely affect the outcome of acute chorioamnionitis. The fetus may be more vulnerable to the consequences of inhaling infected amniotic fluid before 32 weeks of gestation than after 32 weeks because maternal IgG starts to pass the placenta in significant quantities at about the 32nd week of gestation.[306]

Coitus appears to have a role in the genesis of chorioamnionitis in some individuals and populations. In the CPS women who discontinued coitus during pregnancy for a month or more and then resumed it before term had a high rate of preterm labors and deliveries, more than half of which were associated with acute chorioamnionitis. The mechanisms that might be responsible for this finding are as yet uncertain. Coitus could be introducing new organisms into the vagina or seminal fluid and sperm could be facilitating the passage of bacteria through the cervical mucus plug. Seminal fluid has proteolytic enzymes that facilitate the passage of sperm through the cervical mucus plug, but this plug normally becomes resistant to sperm penetration during pregnancy. It remains to be determined if the cervical mucus is always effective in blocking sperm penetration during gestation. It is also known that mycoplasmas and some bacteria can attach themselves to sperm, and thus they might be transported at least some distance through the mucus plug.[334]

In a prospective study we found that chorioamnionitis-associated preterm labor had a timed relationship to coitus. Such labors first increased in frequency about 24 hours after coitus and continued at a frequency higher than expected for about a week (Fig 7–63).[236] Analyses of data from the CPS disclosed that women reporting coitus once a week during pregnancy had a peak frequency of labors starting on Sunday or Monday (Fig 7–64). Women who reported having coitus twice a week had two labor peaks, one on Sunday and Monday and the other on Thursday. Women who reported no coitus for several weeks or longer before delivery had no significant fluctuations in the frequency of the day of the week on which labor started.

In the CPS the frequency of acute chorioamnionitis increased after 12 hours of membrane rupture.[234] Several other factors also predispose to the development of chorioamnionitis. The frequency of acute chorioamnionitis increases with the duration of labor and with the duration of internal fetal monitoring.[242] One study estimated that for each hour increase in the duration of internal monitoring or fetal membrane rupture, the probability of clinically apparent intraamniotic infection increases from 1% to 2%.[242] Acute chorioamnionitis also increases in frequency with gestational age. This increase could be due to a combination of the passage of time giving bacteria and mycoplasmas more opportunities to reach the fetal membrane and to the partial effacement of the cervix in late gestation, which sometimes exposes the fetal membranes to the cervical bacterial flora. Multiparous gravidas are particularly apt

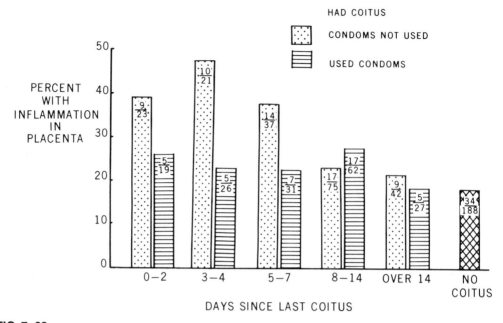

FIG 7–63.
In a prospective study labor increased in frequency 24 hours after coitus and continued at a higher-than-expected frequency for a week.

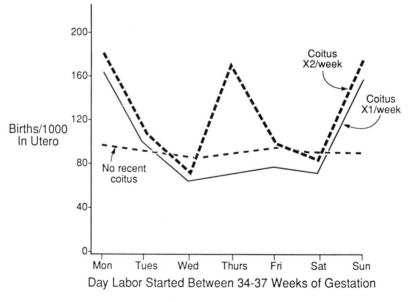

FIG 7–64.
In the CPS women who reported they had coitus once a week had a peak frequency of labors starting on Sunday and Monday. Women who reported coitus twice or more per week had two labor peaks, one on Sunday-Monday and the second on Thursday. Women who reported no recent coitus had no day-of-the-week changes in the frequency on which labor started.

to lose their cervical mucous plugs in late gestation, which also exposes the fetal membranes to cervical organisms.[237] This is probably the reason why the frequency of late gestational chorioamnionitis increases with parity. Overdistention of the uterus, with some dilatation of the cervical canal, may be the reason why acute chorioamnionitis is more frequent with twins after midgestation than with single fetuses.[237,238]

Preventing Acute Chorioamnionitis.— To date, no fully effective means have been discovered to prevent acute chorioamnionitis, but it may be possible to prevent some of its complications. Giving antibiotics to mothers who have an oral temperature of 38° C or higher during labor has been reported to reduce the incidence of neonatal sepsis.[98,100] Preventing chorioamnionitis or controlling it before it initiates labor is a far bigger challenge. Once the infection has started labor, tocolytic agents, rest, and hydration are ineffective in stopping labor.[240,287] Discontinuing coitus or using a condom to keep sperm out of the vagina might reduce the frequency of acute chorioamnionitis if ways could be found to identify the pregnancies that are vulnerable to coitus-initiated chorioamnionitis (see Fig 7–63). Unexplained cervical dilatation is both a well-known risk and a consequence of acute chorioamnionitis. Since a number of days sometimes pass between the time the cervix begins to dilate and the onset of labor, some preterm deliveries might be prevented if antibiotics were given when cervical dilatation is first noted. In one study, administering antibiotics when the cervix had already dilated lengthened from 17 to 30 days the period between the recognition of cervical dilatation and delivery.[203]

Listeriosis

Infection by the gram-positive bacillus *Listeria monocytogenes* is an often unrecognized cause of preterm delivery and perinatal death. It has been estimated that listeriosis infects 1 in 20,000 pregnant women.[315] Maternal infection in the first trimester reportedly leads to abortion.[267] Infection in the second or third trimesters usually leads to either stillbirth or to preterm birth followed by pneumonia and neonatal sepsis.[146,150] Only a few healthy children have been reported after the infection was diagnosed and treated during pregnancy.[53] Some of the survivors have been brain-damaged.[37]

Sporadic human intrauterine listeriosis infections have been reported from many nations and occasional epidemics have been reported in hospitals, suggesting that the agent can be transmitted by interpersonal contacts during or after birth. In epidemics, food is the most frequent mode of transmission. These foods have included milk, cheese, poorly cooked sausage and chicken, and prepacked salads.[37] The organism can multiply in household refrigerators, so food that might be contaminated must be recooked after refrigeration to be safe for consumption. The agent has been found in the soil and many times in human feces. In the majority of sporadic infections the source of the infection is unidentified.

Clinically the infection often presents with a high maternal blood leukocyte count, fetal tachycardia, and neonatal sepsis.[31] A flulike illness in the mother usually starts only a few hours before delivery takes place, so the infection is almost never diagnosed in time to initiate therapy. Boucher and Yonekura found that the combination of a high maternal leukocyte count, fetal tachycardia, decreased fetal heart rate variability, and the absence of intrapartum fetal heart rate accelerations raise the possibility of congenital *Listeria* sepsis.[31] A quick rise in maternal serum levels of antilisteriolysin O after the start of the infection can strongly support the diagnosis.[26]

Placental findings include a necrotizing villitis that sometimes reaches the abscess stage and often affects villi eccentrically (Fig 7–65). Sometimes the abscesses extend into nearby villi. An accompanying acute funisitis and severe acute chorioamnionitis is often present in the chorionic

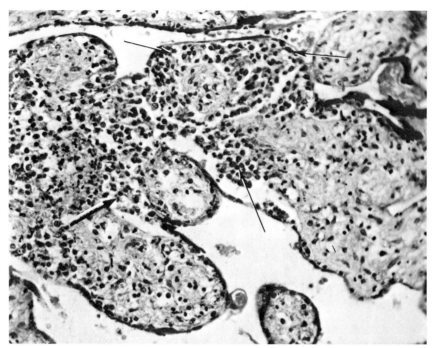

FIG 7–65.
Congenital listeriosis with severe villitis which includes a massive inflammatory infiltrate *(arrows)* and early fusion of villi. (From Blanc WA: Pathology of the placenta, membranes, and umbilical cord in bacterial, fungal and viral infections in man, in Naeye R, Kissane J, Kauffman N: *Perinatal Diseases.* Baltimore, Williams & Wilkins Co, 1981, p 94). Used by permission.)

plate of the placenta. The organism can be demonstrated by Gram's stain. The affected neonates are usually born preterm and often have a rash, pneumonia, and hepatosplenomegaly. Gram's stains of smears and cultures of the placenta, gastric contents, or the skin lesions often help make the diagnosis. The organism is often difficult to culture. In the infants who die the liver is often massively infiltrated by granulomas, with smaller numbers of granulomas in the brain, lymphoid organs, adrenals, lungs, and gastrointestinal tract. Brain lesions are usually most severe in the pons and medulla. If the diagnosis is missed on placental examination, it is sometimes recognized by the finding of tiny granulomas in the skin and posterior pharynx of the neonate. A number of cases have been treated antenatally and scars of the old abscesses identified in the placenta.[24] An infection with *Campylobacter* can produce placental lesions that closely resemble those produced by *Listeria.*[47]

Syphilis

Prenatal infection by *Treponema pallidum* is a major cause of stillbirth and neonatal death in many Third World nations, and it is now increasing in frequency in many North American cities. In one African nation congenital syphilis was reportedly present in 5% to 8% of all neonates.[288]

First-trimester infections by *T. pallidum* occur but are difficult to recognize because the embryo is too immature to mount a tissue reaction to the spirochete.[118] Fetal lesions that are recognizable as syphilis usually first appear in the fifth month of pregnancy. The placenta and fetus can be infected during the primary and secondary stages of the maternal infection but not during its tertiary stage. The later the fetus is infected during

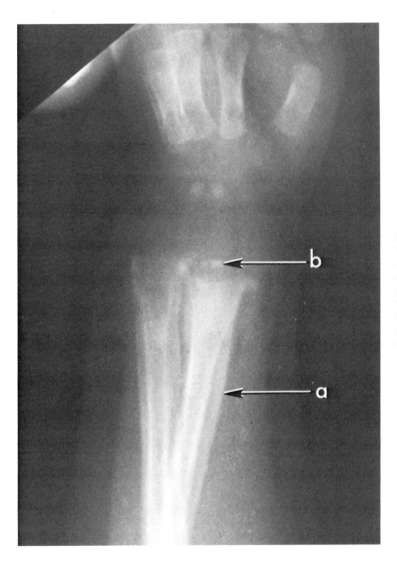

FIG 7–66.
Congenital syphilis. A double line of bone *(arrow a)* indicates periostitis. Also visible are fragmentation of the distal radial epiphysis *(arrow b)* and radiolucent defects adjacent to the zone of provisional calcification.

the course of the maternal disease, the better is the infant's chance of survival. The spirochete often spreads to multiple fetal organs and by this means leads to stillbirth or neonatal death. When the fetus is macerated, the diagnosis can usually be made by radiologic examination of the long bones and a darkfield examination of the amniotic fluid for spirochetes (Fig 7–66).[350] Preterm labor often occurs. Neonatal mortality is high when bullous eruptions or exfoliation is present on the palms and soles of the neonate. Many infected children appear normal until they reach 1 to 3 weeks of age, at which time the development of skin lesions gives the first clinical evidence of the infection. Granu-

lomatous lesions are frequent in the liver, lungs, and pancreas of some newborns with the disease.

The syphilitic placenta is typically enlarged, often exceeding 800 g, while the neonate is often growth-retarded.[185,186] Individual peripheral villi are often larger than normal, which partially explains the large size and immature appearance of some syphilitic placentas (Fig 7–67). Villous edema, sometimes severe, is another factor that often increases the weight of syphilitic placentas. When such edema is both severe and diffuse, neonates are stillborn or are in a severely hypoxic state at birth, which characteristically leads to the development of the neonatal RDS,

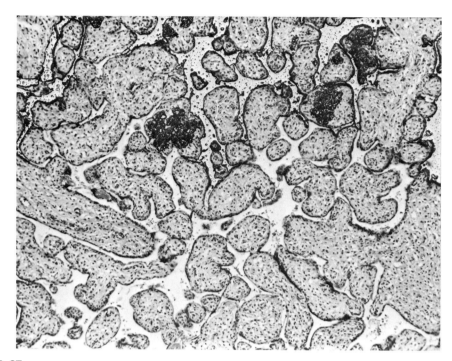

FIG 7–67.
Congenital syphilis. The child died just before birth and had a 986-g placenta. The villi are abnormally large and there is a hyperplasia of villous stromal cells. HE stain, ×94. (From Blanc WA: Pathology of the placenta, membranes, and umbilical cord in bacterial, fungal and viral infections in man, in Naeye R, Kissane J, Kauffman N: *Perinatal Diseases*. Baltimore, Williams & Wilkins Co, 1981, p 95. Used by permission).

necrotizing enterocolitis, and brain damage. Sclerosis sometimes obliterates the arteries in stem villi. The spirochete can be identified in some infected placentas by use of the Warthin-Stary stain (Fig 7–68). Unfortunately, most syphilitic placentas do not have microscopic findings that are diagnostic of the disease when the tissue is stained by hematoxylin-eosin (HE). In a few infected placentas concentric layers of collagen surround the arteries in stem villi and in rare cases endarteritis is present. Focal plasma cell and lymphocyte infiltrates, giant cells, and fibrosis have been described in the villi in a few cases (Fig 7–69).[24,273]

Necrotizing funisitis is sometimes present in congenital syphilis. In a recent analysis 16 out of 35 cases (46%) of congenital syphilis reportedly had this disorder.[77] The lesion was described as often having the gross appearance of a "barber pole" because red and pale blue zones alternated with chalky white streaks in a spiral distribution. In cross section the walls of the umbilical vessels were white and greatly thickened. Focal thrombosis of the umbilical vein was reported to be frequent. Microscopic examination reportedly showed an abscesslike necrosis centered around the umbilical vessels in Wharton's jelly. I have examined scores of syphilitic placentas in two African nations and only two or three cords had these lesions. Syphilis is not the only cause of necrotizing funisitis, so such funisitis is certainly not specific for syphilis.[24]

Leprosy

Infections with *Mycobacterium leprae* reportedly produce no recognizable diagnostic lesions in the placenta.[65] Specifically, no acid-fast bacilli or acid-fast bacillary granules are visible by microscopic examination, electron microscopy, or by immunologic analyses. However, many of the placentas have been reported to be

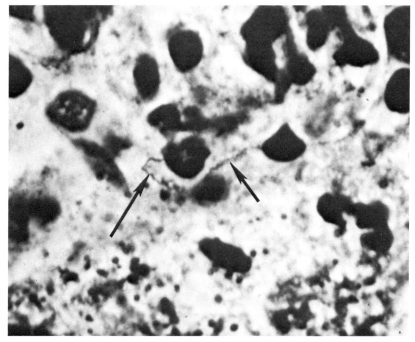

FIG 7–68.
Arrows point to spirochetes in this placenta with congenital syphilis. Warthin-Stary stain, ×2,200.

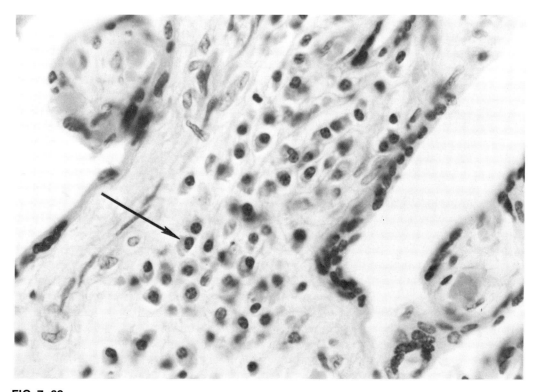

FIG 7–69.
A focal infiltrate of plasma cells *(arrow)* and lymphocytes along with fibrosis are occasionally present in the placental villi in cases of congenital syphilis. HE stain, ×600.

small owing to the small size of their parenchymal cells.[65] This last report originated in an African city where I have studied hundreds of placentas from women who did not have leprosy. Many of these women had small placentas because they were severely undernourished. Undernutrition needs to be considered as an explanation for the small size of the placentas in the women who had leprosy.[65,237]

Fungal Infections

Candida albicans.—This agent usually reaches the amniotic fluid and fetus by way of local infections in the extraplacental membranes near the cervical os. The membranes in such cases are occasionally studded with pinpoint-size yellow-white nodules. The organism can disseminate to many fetal organs, but it is usually confined to the umbilical cord, skin, lungs, and mucous membranes.[351] The characteristic lesions are easily recognized on the surface of the umbilical cord as small clusters of discrete, flat, yellowish plaques varying in diameter from 2 to 5 mm (see Chapter 6).[86] The hyphae are easily identified on the surface of the umbilical cord, and there is usually a zone of neutrophils and occasionally plasma cells just beneath the amnion. These inflammatory cells often can be seen migrating through the walls of nearby umbilical arteries or veins toward the zone of infection. Gastric aspiration is a reliable method for identifying the organism.[351] Infections have been identified in fetuses as early as the start of the second trimester. Stillborn infants infected with *Candida* have sometimes had a giant cell pneumonia.

Those born with the infection often develop skin lesions in intertriginous areas. These skin lesions are usually vesicles with red bases which sometimes evolve into pustules. Lesions in the oral cavity characteristically appear as shallow ulcers covered by a white plaque. When the infection disseminates, microabscesses can develop in the kidneys, liver, spleen, heart, and brain. When the infection is

acquired during passage through the birth canal, mucosal plaques characteristically appear in the mouth 7 to 10 days after birth. *Candida albicans* infections have occasionally been associated with the use of intrauterine contraceptive devices.[316]

Coccidiodes immitis.—Fewer than 100 cases of coccidioidomycosis during pregnancy have been reported. Several have included descriptions of placental infarcts with spherules of *C. immitis* and associated inflammation.[339,342] Only a few newborns have been infected and it may be that the transmission occurred during delivery rather than during pregnancy.[314]

Viral Infections

Cytomegalovirus—The fetus is more often infected by cytomegalovirus than by any other virus.[301] The reported rate of transmission to the fetus after a primary maternal infection is between 20% and 50%.[261,318] An infected fetus has about a 10% risk of being damaged.[254] Ninety percent of the infections are asymptomatic in the neonate. There is strong evidence that gravidas usually acquire the virus from an older child in the family or a close, usually sexual, contact with another adult.[55,251,301] Approximately 3% of the women in one prospective study developed a primary cytomegalovirus infection during pregnancy, a third of which were transmitted to their fetuses.[318] There is a strong possibility that the fetus can be infected and damaged by a recurrent maternal infection.[292,357]

Both the primary and the recurrent infections produce only vague, flulike signs and symptoms. The only fetal infections that produce long-term handicaps appear to be those that are acquired before midgestation.[262,318] There is no need to terminate a pregnancy in which a maternal infection has originated after midgestation. Some of the children infected before midterm are stillborn. There are many preterm births and many neonates with microcephaly, hepatomegaly, chorioretinitis, jaundice, and thrombocytopenia. Twenty percent to 30% of these neonates with clinical evidence of infection die. Of the survivors, 90% have severe handicaps including mental retardation, behavioral disorders, sensorineural hearing defects, and in a few instances cerebral palsy.[294] Hearing defects are reportedly the most frequent adverse outcome of the fetal infections.[294] There is evidence that the placenta may sometimes be a host for a cytomegalovirus infection that is acquired early in gestation but only begins to damage fetal organs at a much later stage of pregnancy.[9,105]

The diagnosis of congenital cytomegalovirus infection depends on a combination of urine examination, rising antibody titers, virus isolation, and placental examination (Figs 7–70, 7–71). Placental lesions are often most severe in preterm born infants, probably because most such infants are infected earlier in gestation than are full-term infants born with the infection.[209] In most instances routine placental examination discloses no more than a chronic villitis with lymphocytes, plasma cells, fibrosis, and sometimes ne-

crosis of villi.[93] Intervillositis, calcification, and cells with intranuclear or cytoplasmic inclusions are found in association with villitis in infected placentas.[93,209] Owl's-eye nuclear inclusions are characteristic of cytomegalic infections and it is usually safe to make the diagnosis if they are present (Fig 7–72).[24]

As term approaches, cytomegalic inclusions become scarce in the placenta, but there is still evidence of the infection in the form of a proliferative villitis. Focal infiltration of the villi by lymphocytes is by far the most frequent finding. When plasma cells are also present, there is a good chance that cytomegalic inclusions can be found.[208] When fetuses are hydropic, the placenta is usually very heavy owing to villous edema.[93,208] Otherwise, cytomegalovirus-infected placentas are usually normal or subnormal in weight. The use of immunofluorescent antibodies sometimes identifies infections in which cytomegalic inclusions are absent.[7,93] In such cases tissue samples from the placental parenchyma and amnion often yield positive viral cultures.

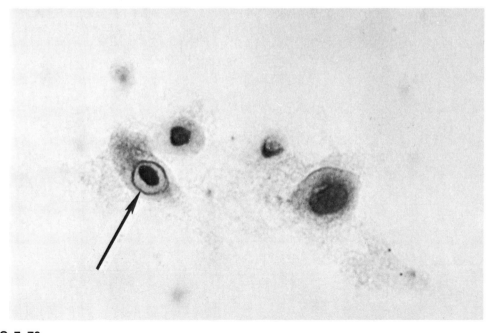

FIG 7–70.
Inclusion-bearing cells in the urine of a 1-month-old infant with generalized cytomegalovirus infection. HE stain, ×1,800. (From Rosenberg HS, et al. in Naeye R, Kissane J, Kauffman N: *Perinatal Diseases.* Baltimore, Williams & Wilkins Co, 1981, p 133. Used by permission.)

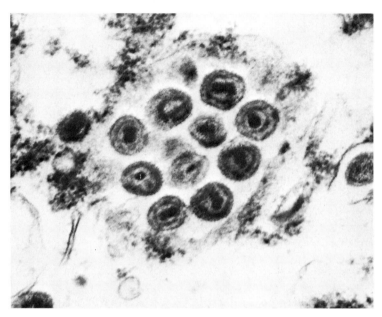

FIG 7–71.
Cytomegalovirus particles with a double envelope are noted in the cytoplasm of a renal tubular cell of a neonate who died of disseminated cytomegalovirus infection. ×66,500.

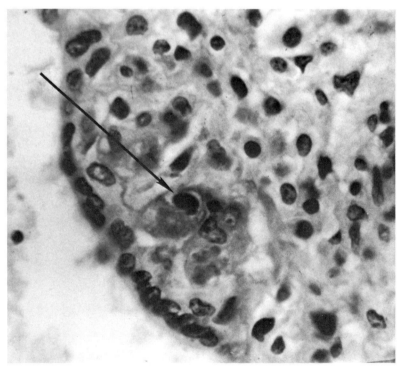

FIG 7–72.
Cytomegalovirus inclusion in the placenta of a late gestational stillbirth. HE stain, ×1,600.

Herpes simplex.—Primary maternal genital herpes infections pose a threat to both the fetus and the newborn. Most of the spread is presumably hematogenous, but a few ascending infections have been reported.[24] With primary genital infections mothers are at high risk to abort, to deliver preterm, or to bear a growth-retarded, infected neonate.[36,239] Two-thirds of these infected neonates are symptomatic by 1 week of age and most of the rest by 3 weeks of age.[157] Four-fifths have seizures and serious neurologic abnormalities (Fig 7–73).[157] Recurrent maternal infections are less of a threat, presumably because maternal antibodies have been passed to the fetus.[36] Mothers are also at risk of transmitting the infection to their infants during labor and delivery, in part because as many as 2.3% of gravidas shed herpes simplex virus during pregnancy.[354]

A variety of lesions have been found in the placenta. They include necrosis of the amnion without inflammation, mononuclear cell infiltrates, coagulative necrosis, and edema in the villi.[5,115] Two placentas had funisitis with infiltrating lymphocytes, plasma cells, and typical herpetic inclusion bodies in amniotic cells (Fig 7–74). In these two cases umbilical vessels had areas of necrosis, medial fibrosis, severe proliferative endovasculitis, and dystrophic calcifications. Benirschke and Kaufmann reported a case with necrotizing chorioamnionitis that included a blister on the surface of the placenta.[24] Very large numbers of plasma cells were present, which is a rare finding. The diagnosis can often be confirmed by viral culture or by fluorescent antibody examination of the amnion and placenta.[275]

Rubella.—Placentas infected during early gestation by the rubella virus have often had multiple foci of villitis with accompanying severe vasculitis. Late gestational placentas have had suppurative

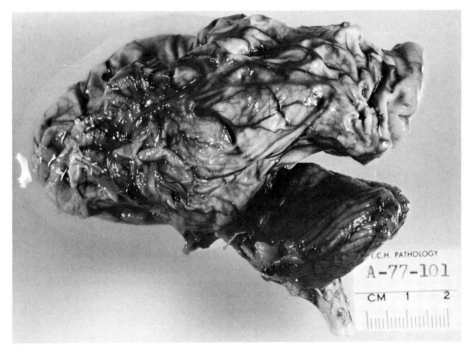

FIG 7–73.
Extensive cortical atrophy is visible in the brain of this 7-week-old male who died of disseminated herpesvirus infection. (From Rosenberg HS, Kohl S, Vogler C: Viral infections of the fetus and the neonate, in Naeye R, Kissane J, Kauffman N: *Perinatal Diseases.* Baltimore, Williams & Wilkins Co, 1981, p 174. Used by permission.)

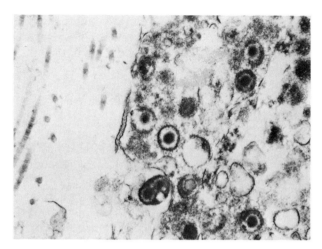

FIG 7–74.
Numerous herpesvirus particles are visible in this tissue from the amnion. ×30,000. (From Blanc WA; Pathology of the placenta, membranes, and umbilical cord in bacterial, fungal and viral infections, in Naeye R, Kissane J, Kauffman N: *Perinatal Diseases.* Baltimore, Williams & Wilkins Co, 1981, p 106. Used by permission.)

villitis, and villous fibrosis of varying severity.[29] In most reported cases the villitis is nonspecific with an infiltration of lymphocytes and a few plasma cells. In such cases rubella villitis resembles the villitis seen with several other viral infections. Inclusions are often hard to find but they have been identified in the trophoblast, the villous stroma, and the endothelial cells of rubella-infected placentas. A necrotizing endarteritis in villous vessels has been reported with recent infection.[32] In term placentas villi have reportedly had a greater-than-normal variation in size, presumably because the infection interferes with villous budding. This produced a marked reduction in the number of terminal villi with a resulting low ratio of terminal to stem villi.[94] Our investigation of antenatal infections has produced strong indirect evidence that the virus exerts many of its effects by inhibiting cell multiplication.[229]

Varicella (Chickenpox).—Only a few placentas infected with varicella have been described in the literature. Severe necrotizing and obliterative villitis and intervillitis have been reported.[92] The most complete descriptions are those of Blanc.[29] None of four placentas that he examined had gross abnormalities. All had

multiple foci of subacute villitis with trophoblastic necrosis, fusing of adjacent villi, lymphocytic infiltrates, occlusion of some villous vessels, and tuberculoid giant cells (Fig 7–75). A fifth placenta had a more chronic infection with plasma cell infiltrates and calcifications in peripheral villi.

Smallpox, Vaccinia.—In the days when smallpox was an active disease the virus often crossed the placenta and produced abortions and stillbirths. Several cases of placental infection with vaccinia were reported. Benirschke and Kaufmann described extensive necrosis of the trophoblast, intervillous fibrin deposits, and focal calcifications with the infection.[24]

Mumps.—The most complete report of placental findings is from three infections that terminated in the first trimester of pregnancy.[95] A diffuse, proliferative, necrotizing villitis was present with severe vasculitis. Cytoplasmic viral inclusions were present in the decidua.

Hepatitis.—A few cases of transplacental infections have been reported. Several placentas have been carefully examined and the only finding has been the presence

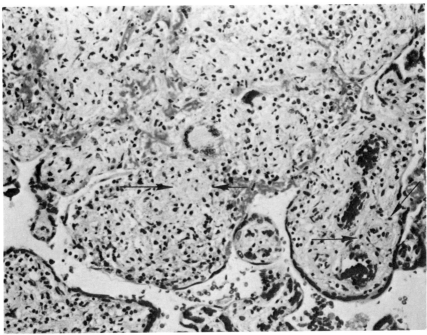

FIG 7–75.
Varicella infection in the placenta. A giant cell is in the center. Between the *arrows* are blood vessels which have been destroyed. The villi are filled with an admixture of chronic inflammatory cells and stromal cells. Much of the trophoblastic covering of the villi has been destroyed and the villi are fused together. HE stain, ×192. (From Blanc WA : Pathology of the placenta, membranes, and umbilical cord in bacterial, fungal and viral infections, in Naeye R, Kissane J, Kauffman N: *Perinatal Diseases.* Baltimore, Williams & Wilkins Co, 1981, p 113. Used by permission.)

of large amounts of bilirubin in Hofbauer cells and in chorionic membrane macrophages.[24] There was no inflammation or necrosis in villi.

Human Immunodeficiency Virus (HIV) (Acquired Immunodeficiency Syndrome).

—It has been estimated that about 1 in 4 maternal infections are transmitted to the fetus, but it is possible that many of these infections were transmitted during delivery.[143] Maury et al. have shown that the placental HIV receptor CD4 is both present and sometimes infected with the virus in the first trimester of pregnancy.[188] Both trophoblastic and endothelial cells appear to synthesize CD4. Other modes of presumed transmission include the transplacental passage of infected maternal lymphocytes to the fetal circulation, contact with maternal blood or other fluids during delivery, and the ingestion of breast milk. Infected mothers who do not transmit the virus to their infants before or

after birth appear to confer some immunologic protection against the virus in their offspring by way of a high-affinity antibody to gp120 epitope.[104] Children who acquire the infection in the perinatal period are usually symptomatic by 1 year of age and have a mean survival of about 3 years.[302] Infants sometimes die before their mothers develop clinical signs of the infection. The most frequent manifestations of the disease in children are lymphoid interstitial pneumonia, encephalopathy, recurrent bacterial infections, and *Candida* esophagitis.[302]

Many presumably HIV-infected placentas have been examined, but only a few reports of placental findings have been published.[133,241] Acute chorioamnionitis and malarial parasites have been reported to be increased in frequency.[241] The nature of these findings suggests that they are secondary disorders rather than primary manifestations of the HIV infection. Their high frequencies could either be the consequence of HIV impairments in defense mechanisms or the result of the lifestyle of those infected with HIV. Gravidas who are seropositive for HIV and have CD4 (helper cell) cell counts under 300/mm^3 are at high risk for serious opportunistic infections during pregnancy.[199] Villitis, the lesion that is characteristic of other viral infections, has not been reported in HIV-infected placentas. It remains to be seen if the hypercellular villi reported in some presumably HIV-infected placentas are the result of the HIV infection. Retrovirus-like particles have been claimed to be present in several of these placentas. This may not be a definitive observation because it is difficult to establish the identity of many viruslike particles that are seen in the placenta. Lewis et al. have demonstrated the presence of HIV by immunocytochemistry and by in situ hybridization in trophoblastic cells, Hofbauer cells, and embryonic blood cell precursors of aborted embryos.[171] Infection in the mother reportedly does not cause preterm birth, fetal growth retardation, or low Apgar scores in liveborn infants.[198]

Parvovirus (Erythema Infectiosum). – Erythema infectiosum (fifth disease) is an infectious disorder caused by a single-stranded DNA virus called parvovirus B19. It is transmitted by respiratory secretions and produces a febrile illness that lasts about a week and is accompanied by a reduced number of reticulocytes in the peripheral blood.[297] In another week a distinctive rash develops which produces a reddish flush on the cheek and a red, lacy appearance on the extremities and trunk. Many of the infections are asymptomatic. Recovery is uneventful without anemia unless the individual has a preexisting hemolytic disorder, in which case an aplastic crisis sometimes develops about a week after the clinical onset of the illness.[297] About half of the adults in the general population have antibodies against the infection and are not susceptible to reinfection. There are many documented cases of abortion and fetal hy

drops, apparently because the virus causes fetal anemia and heart failure. These latter disorders usually develop 4 to 6 weeks after the onset of the acute infection and are most frequent during or before midgestation. A few anemic newborns have been reported after third-trimester infections. The risk of embryonic or fetal death in women infected before midgestation has been estimated to be 3% to 9%.

The placentas of infected infants are large and pale because they are edematous. Microscopically, diffuse villous edema is present with eosinophilic intranuclear inclusions bodies in circulating normoblasts.[10] In some cases the villi are necrotic.[184] The livers of the infants who die have large amounts of hemosiderin, a reflection of the intense hemolysis that can take place before death.[184] Cytomegalovirus and toxoplasmosis are the other two infectious processes that often produce a nonimmune hydropic placenta and fetus.

Parasitic Infections

Malaria.—Malaria is usually limited to low altitude tropical and subtropical areas. It characteristically exists in an environment where there are multiple other factors which also adversely affect mothers and their fetuses. Gravidas who are young and poorly nourished and receive very little antenatal medical care are those most often affected by the malarial parasite because they have the least immunity to it. In such circumstances it is difficult to separate the placental findings of malaria from the findings of other adverse influences. Gravidas who have no immunity to malaria are often anemic after a malarial attack, and this anemia may be the reason why their placentas are sometimes very heavy. As explained earlier in this chapter, maternal anemia often leads to placental hypertrophy. At the present time malaria is on the rise in most locations where it is endemic because it is now very often resistant to chloroquine and to other drugs that until recently were effective in controlling the infection.

The chief microscopic finding in placentas infected with malaria is the presence of plasmodial parasites, sometimes in large numbers, in the intervillous blood.[223] Other reported findings include chronic intervillositis with macrophages and brown pigment in the intervillous space.[349] In areas where malaria is endemic, pregnant women normally have more plasmodial parasites in their blood than nonpregnant women.[191] Whatever its cause, this enhanced parasitemia and the other placental findings are not usually associated with adverse outcomes for the gravida, the fetus, or the neonate.[191,223] In one study of endemic malaria, maternal anemia, which is a good marker for malarial infection, explained only 1% of birth weight variance.[271] Such a finding suggests that malaria may have little or no independent effect on pregnancy outcome in communities where the infection is endemic. Most of the studies that have found heavy parasitemia in placental blood have also found parasites in the blood of the associated newborns.[191] Most such newborns have not had clinical evidence of malaria, presumably because they received antibodies from their mothers before birth.

Nonimmune gravidas who contract malaria, particularly that caused by *Plasmodium falciparum*, sometimes have very poor pregnancy outcomes. In such gravidas the infection often leads to high fever, rapid hemolysis, and severe anemia. This combination presumably accounts for the high rates of maternal mortality, abortions, stillbirths, and preterm deliveries that have occurred in malarial epidemics in nonimmune populations.[194]

Trypanosomes.—The frequency with which the various trypanosomes infect embryos, fetuses, and placentas is unknown. *Trypanosoma cruzi* (Chagas' disease) reportedly produces diagnostic microscopic findings in the placenta that include villitis and parasites that are both outside and inside of macrophages in the villi, in the umbilical cord, and in the chorionic plate of the placenta.[15] The parasites can be present without any associated inflammatory reaction, so the acute chorioamnionitis that is found in some placentas with *T. cruzi* is likely of bacterial or mycoplasmal rather than of parasitic origin. Several neonates who acquired *T. cruzi* before birth have had myocarditis, a granulomatous encephalitis, and a dissemination of the parasite to other organs including the skin.[173] Some placentas with trypanosomes are reported to be larger than normal.[15] It remains to be seen whether this is related to the parasite or to coexisting disorders.

Toxoplasma gondii.—The cat is the definitive host for this intracellular parasite, which is capable of invading any cell in almost every warm-blooded animal. The infections are found throughout the world. The organism has a sexual cycle in the cat's intestinal mucosa, which produces oocytes that pass into the soil with the feces. The oocytes resist many adverse environmental conditions and often survive in the soil for a year or more. Rodents ingest the oocytes, are infected, and the cycle is completed when the rodents are eaten by cats. Children are most often infected by ingesting infected soil during play. Adults are infected when they eat contaminated poorly cooked or uncooked vegetables or meat.[84] Pregnant women are at risk of the infection when they eat unwashed raw vegetables, unwashed fruit, or undercooked meat. They should avoid contact with cats and their litter because some cats are contaminated with *T. gondii*.[323] Cats that hunt their own food are particularly dangerous potential sources of the infection.

The antibodies associated with a chronic maternal infection protect the fetus. New maternal infections can infect the embryo as early as the 7th week of gestation. It has been estimated that about 17% of such maternal infections between the 7th and 14th weeks of gestation are transmitted to the embryo.[58] The lesions in early infected embryos and fetuses are very destructive, often leading to hydranencephaly, hydrops, stillbirth, and occasionally spontaneous abortion. The transmission frequency increases to 67% by the third trimester. Infections acquired in late gestation are less destructive, but the lesions can still be disabling when they include cerebral periaqueductal and periventricular vasculitis, necrosis, and calcifications. Some lesions may not appear until after 5 years of age.[155] There is a high correlation between infection in the placenta and transmission of the infection to the fetus, so the usual route of transmission to the fetus is presumably through the placenta. An occasional infection may be acquired during labor and delivery because a few of the infected infants have not had an elevated serum level of IgM at birth. The avidity–ELISA test (enzyme-linked immunosorbent assay) can identify infections of recent origin.[158]

Infected placentas are often markedly enlarged and show lesions that resemble the characteristic findings of erythroblastosis fetalis. The villi are markedly enlarged, edematous, and often appear immature for their gestational age. They also usually have normoblasts in their blood vessels.[23] Foci of proliferative and necro-

tizing villitis have been observed in some cases. Sometimes the villitis is evidenced by the presence of lymphocytes, plasma cells and fibrosis. The diagnosis is made by identifying the characteristic intracellular organisms (Fig 7–76). The organisms are difficult to find in the placenta, but when they are present they are usually found in typical cysts in the chorion or the subchorionic tissue. Identification is sometimes difficult because degenerated syncytium can mimic the cysts.[24] It is often necessary to inject tissue homogenate into the abdominal cavity of mice and then identify the infection in their organs to be certain of the diagnosis.

Toxoplasma gondii is thought to be spread by macrophages through the lymphatics and the bloodstream of the fetus. Almost no type of cell is immune to being invaded. This rapid spread usually stops when the fetus begins to produce antibodies. The efficiency of antibody production increases as gestation progresses, which probably explains why the early gestational infections produce more tissue damage than later acquired infections. Most neonates who die of the infection

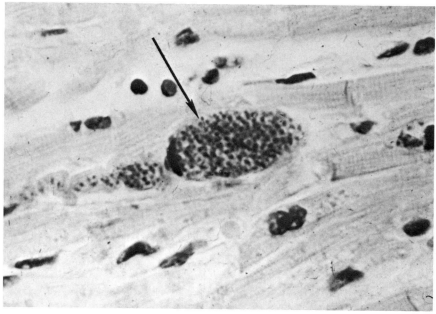

FIG 7–76.
A *toxoplasma* cyst *(arrow)* in a myocardial fiber. HE stain, × 1,200.

have severe brain damage. Damage to blood vessels leads to focal and diffuse necrosis in the cerebral hemispheres, brainstem, and cerebellum. The damage is often most severe in the cortex, periventricular white matter, and basal ganglia. Cysts sometimes form, and their obstruction of the aqueduct can lead to hydrocephalus. Calcifications in the most damaged areas sometimes provide a radiographic clue to the diagnosis (Fig 7–77).

Abruptio Placentae

Causes

The separation of all or part of the placenta from the wall of the uterus before the fetus has been delivered is termed *abruptio placentae.* In one-half or more of the cases in which the placental detachment is sudden the fetus dies.[24] A detachment that occurs in stages or over a period of days or weeks or one that involves less than half of the placenta permits many fetal survivals. The retroplacental hemorrhages that start most placental abruptions presumably originate in the rupture of a decidual vessel (Fig 7–78). This can occur when the vessel is torn by trauma or its wall weakened by necrosis or infection.

The frequency of abruptio placentae is severalfold increased when preeclampsia and eclampsia are present, particularly when the features of the HELP syndrome (Hemolysis, Elevated Liver Enzymes, low platelets) are present.[305] Most textbooks describe the following additional factors as antecedents of abruptio placentae: placenta previa, abdominal trauma, chronic gestational hypertension, uterine neoplasms, uterine malformations, hydramnios, multiple fetuses, high parity, a very short umbilical cord, sudden decompression of the uterus, occlusion or compression of the inferior vena cava, lupus erythematosus, the use of anticoagulants, and fetal malformations.[141,148,237] Placental abruptions are reported to be particularly frequent when a leiomyoma is retroplacental.[274]

Our analyses of data from the CPS identified the following factors as major risks for placental abruptions: an unusually long umbilical cord (91st–100th percentiles), preeclampsia, eclampsia, acute chorioamnionitis, maternal cigarette

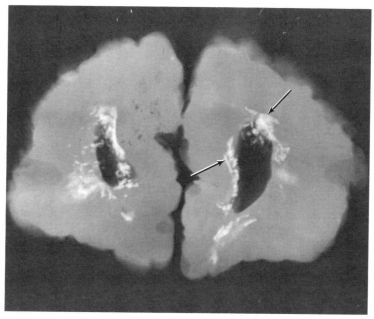

FIG 7–77.
Postmortem radiograph through the frontal lobes of the brain of a neonate with congenital toxoplasmosis.

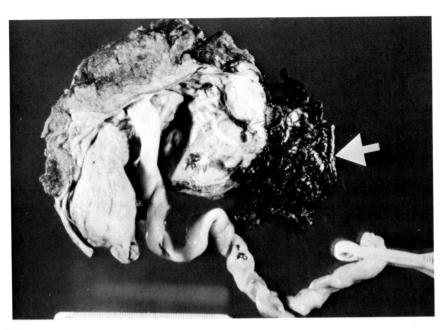

FIG 7–78.
A large retroplacental blood clot was the apparent cause of a placental abruption.

smoking, and advanced maternal age (Table 7–29). Taken together, these risk factors accounted for 40% of the placental abruptions in the CPS (see Table 7–29).[237] The association of long umbilical cords with placental abruptions may indicate that trauma to the placenta by fetal movements is the cause of some abruptions. As explained in Chapter 6 and later in this chapter, unusually long umbilical cords often appear to be the consequence of very vigorous fetal movements that put greater-than-normal tension on the cord. Since there was a strong association of long cords with abruptio placentae in the CPS, trauma to the placenta by fetal movements is an attractive explanation for some abruptions. Ultrasound examination has documented two instances of fetuses striking the placenta at sites where large hemorrhages were present.[67] In both cases the gravidas complained of painful fetal movements followed by vaginal bleeding. This pain coincided with the fetus's striking the placenta.

Spiral artery lesions are frequent with disorders of low uteroplacental blood flow, which may explain their association with abruptions. In the course of acute chorioamnionitis, bacteria often invade the decidua and its blood vessels.[17,237] The resulting damage to blood vessels suggests that hemorrhage from these weakened vessels may explain some placental abruptions (Fig 7–79). An association between premature rupture of the fetal membranes and abruptio placentae in the CPS was due entirely to a greater frequency of acute chorioamnionitis in the premature membrane rupture cases. Acute chorioamnionitis is a major factor in the genesis of both disorders.[344] Cigarette smoking damages the decidua basalis at the edge of the placenta, which is a plausible reason for its association with placental abruptions.[231]

There are many recent reports that the frequency of abruptio placentae increases when women use cocaine or methamphetamines during pregnancy.[41,73,249] The cause may be the sudden uterine vasoconstriction which these drugs appear to induce. The same mechanism may explain why abruptio placentae is increased in frequency when gravidas have functioning pheochromocytomas.[24] Cocaine use is also associated with increased frequencies of preterm birth and fetal growth retarda-

TABLE 7-29.

Risk Estimates for Antecedents to the Development of Fresh Abruptio Placentae*

Risk Factors	No. of Cases of Abruptio Placentae per 1,000 Cases With Risk Factor†	Relative Risks (95% Confidence Intervals)	Attributable Risks (95% Confidence Intervals)
All cases	21 *(1,140)*		
Maternal factors			
Smoked during pregnancy	**27** *(295)*, *P*<.001	**1.5** (1.2, 1.9)	**.07** (.05, .09)
Preeclampsia, eclampsia	**35** *(319)*, *P*<.001	**1.7** (1.4, 2.0)	**.09** (.06, .12)
Age ≥35 yr	**28** *(91)*, *P*<.005	**1.8** (1.2, 2.6)	**.03** (.02, .04)
Fetal factor			
Major fetal malformations	**32** *(160)*, *P*<.001	**1.6** (1.1, 2.2)	**.03** (.02, .04)
Placental factor			
Acute chorioamnionitis	**39** *(269)*, *P*<.001	**1.9** (1.7, 2.2)	**.08** (.05, .11)
Markers for vigorous fetal motor activity			
Unusually long umbilical cord	**24** *(517)*, *P*<.002	**1.6** (1.2, 2.0)	**.11** (.09, .13)
Other indicators			**.01** (.00, .02)
Population attributable risk			**.40** (.36, .45)
Pregnancy outcomes			
Preterm birth	**48** *(558)*, *P*<.001	**1.5** (1.4, 1.8)	
Fetal growth retardation	23 *(110)*, *P*<0.1	1.1 (0.9, 1.3)	
Stillbirth	**190** *(184)*, *P*<.001	**4.1** (3.4, 5.2)	
Neonatal death	**135** *(137)*, *P*<.001	**1.9** (1.0, 3.6)	
Neurologic abnormalities at 7 yr	25 *(42)*, *P*>.1	1.2 (0.4, 2.1)	

*Significant values are in boldface.
†Numbers of cases are in parentheses.

tion, including microcephaly.[113,145] It remains to be seen whether these latter findings are the pharmacologic consequences of using cocaine or have some other cause.

In a few cases nipple stimulation and the administration of prostaglandin E_2 to speed delivery have been followed by a placental abruption.[168,329] Vaginal bleeding, often only spotting, occurs in about 25% of all women during the first half of pregnancy. About half of these bleeds terminate in a spontaneous abortion and most of the rest are related to a dead twin, placenta previa, or to a placental abruption. Sonograms have sometimes identified a subchorionic hematoma at the edge of the placenta as the cause of such bleeding.[2] For unknown reasons blood that originates from a marginal placental abruption before midgestation often works its way behind the chorionic membrane and eventually reaches the vagina. After midgestation such a hematoma is more apt to work its way under the

placenta and cause a major abruption.[2] There is increasing evidence that a major abruption increases vascular resistance in the placenta.[204] As previously mentioned, abruptio placentae can cause maternal death, either by massive blood loss or as the consequence of widespread intravascular coagulation with renal necrosis.[40,353]

Diagnostic Clues

The observer is often uncertain about whether to interpret a retroplacental hematoma as strong evidence of an abruption or whether an abruption could have taken place without a retroplacental clot being present. Clues are sometimes available to help make these difficult decisions. The most frequent manifestation of abruptio placentae is a fresh retroplacental hematoma. If this clot has been present for only a short time, the observer will often not be able to distinguish it from clots that are often normally present on the maternal surface of the placenta at delivery. In

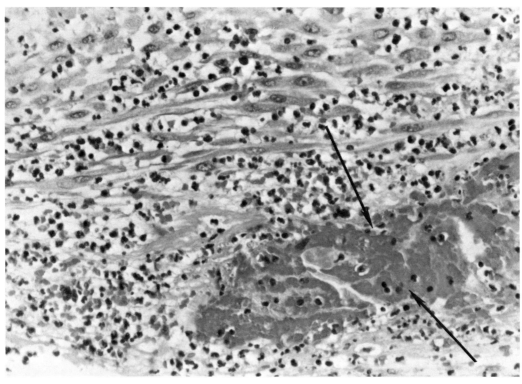

FIG 7–79.
Bacteria have spread into the decidua from an acute chorioamnionitis. Large numbers of acute inflammatory cells infiltrate the edematous decidua. The *arrows* point to a hemorrhage that was the likely cause of a placental abruption. HE stain, ×300.

this situation, clinical information will be needed to make the diagnosis. The following are strong evidence that the clot antedated labor and delivery: (a) lamination of the clot, (b) an infiltration of acute inflammatory cells in the adjacent decidua, (c) necrosis of the adjacent decidua, (d) disappearance of the intervillous space so the villi appear to stick together (Fig 7–80).

If the clot has been present for some days or weeks, it will be firm, brown, and adherent in a compressed area on the maternal surface of the placenta. The area beneath the clot will sometimes be infarcted. In some cases the infarction will have been the nidus that initiated the abruption rather than its consequence. When the clot is old, the underlying infarcted tissue shrinks and the clot may no longer be located in a depressed area.

In the CPS evidences of a very recent placental abruption were associated with a stillbirth rate of 190/1,000 births and a neonatal mortality rate of 135/1,000 (see Table 7–29). These death rates were nearly twice as high when an abruption followed maternal hypertension, smoking during pregnancy, or acute chorioamnionitis as when these latter risk factors were absent. The perinatal mortality rate with a placental abruption in which the placenta completely separated from the uterine wall before delivery was 527/1,000. An abruption with a hematoma at the edge of the placenta had a lower mortality rate than an abruption with a hematoma near the center of the placenta. This was presumably because blood flow to the intervillous space and resulting placental function is less at the edge than at the center of the placenta. Severe placental abruptions can threaten maternal survival, both as the result of hemorrhage and because abruptions sometimes lead to the development of disseminated intravascular coagula-

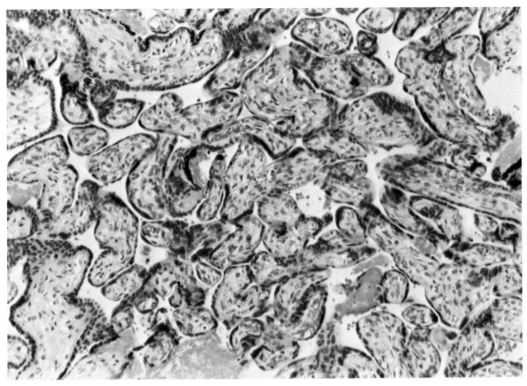

FIG 7–80.
The villi appear to stick together because the intervillous space has disappeared above a placental abruption. HE stain, ×300.

tion.[141] After taking all of the identified risk factors into consideration, recent placental abruptions were associated with increased risks for preterm birth, still-birth, and neonatal death in the CPS (see Table 7–29).

Placental infarcts or severe villous atrophy and fibrosis sometimes develop under the site of an abruption if many days elapse between the time the abruption takes place and delivery. A depressed area on the maternal surface of the placenta, with an underlying infarct or villous atrophy, was associated with a perinatal mortality rate of only 68/1,000 in the CPS, suggesting that most of the fetuses had accommodated to these old abruptions.

Placenta Previa

Placenta previa is the condition in which the placenta is adjacent to the cervical os or covers the cervical os. It is the most frequent cause of bleeding in the third trimester of pregnancy and is life-threatening for both gravida and fetus. Most of the bleeding presumably arises when the placenta detaches from the decidua, but some bleeding could originate from villous disruption or from the edge of the placenta when the cervix begins to dilate in late gestation.[24] The frequency of placenta previa was 0.7% (362) in the CPS, which is in the mid range of published frequencies (Table 7–30). The diagnosis can often be made by sonography. Sonograms undertaken during the second trimester of pregnancy demonstrate a higher frequency of placenta previa than is present at delivery.[90] When the placenta is initially found to cover the cervical os completely, this condition usually persists.

The common view is that placenta previa is the result of defective or absent decidua. This thesis does not explain why the decidua might be abnormal. Risk factors were identified for 36% of the cases

TABLE 7–30.

Risk Estimates for Antecedents to the Development of Placenta Previa*

Risk Factors	No. of Cases of Placenta Previa per 1,000 Cases With Risk Factor†	Relative Risks (95% Confidence Intervals)	Attributable Risks (95% Confidence Intervals)
All cases	7 (*362*)		
Maternal factors			
Leiomyoma or prior gynecologic surgery	**12** (*153*), *P* < .001	**1.9** (1.5, 2.4)	**.13** (.12, .15)
Parity ≥ 5	**14** (*123*), *P* < .001	**2.1** (1.6, 2.6)	**.12** (.10, .14)
Race: white	**7** (*211*), *P* < .02	**1.3** (1.0, 1.6)	**.07** (.06, .09)
Smoked during early pregnancy	**10** (*107*), *P* < .001	**1.5** (1.2, 1.9)	**.06** (.05, .07)
Age ≥ 35 yr	**16** (*52*), *P* < .001	**1.7** (1.2, 2.3)	**.03** (.02, .04)
Fetal factor			
Twins	**14** (*16*), *P* < .005	**1.8** (1.2, 2.5)	**.02** (.00, .04)
Population attributable risk			**.36** (*.34, .39*)
Pregnancy outcomes			
Preterm birth	**17** (*201*), *P* < .001	**4.7** (3.8, 5.8)	
Fetal growth retardation	7 (*33*), *P* > .1	1.1 (0.8, 1.4)	
Stillbirth	**26** (*25*), *P* < .001	1.0 (0.6, 1.5)	
Neonatal death	**46** (*45*), *P* < .001	**3.0** (2.2, 4.0)	
Neurologic abnormalities at 7 yr	**10** (*17*), *P* < .01	**1.6** (1.0, 2.5)	
Motor abnormalities + severe mental retardation		**4.0** (2.2, 6.0)	
Cerebral palsy		**3.2** (1.3, 5.2)	

Significant values are in boldface.
†Numbers of cases are in parentheses.

of placenta previa in the CPS. These were uterine leiomyoma, prior uterine surgery, high parity, cigarette smoking during early pregnancy, advanced maternal age, and multiple fetuses (see Table 7–30 and Fig 7–81).[214] Uneven blood flow to the endometrium along the route which the fertilized egg must travel might explain why leiomyomas, old surgical scars, cigarette smoking, and maternal advanced age are risks for placenta previa. Both cigarette smoking and advanced maternal age are associated with marked sclerosis in the walls of small arteries and arterioles in many organs including the myometrium.[215,237] These lesions are unevenly distributed, which could restrict blood flow to some but not to all areas of the endometrium. The poorly perfused endometrial sites associated with leiomyomas and old surgical scars may be inhospitable to implantation so that embryos

are forced to implant at sites in the uterine wall that are lower than normal.

After taking all of the aforementioned risk factors into consideration, placenta previa was associated in the CPS with increased risks for preterm birth, neonatal death, and neurologic abnormalities at 7 years of age (see Table 7–30). The neurologic abnormalities include cerebral palsy and lesser motor abnormalities accompanied by mental retardation. Sixty-nine of the 362 cases (19%) of placenta previa in the CPS ended with placental abruptions. The perinatal mortality rate was 320/1,000 when an abruption took place vs. 99/1,000 when no abruption occurred (*P* < .001). Forty-seven percent (171) of the deliveries with placenta previa occurred preterm.

Disruption of villi during labor and delivery with resultant loss of fetal blood is frequent with placenta previa. This fetal blood loss is reported to be most severe

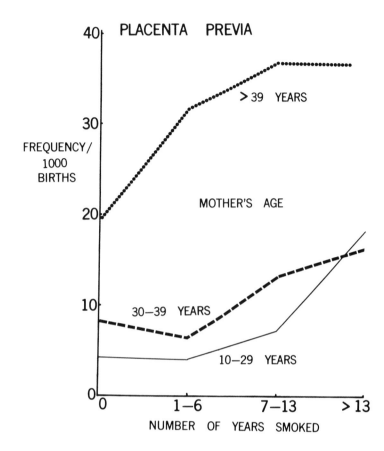

FIG 7–81.
Placenta previa increased in frequency with both the mother's age and with the number of years she had smoked cigarettes.

when there has been severe maternal bleeding.[193] Among CPS children the mean hemoglobin value 48 hours after full-term birth with a placenta previa was 17.0 ± 2.7 g/dL vs. 18.2 ± 2.7 g/dL without placenta previa (P < .001). As previously mentioned, placenta accreta is increased in frequency with placenta previa.

Nonchromosomal Congenital Malformations in the Fetus

When the fetus has malformations without a recognized chromosomal disorder, the placenta is usually subnormal in size if the fetus is growth-retarded. Placental villous structure varies widely with fetal malformations. In most cases villous structure appears to be normal. In an occasional case the villi vary greatly in size and shape (Figs 7–82, 7–83). The finding of unusually large villi that are markedly irregular in shape should raise the possi-

bility of major congenital malformations in the newborn.

Chromosomal Disorders

Placentas are often subnormal in weight for gestational age when fetuses have chromosomal abnormalities (Table 7–31). Trisomy 21 is an exception in that placental weights are usually normal. A single umbilical artery is frequent with trisomic chromosomal disorders. The most easily recognized microscopic abnormalities in the villi with chromosomal disorders are hydrops and hydatidiform changes (Fig 7–84; see Table 7–31).[290] Another easily recognized finding is the presence of enlarged villi with marked invaginations and infoldings (Fig 7–85). Giant cells are present in the cytotrophoblast in several trisomic disorders. Various authors think they originate from villous stromal cells, from the cytotropho-

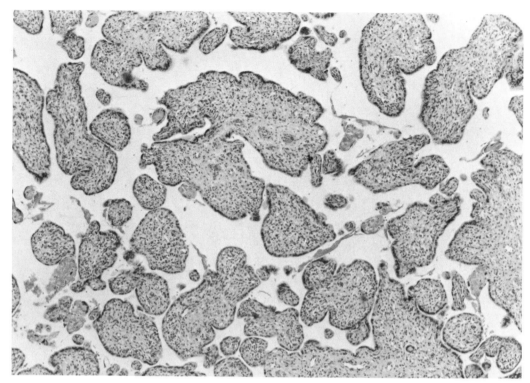

FIG 7–82.
Villi are abnormally large and have markedly abnormal shapes in this placenta from a child with the VATER syndrome. HE stain, ×120.

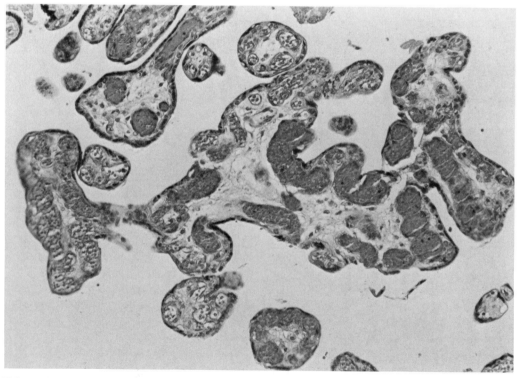

FIG 7–83.
The abnormally large and abnormally shaped villi from the placenta of a neonate with cyclopia. HE stain, ×300.

TABLE 7–31.

Placental, Embryo, and Fetal Findings With Various Chromosomal Abnormalities

	Trisomies					Other Trisomies	Triploidy	Tetraploidy
	8	13	16	18	21			
Embryo present	+	+	0	±	+	±	±	0
Fetal hydrops		±		±	±	±		
Growth-retarded placenta	+	+	+	+	0	Variable	Large	+
Hydropic villi	±	+		+		+	+	+
Hydatidiform changes				0			+	+
Scattered vesicles			0	0			+	
Invaginations in villi				0			+	
Paucity of blood vessels	±	+	+	+	0			+
Cytotrophoblastic giant cells	+	+	+		0			
Hypoplastic trophoblast					0		+	
Immature villi in some areas	+	+			0		+	
Some very large villi					0		+	+

+ = present or frequently present; ± = occasionally present; 0 = absent or usually absent.

blast itself, or from Hofbauer cells.[24] Other placental findings associated with the various chromosomal disorders are found in Table 7–31.

Third-trimester fetuses with trisomies 13, 18, or 21 have been reported to have placentas with a high vascular resistance owing to the small size, reduced number, and sclerotic obliteration of arteries in the stem and peripheral villi (Fig 7–86).[277] These vascular findings correlate with Doppler waveform patterns that suggest low umbilical arterial blood flow. This raises a question about whether low blood flow from the fetus to the placenta contributes to the fetal growth retardation

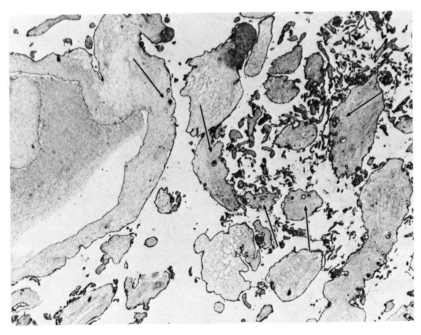

FIG 7–84.
This is the histologic picture of a typical triploid (69,XXY) partial hydatidiform mole. The enlarged villus on the left contains a large fluid-filled cyst. Other villi vary greatly in size and shape. The *arrows* point to characteristic syncytial villous inclusions. HE stain, ×16.

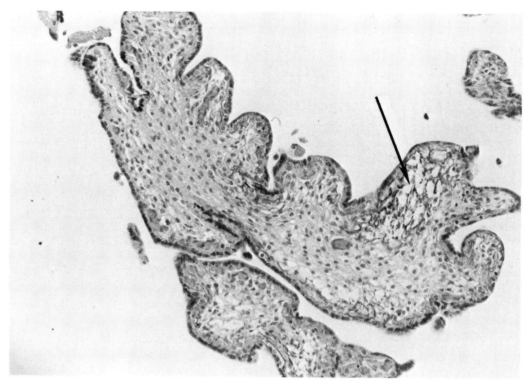

FIG 7–85.
The placenta of a 20-week fresh stillbirth with chromosome XO shows large, abnormally shaped villi and foci of degeneration *(arrow).*

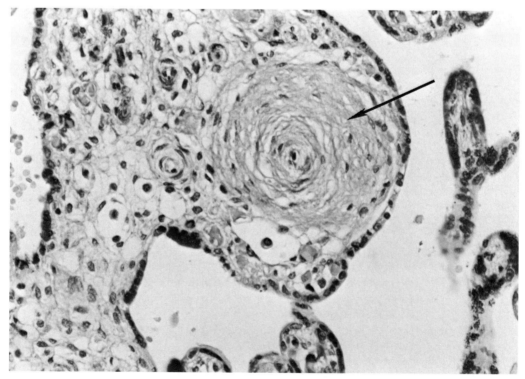

FIG 7–86.
The sclerotic obliteration of an artery in a stem villus associated with trisomy 13.

that is usually present in these trisomic disorders. However the major cause of this fetal growth retardation is presumed to be a slow rate of DNA synthesis which leads to a subnormal number of cells in most organs (see Chapter 4).[139,172,211,253]

There is some evidence that chromosomal mosaicism in placental villous cells can produce placental abnormalities that contribute to the death of otherwise normal embryos and fetuses. Chromosomal mosaicism was present in 1.3% of the villous biopsies in a large study.[136] When the mosaicism was limited to the cytotrophoblast there was no corresponding mosaicism in the fetus. However, there was a 17% mortality rate in such cases vs. a 3% mortality rate in the nonmosaics. Every mosaic abnormality that was associated with perinatal death involved an autosome. This makes it likely that cytotrophoblastic mosaicism predisposes to perinatal death. This possibility receives support from the fact that villous maturational arrest with resultant villous immaturity is often present in placentas with trisomic chromosomal abnormalities.[247]

How great is the role of chromosomal disorders in recurrent pregnancy loss? Cytogenetic studies of tissues from spontaneous abortions have found chromosomal abnormalities in 45% to 60% of the tissue specimens.[52,60] A balanced translocation is diagnosed in about 2% of couples affected by repeated losses and it is estimated that their offspring will have a 10% to 15% risk of an unbalanced translocation.[52,60] The risk for a subsequent aneuploid conception has not been completely defined in cases in which parental karyotypes are normal, but it appears that the risk is not significantly increased.[206] Therefore, other explanations must be found for most repeat spontaneous abortions and later pregnancy losses.

Erythroblastosis Fetalis

This is a hemolytic disorder caused by specific maternal antibodies that are directed against fetal red cell antigens. Most of the antibodies are anti-D but occasionally they are anti-c, anti-Kell, or against one of the other weak erythrocyte antigens. The ABO antigens are not as well differentiated before birth as the Rh antigens, so ABO erythroblastosis fetalis is much less frequent than Rh erythroblastosis. In the disorder Rh-incompatible fetal erythrocytes enter the maternal circulation, sensitize the mother, and resulting maternal antibodies cross the placenta and produce hemolysis in the fetus. Hematopoietic activity is greatly stimulated in several fetal organs in addition to the bone marrow and liver with the result that immature erythrocyte precursors circulate in the fetus. Fetal anemia, when severe, results in fetal heart failure and sometimes placental villous edema. The edema compresses blood vessels in the villi, reduces fetal blood flow into the placenta, and thereby further deprives the fetal organs of oxygen. When these processes are severe the result is fetal hydrops and a very edematous placenta with nucleated red blood cells in the fetal blood vessels (Fig 7–87).[244]

There is great variability in the placental findings that are associated with Rh erythroblastosis fetalis. Some of the placentas are normal in structure and others very abnormal, particularly when the fetus had experienced severe hemolysis. This disorder is one of the well-known causes of a very large placenta. In many cases the large size is due to severe fetal anemia, which produces abnormally large villi and eventually severe, diffuse villous edema. In many such placentas the villi appear immature in addition to being overgrown and edematous (see Fig 7–87). The villi often have few syncytial knots, a subnormal number of small terminal villi, and many normoblasts in their fetal blood vessels (see Fig 7–87). The villi in such placentas often have numerous constrictions and U-shaped undulations in their veins and H-shaped anastomoses between their arteries.[165] The venous undulations have been postulated to be the result of fetal venous hypertension which raises

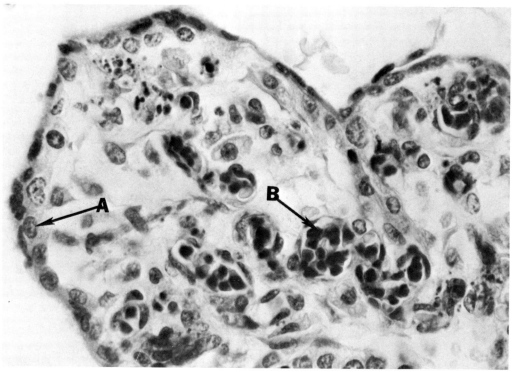

FIG 7–87.

Rh erythroblastosis fetalis. The villi are edematous and structurally immature for 35 weeks of gestation. Note the retained cytotrophoblast cells which usually disappear many weeks earlier *(arrow A)*. Nucleated red blood cells are present within the fetal blood vessels *(arrow B)*. HE stain, ×1,200.

pressure in the capillaries and arteries. These same villous vascular abnormalities are also sometimes present in placentas that have been chronically underperfused from the uterus. Perhaps these vascular abnormalities are a compensatory response to a placental capillary exchange surface that is inadequate to meet fetal needs.

The fetal liver is markedly enlarged in Rh erythroblastosis fetalis, mainly due to a great increase in erythroblastic hematopoietic tissue. Plasma levels of albumin are low in the neonate and some degree of thrombocytopenia is often present. A study of organ structure in neonates who died with Rh erythroblastosis fetalis has disclosed that both cell number and size were usually normal, suggesting that fetal tissue hypoxia, without an accompanying deficiency of glu-

cose and other nutrients, does not usually retard fetal growth.[210,237]

Nonimmune Fetal Hydrops

There is now a long list of nonimmune disorders that are associated with fetal hydrops and an edematous placenta. Jauniaux et al. recently reported that at least 35% of such cases are genetic in origin. Nearly half of the identified genetic disorders were chromosomal abnormalities, 11% were α-thalassemia, and the rest were small numbers of other genetic disorders. The chromosomal disorders are listed in Table 7–31. In α-thalassemia the abnormal hemoglobin is defective in releasing its oxygen. As a result, fetal cardiac failure is frequent and sometimes leads to severe, diffuse placental edema, a heavy placenta, and fetal hydrops.[248] Some of the other common hemoglobinopathies produce placental villous edema without fetal hydrops.[156]

There are a number of disorders that lead to fetal heart failure, which in turn sometimes produces placental villous edema and fetal hydrops. They include fetal hemorrhage into the maternal circulation, large chorangiomas of the placenta, angiomas in the fetus, sacrococcygeal teratomas, many different cardiac malformations, and cardiac arrhythmias of different origins.[24,108,129,154,164] Cystic-adenomatoid malformations of the lung and several other fetal malformations have also been associated with placental edema and fetal hydrops.[24,343] Fetal neuroblastomas have been described with placental villous edema and fetal hydrops.[320] The responsible mechanisms are the subject of speculation. Fetal hypoproteinemia is the probable mechanism responsible for the placental edema and fetal hydrops that is sometimes found with the congenital nephrotic syndrome.[124] Fetal infections with parvovirus, cytomegalovirus, Chagas' disease, and *L. monocytogenes* have occasionally produced placental edema and fetal hydrops.[24]

MATERNAL DISORDERS AND CONDITIONS

Diabetes Mellitus

Diabetic gestations have long been known to be at high risk with an excess of spontaneous abortions, fetal malformations, macrosomia, and fetal and neonatal death.[119] The diabetic placenta is well known for its large size. This size tends to be greatest when diabetes is of recent origin and poorly controlled.[64] In general, the greater the macrosomia of the baby, the larger the size of the placenta. Many of these very large placentas have a mass of cells and villous surface area for gas and nutrient exchange that is greater than normal.[331] Not all of the large size is directly due to the diabetes. The frequency of diabetes increases with maternal pregravid fatness, so there is a relatively high frequency of obesity among diabetic gravi-

das. Obese gravidas have larger placentas than the nonobese, with or without the presence of diabetes mellitus. The villi in the large placentas of diabetic gravidas often appear immature in addition to being large for gestational age, and villous edema is often present.[33] Ultrastructural analysis of the trophoblast often reveals increases in cytotrophoblastic thickness and foci of necrosis in the syncytial trophoblast.[138] All of the aforementioned abnormalities have become much less frequent in recent years as the control of diabetes during pregnancy by diet, exercise, and insulin has improved. When diabetes is well controlled, placental weights and structure are normal or nearly normal.[45]

Placental findings are variable in the placentas of women who have longstanding diabetes mellitus. When diabetes is complicated by nephropathy, arterial and arteriolar disease is often advanced in the uterus and the associated fetuses are sometimes growth-retarded. These uterine vascular lesions often restrict blood flow from the uterus to the placenta, which leads to infarcts and an unevenly accelerated maturation of placental villi. When this uterine vascular disease is severe, placental size can be normal, even when diabetic control has been uneven during pregnancy. The placentas associated with growth-retarded babies of diabetic mothers reportedly have a reduced number of insulin-binding receptors.[259] Both the placentas and the fetuses of diabetic gravidas have an increased frequency of vascular thromboses.[24] Maintaining blood glucose levels at too low a level during the pregnancies of diabetic women can lead to a subnormal-sized placenta.

Cigarette Smoking

A long list of abnormalities have been reported in the pregnancies, fetuses, and placentas of cigarette smokers (see Chapter 5). The most widely known is fetal growth retardation, which was first reported by Simpson in 1957.[311] The placenta is usually not as growth-retarded as the fetus, so the placental-fetal weight ratio is characteristically increased in smokers. There are several nonspecific abnormalities that are more frequent in the placentas of cigarette smokers than of nonsmokers.[231,237] The most important of these are decidual necrosis at the edge of the placenta and small placental infarcts.[231] Maternal smoking causes vasoconstriction in the uterus, which is a likely cause of these lesions. Both of these lesions may serve as the nidus for placental abruptions, which are more frequent in smokers than in nonsmokers.[237,252] Both the decidual necrosis and the infarcts are presumably the result of reductions in blood flow from the uterus to the placenta, which is a characteristic consequence of smoking. Studies have shown that smoking a single cigarette reduces uteroplacental blood flow for up to 15 minutes, which is probably long enough to produce decidual necrosis and infarcts.[166]

The other placental findings in cigarette smokers that might have significance are an increased thickening of the basal lamina beneath the trophoblastic covering of the villi and a decreased density of blood vessels inside the terminal villi.[341] Both may pose a barrier to the passage of oxygen and nutrients from the placenta to the fetus and thus explain why the children of cigarette smokers have higher hemoglobin levels at birth than the newborns of nonsmokers.[237] Finally, lesions of unknown significance are present in the intima of the umbilical arteries when women smoke during pregnancy.[13] The intimal cells have been described as having a "cobblestone" appearance, with leakage of plasma and red blood cells into the subendothelial spaces.

Autoimmune Reproductive Failure Disorders

Endometriosis has long been known to be associated with increased pregnancy wastage, and recently it has been discovered that more than two-thirds of women with endometriosis have evidence of abnormal polyclonal B cell activation with resultant increases in circulating levels of autoantibodies.[102] These same findings are present in many women with unexplained pregnancy losses and unexplained infertility, so the possibility arises that polyclonal B cell activation is in some manner responsible for some infertility and pregnancy wastage.[103] These findings usually occur without increased circulating levels of the lupus anticoagulants or anticardiolipin antibody. The affected women characteristically have a successful first pregnancy followed by repeated pregnancy losses.[103] There are reports that abnormal autoantibodies can interfere with pregnancy success after in vitro fertilization.[71] This would support the thesis that polyclonal B cell antivation might have a role in some infertility and pregnancy wastage. It is still not known whether the autoantibodies are directly responsible for infertility and pregnancy losses or whether they are a response to other, currently unidentified disorders.

Renal Failure

The major risk factor for pregnancy outcome with chronic maternal renal disease is a marked attenuation of maternal blood volume expansion when the renal disease is severe.[54] A very low blood volume expansion leads to low uteroplacental blood flow, which in turn produces unevenly accelerated placental villous maturation, placental and fetal growth retardation, preterm births, and an increase in fetal and neonatal deaths.[313] If the renal failure is treated appropriately, the fetus can survive and be well at birth. However, pregnancy is an unusual occurrence in women with end-stage renal disease. When it occurs, 75% to 80% reportedly end spontaneously with abortion, stillbirth, or neonatal death.[122] Premature labor sometimes begins during dialysis, but it also occurs in women with renal insufficiency who are not being dialyzed. Nearly half of the newborns of mothers with renal failure are growth-retarded at birth and they often have low 1-minute Apgar scores. Gravidas who are in renal failure with end-stage renal disease have a high frequency of life-threatening hypertension, which is particularly difficult to control when the gravida is on dialysis. Gravidas on dialysis also seem unable to increase their erythrocyte production, so most experience a worsening of their chronic anemia during pregnancy. Administered erythropoietin ameliorates this anemia. As might be expected, the placentas from women with renal failure are usually abnormal, showing the characteristic gross and microscopic findings of chronic low uteroplacental blood flow. These include high frequencies of infarcts and abruptions.

Liver Transplantation

Liver transplantation is becoming more frequent and some young women with these transplants have become pregnant. A mild fetal growth retardation was described in two of four children whose births followed such transplants.[243] The placenta from a third posttransplant gravida reportedly showed the findings of an abruption.

MISCELLANEOUS DISORDERS

The Sudden Infant Death Syndrome (SIDS)

There is nothing distinctive about the placental findings of children who becomes SIDS victims. Preterm birth is a strong risk factor for SIDS, and the placentas of preterm born SIDS victims display about the same frequencies of disorders that cause preterm birth as do the placentas of non-SIDS preterm born children.[57] The placentas of full-term born SIDS victims have an excess of the lesions that are associated with maternal cigarette smoking during pregnancy and the lesions that are characteristic of chronic low uteroplacental blood flow. This is not surprising because both maternal cigarette smoking and the disorders that produce low uteroplacental blood flow are major risk factors for SIDS.[224,228,237]

Maternal Neoplasms

More than half of the placentas that implant over uterine leiomyomas are reported to abrupt. Nonplacental maternal neoplasms rarely metastasize to the placenta. When it occurs, the neoplasm is almost always a melanoma, a lymphoma, a leukemia, a breast carcinoma, or a sarcoma.[56,81] Melanomas constitute about 30% of these metastatic neoplasms and breast carcinoma and hematopoietic malignancies another 30%. Melanomas are the only maternal neoplasm that has metastasized to the fetus.[24,81] With one exception all of the metastases have spontaneously disappeared in the child before 1 year of age.[24] The one exception was fatal to the infant.[35]

Trauma to the Placenta, Umbilical Cord, and Fetal Membranes by Fetal Movements

Trauma to the uterus and placenta as the result of automobile accidents, falls, and domestic violence is a well-known cause of placental abruptions, fetomaternal hemorrhage, and fetal skull fractures.[38,148,317] We have recently found indirect evidence that trauma to the placenta, umbilical cord, and fetal membranes by fetal movements sometimes seriously damages these structures. The evidence for such trauma started with the 1981–1982 discovery by Miller et al.[196,197] and Moessinger et al.[201] that tension applied to the umbilical cord by fetal movements has a strong, positive influence on umbilical cord length. Taking this finding into account we found that unusually long umbilical cords were associated with hyperactive behavior and above-normal IQ values in children at 7 years of age.[221] These correlations were derived from multiple regression analyses that took into consideration race; birth order; maternal IQ; maternal and paternal education; family income; whether or not the child's father was living with the family; the number, sex, and spacing of siblings; children's sex; and gestational age at birth. We also found that short umbilical cords were associated with low IQ values and with disorders of low motor activity and muscle tone, specifically neonatal hypotonia, neonatal lethargy, muscular dystrophy, a child being mongoloid, breech presentation at delivery, and a child having central nervous system malformations.[221] Unusually short cords were associated with a high perinatal mortality rate (see Chapter 6). Normal values for umbilical cord length are found in Chapter 6.

All of these findings led us to wonder if vigorous fetal movements might sometimes damage the placenta, the umbilical cord, or the fetal membranes. To explore this possibility, we used the nearly 35,000 umbilical cords, placentas, and fetal membranes in the CPS to see if umbilical cord length correlated with placental, umbilical cord, and fetal membrane disorders that logically could have a traumatic origin. Such a correlation was found between umbilical cord length and umbilical cord knots, umbilical cord hematomas, umbil-

ical cord around the neck, maternal floor placental infarcts, placental intervillous thrombi, diffuse fibrin beneath the chorionic plate of the placenta, fresh placental abruptions, premature rupture of the fetal membranes, and lacerations of the maternal surface of the placenta (Table 7–32).[226] Children with these disorders were less often hypoactive as neonates than were other children in the CPS (Table 7–33). These disorders were associated with a high rate of stillbirths and a normal or low rate of neonatal deaths (see Table 7–32). From these findings it is plausible to postulate that all of these disorders are sometimes the consequence of trauma administered by a physically vigorous fetus.

Could this physical vigor of the fetus that we postulate sometimes be the reflection of superior brain development? This is likely because children who survived the antenatal disorders associated with long umbilical cords had superior IQ and achievement test scores in later childhood (see Table 7–33). It can be deduced from these findings that some potentially very bright and vigorous children self-destruct before birth. If this is true, why hasn't this self-destructive behavior reduced the frequency of the responsible genes in the general population? An attractive possibil-

TABLE 7–32.

The Relationship of Umbilical Cord Length to Various Disorders That May Be Caused by Fetal Trauma to the Placenta*

		Relative Risks	
	Attributable Risks	Stillbirth	Neonatal Death
Umbilical cord disorders			
Tight knot	**.46** (.43, .49)	**19.1** (9.9, 29.4)	0.8 (0.5, 1.3)
Hematoma	**.25** (.18, .31)	**7.4** (6.0, 9.0)	0.9 (0.6, 1.2)
Loose around neck	**.16** (.12, .21)	1.1 (0.8, 1.4)	**0.4** (0.2, 0.6)
Placental and fetal membrane disorders			
Floor infarcts	**.18** (.13, .22)	**26.2** (7.2, 96.3)	1.0 (0.2, 2.3)
≥5 intervillous thrombi	**.19** (.16, .22)	1.0 (0.4, 1.9)	1.5 (0.7, 2.4)
Fresh abruption	**.11** (.09, .13)	**4.1** (3.4, 5.2)	**1.9** (1.0, 3.6)
Premature membrane rupture	**.02** (.01, .03)	0.7 (0.5, 1.0)	0.7 (0.5, 1.0)
Laceration of maternal surface of the placenta	**.02** (.01, .03)	1.2 (1.0, 1.4)	1.2 (1.0, 3.6)

*Significant intervals are in boldface; 95% confidence intervals are in parentheses.

ity is that the gene losses due to the self-destructive behavior have been balanced by the reproductive success of the survivors with their superior physical and cognitive vigor.

Low Blood Flow to the Placenta

Blood flow to the placenta can be low from either the fetus or the gravida. There are both similarities and differences in the outcomes of the two types of low blood flow. The main similarity is a high risk for stillbirth (Table 7–34). With either type of low flow the fetus is deprived of needed oxygen and nutrients. The risk for neonatal death and for long-term developmental

disorders was increased only when blood flow was low from the mother to the placenta (see Table 7–34). In the CPS these poor outcomes consisted of increased frequencies of mild mental retardation and learning disorders (see Chapter 11). Low uteroplacental blood flow is usually a chronic condition and this may be the reason why the brain is affected. The fetal brain is also affected by acute hypoxia and asphyxia but it is not the most vulnerable organ. The kidneys, lungs, and heart are all more vulnerable so hypoxia or asphyxia that is severe enough to damage the brain usually kills the fetus or leads to early neonatal death. Children who have enough heart, lung, and kidney function to

TABLE 7–33.
The Relationship of Umbilical Cord and Placental Findings to Neonatal Activity and to Cognitive Test Scores at 7 Years of Age*

	Hypoactive as Neonate	High Scores on Spelling Tests	IQ > 120
Umbilical cord findings			
True knot	**0.1** (0.0, 0.7)	**2.1** (1.0, 3.3)	**1.4** (1.0, 1.9)
Hematoma	**0.1** (0.0, 0.5)	**1.9** (1.2, 2.7)	1.2 (0.8., 1.6)
Loose around neck	**0.8** (0.5, 1.0)	**1.2** (1.0, 1.4)	**1.1** (1.0, 1.3)
Abnormally long cord	**0.8** (0.6, 1.0)	**2.1** (1.5, 3.0)	**2.1** (1.7, 2.7)
Placental findings			
Diffuse subchorionic fibrin	**0.7** (0.5, 1.0)	**2.9** (2.2, 3.9)	**2.1** (1.7, 2.7)
Maternal floor infarcts	**0.0** (0.0, 1.0)	0.9 (0.5, 1.4)	**1.1** (1.0, 1.3)
≥5 intervillous thrombi	1.4 (0.4, 2.5)	**2.4** (1.1, 5.4)	**2.0** (1.1, 3.4)
Fresh abruption	1.0 (0.3, 1.8)	**1.6** (1.2, 2.1)	**1.4** (1.0, 1.9)
Lacerations of maternal surface	**0.6** (0.4, 0.9)	**2.5** (2.1, 2.9)	**2.1** (1.8, 2.5)

Significant values are in boldface. Relative risks; 95% confidence intervals are in parentheses.

TABLE 7–34.
The Relationship of Disorders That Reduce Blood Flow to the Placenta to Perinatal Death and Neurologic Abnormalities at 7 Years of Age

	Relative Risks		
	Stillbirths	Neonatal Deaths	Neurologic Abnormalities
Low blood flow from fetus to placenta			
Umbilical cord			
Thrombosis	2.8, $P<.01$	2.8, $P<.01$	1.1
Hematoma	7.4, $P<.01$	0.9	0.6
Tight knot	19.1, $P<.01$	0.8	0.7
Prolapse	2.9, $P<.01$	1.9, $P<.01$	0.7
Placental artery thrombosis	21.4, $P<.01$	1.0	1.0
Low blood flow from gravida to placenta			
Unevenly accelerated placental maturation	1.6, $P<.01$	1.3, $P<.01$	1.2, $P<.01$
Maternal floor infarction	26.2, $P<.01$	1.0	1.6, $P<.01$

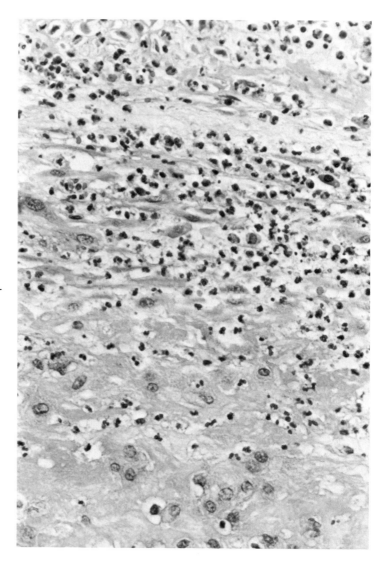

FIG 7–88.
The bacterial infection that causes acute chorioamnionitis has spread into the decidua. HE stain, × 600.

survive acute severe antenatal hypoxia or asphyxia rarely have brain damage (see Chapter 11).

DISORDERS OF THE DECIDUA

Acute Inflammation

Acute inflammation is frequent in the decidua. It is usually focal and varies from the presence of a few neutrophils to abscess formation. It is most often associated with acute chorioamnionitis and in that setting is presumed to be the consequence of infection caused by bacteria or mycoplasmas that have spread from the chorion into the decidua (Fig 7–88). This interpretation is supported by the finding of Salafia et al. that in every case where acute inflammation was present in the chorionic plate of the placenta, acute inflammation was also present in the decidua.[296] The reverse is not true. There are many cases in which acute inflammation is present in the decidua without similar inflammation being present in the placenta or the umbilical cord. In these latter cases the decidual inflammation is seldom associated with an unfavorable pregnancy outcome. As previously mentioned, acute deciduitis is one of the risk factors for placental abruptions, particularly when it is associated with evidence of acute chorioamnionitis in the chorionic plate of the placenta and the umbilical cord.[216,237,252] Acute deciduitis is sometimes striking with infection by *L. monocytogenes.*

Chronic Inflammation

Chronic inflammation in the decidua has been given little attention because small numbers of chronic inflammatory cells, mainly lymphocytes, are normally present in both the decidua basalis and the decidua capsularis. Of the placentas in the CPS, 1.5% (305) had a heavy infiltration of lymphocytes in the decidua basalis. The only risk factor identified was being white (Table 7–35). Taking this risk factor into consideration, a heavy infiltration of lymphocytes in the decidua basalis was not a risk factor for any unfavorable pregnancy outcome. Tuberculosis sometimes manifests as a chronic inflammation in the decidua. Caseous necrosis is a characteristic finding.

Necrosis of the Decidua Basalis

Necrosis of the decidua basalis had a frequency of 2.4% (765) in the CPS. The frequency of small areas of such necrosis is much higher and is presumably a normal finding.[189] Two risk factors for decidual necrosis in the CPS, acute chorioamnionitis and disorders that cause low uteroplacental blood flow, were likely common causes of the necrosis (Table 7–36). Acute chorioamnionitis is an infection caused by bacteria and mycoplasmas. The extension of the infection into the decidua likely explains its association with decidual necrosis (Fig 7–89). Decidual necrosis is presumably associated with disorders that produce low uteroplacental blood flow because these latter disorders also reduce blood flow to the decidua. Markers for vigorous fetal motor activity were the most frequent risk factor for necrosis in the decidua basalis.

After antecedent risk factors had been taken into account, decidual necrosis was independently associated with an increased risk for preterm birth (see Table 7–36).

Decidual necrosis at the edge of the placenta, where the decidua capsularis joins the decidua basalis, is a characteristic finding in cigarette smokers.[237] Normally, uteroplacental blood flow is lower at the edge than at the center of the placenta. With each cigarette smoked, maternal blood pressure decreases for 5 to 15 minutes.[166] Resulting decreases in uteroplacental blood flow are a plausible explanation for the decidual necrosis at the edge of the placenta.[215] In the CPS decidual necrosis at this site was four

TABLE 7–35.

Risk Estimates for Antecedents to Large Numbers of Lymphocytes in the Decidua Basalis*

Risk Factors	No. of Placentas With Many Decidual Lymphocytes per 1,000 Cases With Risk Factor†	Relative Risks (95% Confidence Intervals)	Attributable Risks (95% Confidence Intervals)
All cases	5 *(130)*		
Maternal factor			
Race: white	**6** *(87), P < .02*	**1.6** (1.3, 1.9)	**.16** (.14, .18)
Population attributable risk			*.16 (.14, .18)*
Pregnancy outcomes			
Preterm birth	**24** *(94), P < .001*	1.3 (0.9, 1.7)	
Fetal growth retardation	11 *(29), P > .1*	0.8 (0.5, 1.1)	
Stillbirth	**71** *(20), P < .001*	1.2 (0.3, 4.0)	
Neonatal death	**36** *(11), p < .001*	1.3 (0.7, 2.6)	
Neurologic abnormalities at 7 yr	12 *(12), P > .1*	0.7 (0.3, 1.1)	

*Significant values are in boldface.
†Numbers of cases are in parentheses.

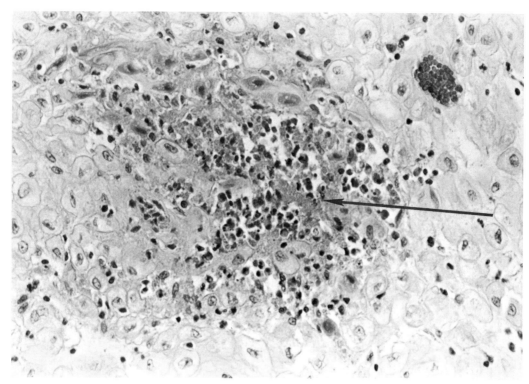

FIG 7–89.
Necrosis in the decidua due to the spread of acute chorioamnionitis. HE stain, ×600.

TABLE 7–36.

Risk Estimates for Antecedents to the Development of Necrosis in the Decidua Basalis*

Risk Factors	No. of Cases of Decidual Necrosis per 1,000 Cases With Risk Factor†	Relative Risks (95% Confidence Intervals)	Attributable Risks (95% Confidence Intervals)
All cases	24 *(1,325)*		
Maternal factor			
Preeclampsia, eclampsia	**37** *(603)*, P < .001	**1.9** (1.7, 2.2)	**.16** (.14, .20)
Fetal factor			
Race: black	**30** *(870)*, P < .001	**1.5** (1.3, 1.8)	**.17** (.15, .18)
Placental factor			
Acute chorioamnionitis	**30** *(559)*, P < .001	**1.3** (1.1, 1.5)	**.07** (.06, .08)
Markers for vigorous fetal motor activity	**31** *(568)*, P < .001		**.20** (.17, .25)
Population attributable risk			**.59** *(.57, .62)*
Pregnancy outcomes			
Preterm birth	**30** *(398)*, p < .001	**1.2** (1.0, 1.5)	
Fetal growth retardation	**33** *(192)*, P < .001	1.3 (0.9, 1.7)	
Stillbirth	**92** *(87)*, P < .001	1.4 (0.8, 2.7)	
Neonatal death	**47** *(50)*, P < .001	0.8 (0.3, 1.8)	
Neurologic abnormalities at 7 yr	22 *(42)*, P > .1	0.9 (0.6, 1.2)	

Significant values are in boldface.
†Numbers of cases are in parentheses.

times more frequent in blacks than in whites and two times more frequent when the fetus had major malformations than when such malformations were absent.

Necrosis of the Decidua Capsularis

Necrosis of the decidua capsularis often has a different significance from necrosis in the decidua basalis. Necrosis of the decidua capsularis is usually focal and much more frequent than necrosis in the decidua basalis. In many instances there is no associated acute inflammation (Fig 7–90). In some instances necrosis of the decidua capsularis is the consequence of acute chorioamnionitis. However, the cause of most necrosis in the decidua capsularis is unknown, and when acute chorioamnionitis was taken into consideration it did not increase the risk of any unfavorable pregnancy outcome in the CPS.

Thrombosis of Blood Vessels in the Decidua Basalis

Thrombosis of blood vessels in the decidua basalis had a frequency of 0.9% (288) in the CPS (Table 7–37). Its risk factors were the same as those for necrosis in the decidua basalis and it is likely that these thromboses are sometimes the cause of the necrosis (see Table 7–37). After taking all of its associated risk factors into account, blood vessel thrombosis in the decidua basalis was associated with an increased risk for preterm birth (see Table 7–37).

ULTRASONIC IDENTIFICATION OF GROSS ABNORMALITIES

There is now more than 20 years of international experience with ultrasound as a technique to diagnose placental dis-

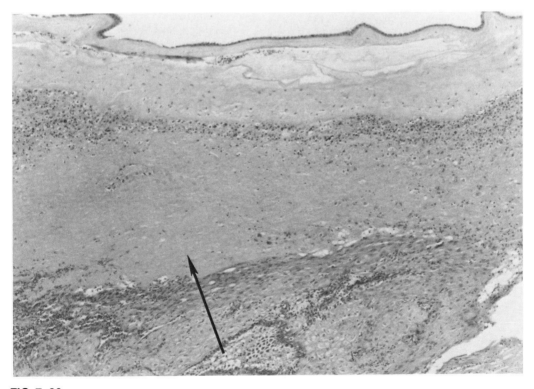

FIG 7–90.
Bland necrosis in the decidua capsularis. HE stain, ×120.

TABLE 7–37.

Risk Estimates for Antedcedents to the Development of Blood Vessel Thrombosis in the Decidua Basalis*

Risk Factors	No. of Cases of Decidual Blood Vessel Thrombosis per 1,000 Cases With Risk Factor†	Relative Risks (95% Confidence Intervals)	Attributable Risks (95% Confidence Intervals)
All cases	**9** *(571)*		
Maternal factors			
Race: black	**12** *(344), P* < .001	**1.7** (1.3, 2.1)	**.20** (.18, .23)
Preeclampsia, eclampsia	**14** *(226), P* < .001	**1.9** (1.5, 2.4)	**.16** (.13, .18)
Placental factor			
Acute chorioamnionitis	**11** *(205), P* < .01	**1.2** (1.0, 1.6)	**.06** (.04, .08)
Markers for vigorous fetal motor activity			**.30** (.27, .35)
Population attributable risk			**.71** *(.68, .75)*
Pregnancy outcomes			
Preterm birth	**13** *(120), P* < .01	**1.3** (1.0, 1.7)	
Fetal growth retardation	9 *(51) P* > .1	1.2 (0.8, 1.6)	
Stillbirth	**29** *(26), P* < .001	1.0 (0.5, 2.2)	
Neonatal death	16 *(14), P* > .1	1.2 (0.5, 2.1)	
Neurologic abnormalities at 7 yr	6 *(12), P* > .1	0.7 (0.4, 1.1)	

*Significant values are in boldface.
†Numbers of cases are in parentheses.

orders. There were many failures in the early years to make correct diagnoses because of primitive equipment, lack of experience, and failure to make detailed comparisons between the ultrasound images and placental findings at delivery. Jauniaux and Campbell have critically reviewed the literature and reported on the efforts to identify circumvallate placenta, circummarginate placenta, placental cysts, hemorrhages, chorioangiomas, infarcts, hydatidiform transformations, and retroplacental hemorrhages.[132]

REFERENCES

1. Abramowsky CR, Vegas ME, Swinehart G, Gyues MT: Decidual vasculopathy of the placenta in lupus erythematosus. *N Engl J Med* 1980; 303:668–672.

2. Abu-Yousef MN, Bleicher JJ, Williamson RA, Weiner CP: Subchorionic hemorrhage: Sonographic diagnosis and clinical significance. *AJR* 1987; 149:737–740.

3. Aherne A: Morphometry, in Gruenwald P (ed): *The Placenta and Its Maternal Supply Line.* Lancaster, Penn, MTP Press, 1975, pp. 80–97.

4. Althabe O, Labarrere C: Chronic villitis of unknown aetiology and intrauterine growth-retarded infants of normal and low ponderal index. *Placenta* 1985; 6:369–373.

5. Altshuler G: Pathogenesis of congenital herpesvirus infection: Case report including a description of the placenta. *Am J Dis Child* 1974; 127:427–429.

6. Altshuler G: Chorangiosis: An important placental sign of neonatal morbidity and mortality. *Arch Pathol Lab Med* 1984; 108: 71–74.

7. Altshuler G: Placental infection and inflammation, in Perrin EVDK (ed): *Pathology of the Placenta.* New York, Churchill Livingstone, Inc, 1984, pp 150–152.

8. Altshuler G, Hyde S: Clinicopathologic considerations of fusobacteria chorioamnionitis. *Acta Obstet Gynecol Scand* 1988; 67:513–517.

9. Amirhessami-Aghili N, Manalo P, Hall MR, Tibbitts FD, Ort CA, Afsari A: Human cytomegalovirus infection of human placental explants in culture: Histologic and immunohistochemical studies. *Am J Obstet Gynecol* 1987; 156:1365–1374.

10. Anand A, Gray ES, Brown T, Clewley JP, Cohen BJ: Human parovirus infection in pregnancy and hydrops fetalis. *N Engl J Med* 1987; 316:183–186.

11. Appelbaum PC, Holloway Y, Ross SM, Dhupelia I. The effect of amniotic fluid on bacte-

rial growth in three population groups. *Am J Obstet Gynec* 1977; 128:868–871.

12. Aquino TI, Zhang J, Kraus FT, Knefel R, Taff T: Subchorionic fibrin cultures for bacteriologic study of the placenta. *Am J Clin Pathol* 1984; 81:482–486.

13. Asmussen I, Kjeldsen K: Intimal ultrastructure of human umbilical arteries. Observations on arteries of newborn children of smoking and nonsmoking mothers. *Circ Res* 1975; 36:579–589.

14. Averbuch M, Koifman B, Levo Y: Lupus anticoagulant, thrombosis and thrombocytopenia in systemic lupus erythematosus. *Am J Med Sci* 1987; 293:2–5.

15. Azogue E, LaFuente C, Darros C: Congenital Chagas disease in Bolivia, epidemiologic aspects and pathologic findings, *Trans R Soc Trop Med* 1985; 79:176–180.

16. Azzarelli B, Lafuze J: Amniotic basement membrane: A barrier to neutrophil invasion. *Am J Obstet Gynecol* 1987; 156:1130–1136.

17. Azziz R, Cumming J, Naeye R. Acute myometritis and chorioamnionitis during cesarean section of asymptomatic women. *Am J Obstet Gynecol* 1988; 159:1137–1139.

18. Barss P, Misch KA: Epidemic placenta accreta in a population of remote villagers in Papua, New Guinea. *Br J Obstet Gynaecol* 1990; 97:167–174.

19. Batcup G, Tovey LAD, Longster G: Fetomaternal blood group incompatibility studies in placental intervillous thrombosis. *Placenta* 1983; 4:449–454.

20. Battaglia FC, Wollevor CA: Fetal and neonatal complications associated with recurrent chorioangiomas. *Pediatrics* 1968; 41:62–66.

21. Bejar R, Curbelo V, Davis C, Gluck L: Premature labor: II. Bacterial sources of phospholipase. *Obstet Gynecol* 1981; 57:479–482.

22. Benirschke K, Altschuler G: The future of perinatal physiopathology, H. Abramson (ed): *Symposium on the Functional Physiopathology of the Fetus and Neonate.* St Louis, CV Mosby Co, 1971, pp 158–168.

23. Benirschke K, Driscoll SG: *The Pathology of the Human Placenta.* New York, Springer-Verlag, 1967.

24. Benirschke K, Kaufmann P: *Pathology of the Human Placenta.* New York, Springer-Verlag, 1990.

25. Benirschke K, Mendoza GR, Bazeley PL: Placental and fetal manifestations of cytomegalovirus infection. *Virchows Arch [Cell Pathol]* 1974; 16:121–139.

26. Berche P, Reich KA, Bonnichon M, Beretti JL, Geoffroy C, Raveneau J, Cossart P, Gaillard JL, Geslin P, Kreis H, Veron M: Detection of anti-listeriolysin O for serodiagnosis of human listeriosis. *Lancet* 1990; 335:624–627.

27. Berkowitz GS, Mehalek KE, Chitkara U, Rosenberg J, Cogswell C, Berkowitz RL: Doppler umbilical velocimetry in the prediction of adverse outcome in pregnancies at risk for intrauterine growth retardation. *Obstet Gynecol* 1988; 71:742–746.

28. Bernal AL, Hansell DJ, Soler RC, Keeling JW, Turnbull AC: Prostaglandins, chorioamnionitis and preterm labour. *Br J Obstet Gynaecol* 1987; 94:1156–1158.

29. Blanc W: Pathology of the placenta, membranes, and umbilical cord in bacterial, fungal and viral infection in man, in Naeye RL, Kissane JM, Kaufman N (eds): *Perinatal Diseases.* Baltimore, Williams & Wilkins Co, 1981, pp 67–132.

30. Bloxam DL, Bullen BE, Walters BNJ, Lao TT: Placental glycolysis and energy metabolism in preeclampsia. *Am J Obstet Gynecol* 1987; 157:97–101.

31. Boucher M, Yonekura ML: Perinatal listeriosis (early onset): Correlation of antenatal manifestations and neonatal outcome. *Obstet Gynecol* 1986; 68:593–597.

32. Boyd PA: Placenta and umbilical cord, in Keeling JW (ed): *Fetal and Neonatal Pathology.* London, Springer-Verlag, 1987, pp 45–76.

33. Boyd PA, Scott A, Keeling JW: Quantitative structural studies on human placentas from pregnancies complicated by diabetes mellitus. *Br J Obstet Gynaecol* 1986; 93:31–35.

34. Bret AJ, Legros R, Toyoda S: Les kystes placentaires. *Presse Med* 1960; 68:1552–1560.

35. Brodsky I, Baren M, Kahn SB, Lewis G Jr, Tellem M: Metastatic malignant melanoma from mother to fetus. *Cancer* 1965; 18:1048–1054.

36. Brown ZA, Vontver LA, Benedetti J, Critchlow CW, Sells CJ, Berry S, Corey L: Effects on infants of a first episode of genital herpes during pregnancy. *N Engl J Med* 1987; 317:1246–1251.

37. Buchdahl R, Hird M, Gamsu H, Tapp A, Gibb D, Tzannatos C: Listeriosis revisited: The role of the obstetrician. *Br J Obstet Gynaecol* 1990; 97:186–189.

38. Buchsbaum HJ: *Trauma in Pregnancy.* Philadelphia, WB Saunders Co, 1979.

39. Bussolino F, Benedetto C, Massobrio M, Camussi G: Maternal vascular prostacyclin activity in pre-eclampsia. *Lancet* 1980; 2:702.

40. Carter B: Premature separation of the normally implanted placenta: Six deaths due to gross bilateral cortical necrosis of the kidneys. *Obstet Gynecol* 1967; 29:30–33.

41. Chasnoff IJ, Burns WJ, Schnoll SH, Burns KA: Cocaine use in pregnancy. *N Engl J Med* 1985; 313:666–669.

42. Chasnoff IJ, Griffith DR, MacGregor S, Dirkes K, Burns KA: Temporal patterns of cocaine use in pregnancy: Perinatal outcome. *JAMA* 1989; 261:1741–1744.

43. Chiswick M, D'Souza SW, Occleshaw JV: Computerized transverse axial tomography in the newborn. *Early Hum Dev* 1977; 1:17–80.

44. Clark SL, Koonings PP, Phelan JP: Placenta previa/accreta and prior cesarean section. *Obstet Gynecol* 1985; 66:89–92.

45. Clarson C, Tevaarwerk GJM, Harding PGR, Chance GW, Haust MD: Placental weight in diabetic pregnancies. *Placenta* 1989; 10:275–281.

46. Clewell WH, Manchester DK: Recurrent maternal floor infarction: A preventable cause of fetal death. *Am J Obstet Gynecol* 1983; 147:346–347.

47. Coid DR, Fox H: Short review: Campylobacters as placental pathogens. *Placenta* 1983; 4:295–306.

48. Confino E, Friberg J, Silverman S, Dudkiewicz AB, Goldin M, Gleicher N: Penetration of bacteria and spermatozoa into bovine cervical mucus. *Obstet Gynecol* 1987; 70:134–136.

49. Cooperman NR, Kasim M, Rajashekaraiah KR: Clinical significance of amniotic fluid, amniotic membranes, and endometrial biopsy cultures at the time of cesarean section. *Am J Obstet Gynecol* 1980; 137:536–541.

50. Cooperstock M, England JE, Wolfe RA: Circadian incidence of labor onset hour in preterm birth and chorioamnionitis. *Obstet Gynecol* 1987; 70:852–855.

51. Cotran RS: New roles for the endothelium in inflammation and immunity. *Am J Pathol* 1987; 129:407–413.

52. Coulam CB: Unexplained recurrent pregnancy loss: Epilogue. *Clin Obstet Gynecol* 1986; 29:999–1004.

53. Cruikshank DP, Warenski JC: First-trimester maternal *Listeria monocytogenes* sepsis and chorioamnionitis with normal neonatal outcome. *Obstet Gynecol* 1989; 73:469–471.

54. Cunningham FG, Cox SM, Harstad TW, Mason RA, Pritchard JA: Chronic renal disease and pregnancy outcome. *Am J Obstet Gynecol* 1990; 163:453–459.

55. Dehner LP, Askin FB: Cytomegalovirus endometritis: Report of a case associated with spontaneous abortion. *Obstet Gynecol* 1975; 45:211–214.

56. Delerive C, Locquet F, Mallart A, Janin A, Gosselin B: Placental metastasis from maternal bronchial oat cell carcinoma. *Arch Pathol Lab Med* 1989; 113:556–558.

57. Denmead DT, Ariagno RL, Carson SH, Benirschke KB: Placental pathology is not predictive for sudden infant death syndrome (SIDS). *Am J Perinatol* 1987; 4:308–312.

58. Desmonts G, Couvreur J: Toxoplasmosis, epidemiologic and serologic aspects of perinatal infection, in Krugman S, Gershon AA (eds): *Infections of the Fetus and Newborn: Progress in Clinical and Biologic Research.* New York, Alan R Liss Inc. 1975, p 115.

59. DeVries LS, Wigglesworth JS, Regev R, Dubowitz LMS: Evolution of periventricular leukomalacia during the neonatal period and infancy: Correlation of imaging and postmortem findings. *Early Hum Dev* 1988; 17:205–219.

60. DeWald GW, Michels VV: Recurrent miscarriages: Cytogenetic causes and genetic counseling of affected families. *Clin Obstet Gynecol* 1986; 29:865–885.

61. De Wolf F, Brosens I, Renaer M: Fetal growth retardation and the maternal arterial supply of the human placenta in the absence of sustained hypertension. *Br J Obstet Gynaecol* 1980; 87:678–685.

62. De Wolf F, Carreras LO, Moerman P, Vermylen J, Van Assche A, Renaer M: Decidual vasculopathy and extensive placental infarction in a patient with repeated thromboembolic accidents, recurrent fetal loss, and a lupus anticoagulant. *Am J Obstet Gynecol* 1982; 142:829–834.

63. Dong Y, St Clair PJ, Ramzy I, Kagan-Hallet KS, Gibbs RS: A microbiologic and clinical study of placental inflammation at term. *Obstet Gynecol* 1987; 70:175–182.

64. Driscoll SG: The pathology of pregnancy complicated by diabetes mellitus. *Med Clin North Am* 1965; 49:1053–1067.

65. Duncan ME, Fox H, Harkness RA, Rees RJW: The placenta in leprosy. *Placenta* 1984; 5:189–198.

66. Earl U, Bulmer JN, Briones A: Placenta accreta: An immunohistological study of trophoblast populations. *Placenta* 1987; 8:273–282.

67. Eden JA: Fetal-induced trauma as a cause of antepartum hemorrhage. *Am J Obstet Gynecol* 1987; 157:830–831.

68. Edwards LE, Barrada MI, Hamann AA, Hakanson EY: Gonorrhea in pregnancy. *Am J Obstet Gynecol* 1978; 132:637–641.

69. Egley CC, Katz VL, Herbert WNP: Leukocyte esterase: A simple bedside test for the detection of bacterial colonization of amniotic fluid. *Am J Obstet Gynecol* 1988; 159:120–122.

70. Eldar-Geva T, Hochner-Celnikier D, Ariel I, Ron M, Yagel S: Fetal high output cardiac failure and acute hydramnios caused by large placental chorioangioma. Case report. *Br J Obstet Gynecol* 1988; 95:1200–1203.

71. El-Roeiy A, Gleicher N, Friberg J, Confino E, Dudkiewicz A: Correlation between peripheral blood and follicular fluid autoantibodies and impact on invitro fertilization. *Obstet Gynecol* 1987; 70:163–170.

72. El-Roeiy A, Myers SA, Gleicher N: The prevalence of autoantibodies and lupus anticoagulant in healthy pregnant women. *Obstet Gynecol* 1990; 75:390–396.

73. Eriksson M, Larsson G, Zetterstrom R: Amphetamine addiction and pregnancy, *Acta Obstet Gynecol Scand* 1981; 60:253–259.

74. Erskine RLA, Ritchie JWK. Umbilical artery blood flow characteristics in normal and growth retarded fetuses. *Br J Obstet Gynaecol* 1985; 92:605–610.

75. Feinstein DI: Lupus anticoagulant, thrombosis, and fetal loss. *N Engl J Med* 1985; 313:1348–1350.

76. FitzSimmons J, Callahan C, Shanahan B, Jungkind D: Chlamydial infections in pregnancy. *J Reprod Med* 1986; 31:19–22.

77. Fojaco RM, Hensley GT, Moskowitz L: Congenital syphilis and necrotizing funisitis. *JAMA* 1989; 261:1788–1790.

78. Fok RY, Pavlova Z, Benirschke K, Paul RH, Platt LD: The correlation of arterial lesions with umbilical artery Doppler velocimetry in the placentas of small-for-dates pregnancies. *Obstet Gynecol* 1990; 75:578–583.

79. Fox H: The significance of placental infarction in perinatal morbidity and mortality. *Biol Neonate* 1967; 11:87–105.

80. Fox H: Fibrinoid necrosis of placental villi. *J Obstet Gynaecol Br Commonw* 1968; 75:448–452.

81. Fox H: *Pathology of the Placenta.* Philadelphia, WB Saunders Co, 1978.

82. Fox H, Jones CJP: Pathology of trophoblast, in Loke YW, White A (eds): *Biology of Trophoblast.* New York, Elsevier, 1983, pp 137–185.

83. Frank DA, Zuckerman BS, Amaro H, Aboagye K, Bauchner H, Cabral H, Fried L, Hingson R, Kayne H, Levenson SM, Parker S, Reece H, Vinci R: Cocaine use during pregnancy: Prevalence and correlates. *Pediatrics* 1988; 82:888–895.

84. Frenkel JK: Toxoplasmosis: Mechanisms of infection, laboratory diagnosis and management. *Curr Top Pathol* 1971; 28–75.

85. Friedman A, DeFazio J, DeCherney A: Severe obstetric complications after aggressive treatment of Asherman syndrome. *Obstet Gynecol* 1986; 67:864–867.

86. Friedman EA: Obstetric infections in labor, in Charles D, Finland M (eds): *Obstetric and Perinatal Infections.* Philadelphia, Lea & Febiger, 1973, pp 501–516.

87. Friedman SA: Preeclampsia, a review of the role of prostaglandins, *Obstet Gynecol* 1988; 71:122–130.

88. Fujikura T: Placental calcification and maternal age. *Am J Obstet Gynecol* 1963; 87:41–45.

89. Fujimura M, Takeuchi T, Kitajima H, Nakayama M: Chorioamnionitis and serum IgM in Wilson-Mikity syndrome. *Arch Dis Child* 1989; 64:1379–1383.

90. Gallagher P, Fagan CJ, Bedi DG, Winsett MZ, Reyes RN: Potential placenta previa: Definition, frequency, and significance. *AJR* 1987; 149:1013–1015.

91. Gant NF, Daley GL, Chand S, Whalley PJ, MacDonald PC: A study of angiotensin II pressor response throughout primigravid pregnancy. *J Clin Invest* 1973: 52:2682–2689.

92. Garcia AGP: Fetal infection in chickenpox and alastrim, with histopathologic study of the placenta. *Pediatrics* 1963; 32:895–901.

93. Garcia AGP, Fonesca EF, Marques RLS, Lobato YY: Placental morphology in cytomegalovirus infection. *Placenta* 1989; 10:1–18.

94. Garcia AGP, Marques RLS, Lobato YY, Fonesca MEF, Wigg MD: Placental pathology in congenital rubella. *Placenta* 1985; 6:281–295.

95. Garcia AGP, Pereira JMS, Vidigal N, Lobato YY, Pegado CS, Branco JPC: Intrauterine infection with mumps virus. *Obstet Gynecol* 1980; 56:756–759.

96. Garrow JS, Hawes SF: The relationship of the size and composition of the human placenta to its functional capacity. *J Obstet Gynaecol Br Commw* 1971; 78:22–28.

97. Gibbs RS, Cassell GH, Davis JK, St Clair PJ: Further studies on genital mycoplasmas in intra-amniotic infection: Blood cultures and serologic response. *Am J Obstet Gynecol* 1986; 154:717–726.

98. Gibbs RS, Dinsmoor MJ, Newton ER, Rama-murthy RS: A randomized trial of intrapar-tum versus immediate postpartum treatment of women with intra-amniotic infection. *Obstet Gynecol* 1988; 72:823–828.

99. Giles WB, Trudinger BJ, Baird PJ: Fetal um-bilical artery flow velocity waveforms and placental resistance: Pathological correlation. *Br J Obstet Gynaecol* 1985; 92:31–38.

100. Gilstrap LC, Leveno KJ, Cox SM, Burris JS, Mashburn M, Rosenfeld CR: Intrapartum treatment of acute chorioamnionitis: Impact on neonatal sepsis. *Am J Obstet Gynecol* 1988; 159:579–583.

101. Gilstrap LC, Leveno KJ, Cunningham FG, Whalley PJ, Roark ML: Renal infection and pregnancy outcome. *Am J Obstet Gynecol* 1981; 141:709–716.

102. Gleicher N, El-Roeiy A, Confino E, Friberg J: Is endometriosis an autoimmune disease? *Obstet Gynecol* 1987; 70:115–122.

103. Gleicher N, El-Roeiy A, Confino E, Friberg J: Reproductive failure because of autoanti-bodies: Unexplained infertility and pregnancy wastage. *Am J Obstet Gynecol* 1989; 160: 1376–1385.

104. Goedert JJ, Mendez H, Drummond JE, Robert-Guroff M, Minkoff HL, Holman S, Stevens R, Rubinstein A, Blattner WA, Willoughby A, Landesman SH: Mother-to-infant transmission of human immunodefi-ciency virus type 1: Association with prema-turity or low Anti-gp 120. *Lancet* 1989; 2:1351–1354.

105. Goff E, Griffith BP, Booss J: Delayed amplifi-cation of cytomegalovirus infection in the placenta and maternal tissues during late gestation. *Am J Obstet Gynecol* 1987; 156: 1265–1270.

106. Golding J, Shenton T, Thomas P, MacGillivray I: Geographic variation in the incidence of hypertension in pregnancy. *Am J Obstet Gynecol* 1988; 158:80–83.

107. Goldstein I, Romero R, Merrill S, Wan M, O'Connor TZ, Mazor M, Hobbins JC: Fetal body and breathing movements as predictors of intraamniotic infection in preterm pre-mature rupture of membranes. *Am J Obstet Gynecol* 1988; 159:363–368.

108. Gonen R, Fong K, Chiasson DA: Prenatal sonographic diagnosis of hepatic heman-gioendothelioma with secondary nonimmune hydrops fetalis. *Obstet Gynecol* 1989; 73:485–487.

109. Gravett MG, Nelson HP, DeRouen T, Critchlow C, Eschenbach DA, Holmes KK: Independent associations of bacterial vagino-sis and *Chlamydia trachomatis* infection with adverse pregnancy outcome. *JAMA* 1986; 256:1899–1903.

110. Grimmer D, Landas S, Kemp JD: IgM anti-trophoblast antibodies in a patient with a pregnancy-associated lupus like disorder, vas-culitis, and recurrent intrauterine fetal de-mise. *Arch Pathol Lab Med* 1988; 112:191–193.

111. Guidetti DA, Divon MY, Cavalieri RL, Langer O, Merkatz IR: Fetal umbilical artery flow ve-locimetry in postdate pregnancies. *Am J Ob-stet Gynecol* 1987; 157:1521–1523.

112. Guzman L, Avalos E, Ortiz R, Gurrola R, Lo-pez E, Herrera R: Placental abnormalities in systemic lupus erythematosus: in situ depo-sition of antinuclear antibodies. *J Rheumatol* 1987; 14:924–929.

113. Hadeed AJ, Siegel SR: Maternal cocaine use during pregnancy: Effect on the newborn in-fant. *Pediatrics* 1989; 84:205–210.

114. Hager WD, Pauly TH. Fetal tachycardia as an indicator of maternal and neonatal morbidity. *Obstet Gynecol* 1985; 66:191–194.

115. Hain J, Doshi N, Harger JH: Ascending transcervical herpes simplex infection with intact fetal membranes. *Obstet Gynecol* 1980; 56:106–109.

116. Hanly JG, Gladman DD, Rose TH, Laskin CA, Urowitz MB: Lupus pregnancy. A prospective study of placental changes. *Arthritis Rheumat* 1988; 31:358–366.

117. Harman CR, Manning FA, Stearns E, Morrison I: The correlation of ultrasonic placental grading and fetal pulmonary matu-ration in five hundred sixty-three pregnan-cies. *Am J Obstet Gynecol* 1982; 143: 941–943.

118. Harter CA, Benirschke K: Fetal syphilis in the first trimester. *Am J Obstet Gynecol* 1976; 124:705–711.

119. Haust MD: Maternal diabetes mellitus, effects on the fetus and placenta, in Naeye RL, Kis-sane JM, Kaufman N (eds): *Perinatal Dis-eases.* Baltimore, Williams & Wilkins Co, 1981, pp 201–285.

120. Heggtveit HA, de Carvalho R, Nuyens AJ: Chorioangioma and toxemia of pregnancy. *Am J Obstet Gynecol* 1965; 91:291–292.

121. Hiller SL, Martius J, Kronn M, Kiviat N, Holmes KK, Eschenback DA: A case-controlled study of chorioamnionitic infection and histologic chorioamnionitis in prematu-rity. *N Engl J Med* 1988; 319:972–978.

122. Hou S: Pregnancy in women requiring dialysis for renal failure. *Am J Kidney Dis* 1987; 9:368–373.

123. Howard RB, Hosokawa T, Maguire MH: Hypoxia-induced fetoplacental vasoconstriction in perfused human placental cotyledons. *Am J Obstet Gynecol* 1987; 157:1261–1266.

124. Hung PL, Huang CC, Huang TS: Nephrotic syndrome in a Chinese infant. *Am J Dis Child* 1977; 131:557–559.

125. Hurley VA, Beischer NA: Placenta membranacea. Case reports. *Br J Obstet Gynaecol* 1987; 94: 798–802.

126. Hurwitz A, Milwidsky A, Yarkoni S, Palti Z: Severe fetal distress with hydramnios due to chorangioma. *Acta Obstet Gynecol Scand* 1983; 62:633–635.

127. Hytten FE, Chamberlain GVP: *Clinical Physiology of Obstetrics.* Oxford, England, Blackwell Scientific Publications, 1980.

128. Hytten FE, Leitch I: *The Physiology of Human Pregnancy*, ed 2. Oxford, England, Blackwell Scientific Publications, 1971.

129. Imakita M, Yutani C. Ishibashi-Ueda H, Murakami M, Chiba Y: A case of hydrops fetalis due to placental chorioangioma. *Acta Pathol Jpn* 1988; 38:941–945.

130. Jackson MR, Mayhew TM, Haas JD: On the factors which contribute to thinning of the villous membrane in human placeantae at high altitude. *Placenta* 1988; 9:1–18.

131. Jaffe R, Siegal A, Rat L, Bernheim J, Gruber A, Feigin M: Placental chorioangiomatosis, a high risk pregnancy. *Postgrad Med J* 1985; 61:453–455.

132. Jauniaux E, Campbell S: Fetal growth retardation with abnormal blood flows and placental sonographic lesions. *J Clin Ultrasound* 1990; 18:210–214.

133. Jauniaux E, Nessmann C, Imbert MC, Meuris S, Puissant F, Hustin J: Morphological aspects of the placenta in HIV pregnancies. *Placenta* 1988; 9:633–642.

134. Jeacock MK, Scott J, Plester JA: Calcium content of the human placenta. *Am J Obstet Gynecol* 1963; 87:34–40.

135. Jogee M, Myatt L, Elder MG: Decreased prostacyclin production by placental cells in culture from pregnancies complicated by fetal growth retardation. *Br J Obstet Gynaecol* 1983; 90:247–250.

136. Johnson A, Wapner RJ, Davis GH, Jackson LG: Mosaicism in chorionic villus sampling: An association with poor perinatal outcome. *Obstet Gynecol* 1990; 75:573–577.

137. Johnson N, Moodley J, Hammond MG: Human leucocyte antigen status in African women with eclampsia. *Br J Obstet Gynaecol* 1988; 95:877–879.

138. Jones CJP, Fox H: An ultrastructural and ultrahistochemical study of the human placenta of the diabetic woman. *J Pathol* 1976; 119:91–99.

139. Kaback MM, Bernstein LH: Biologic studies of trisomic cells growing in vitro. *Ann NY Acad Sci* 1970; 171:526–536.

140. Kanbour-Shakir A, Zhang X, Rouleau A, Armstrong DT, Kunz HW, Macpherson TA, Gill TJ: Gene imprinting and major histocompatibility complex class I antigen expression in the rat placenta. *Immunology* 1990; 87: 444–448.

141. Karegard M, Gennser G: Incidence and recurrence rate of abruptio placentae in Sweden. *Obstet Gynecol* 1986; 67:523–528.

142. Katz VL, Bowes WA Jr, Sierkh AE: Maternal floor infarction of the placenta associated with elevated second trimester serum alphafetoprotein. *Am J Perinatol* 1987; 4:225–228.

143. Katz SL, Wilfert GM: Human immunodeficiency virus infection of newborns. *N Engl J Med* 1989; 320:1687–1689.

144. Kaufman P: Influence of ischemia and artificial perfusion on placental ultrastructure and morphometry. *Contrib Gynecol Obstet* 1985; 13:18–26.

145. Keith LG, MacGregor S, Friedell S, Rosner M, Chasnoff IJ, Sciarra JJ: Substance abuse in pregnant women: Recent experience at the Perinatal Center for Chemical Dependence of Northwestern Memorial Hospital. *Obstet Gynecol* 1989; 73:715–720.

146. Kelly CS. Gibson JL: Listeriosis as a cause of fetal wastage. *Obstet Gynecol* 1972; 40:91–97.

147. Kessel SS, Villar J, Berendes HW, Nugent RP: The changing pattern of low birth weight in the United States, 1970–1980. *JAMA* 1984; 251:1978–1982.

148. Kettel LM, Branch DW, Scott JR: Occult placental abruption after maternal trauma. *Obstet Gynecol* 1988; 71:449–453.

149. Khong TY, DeWolf F, Robertson WB, Brosens I: Inadequate maternal vascular response to placentation in pregnancies complicated by pre-eclampsia and by small-for-gestational age infants. *Br J Obstet Gynaecol* 1986; 93:1049–1059.

150. Khong TY, Frappell JM, Steel HM, Stewart CM, Burke M: Perinatal listeriosis. A report of six cases. *Br J Obstet Gynaecol* 1986; 93:1083–1087.

151. Khong TY, Robertson WB: Placenta creta and placenta praevia creta. *Placenta* 1987; 8:399–409.

152. Kitzmiller JL, Watt N, Driscoll SG: Decidual arteriopathy in hypertension and diabetes in pregnancy: Immunofluorescent studies. *Am J Obstet Gynecol* 1981; 141:773–779.

153. Knox WF, Fox H: Villitis of unknown etiology: Its incidence and significance in placentae from a British population. *Placenta* 1984; 5:395–402.

154. Kohga S, Nambu T, Tanaka K, Benirschke K, Feldman BH, Kishikawa T: Hypertrophy of the placenta and sacrococcygeal teratoma: Report of two cases. *Virchows Arch [Pathol Anat]* 1980; 386:223–229.

155. Koppe JG, Loewer-Sieger DH, de Roever-Bonnet H: Results of 20-year follow-up of congenital toxoplasmosis. *Lancet* 1986; 1:254–256.

156. Koshy M, Burd L, Wallace D, Moawad A, Baron J: Prophylactic red-cell transfusions in pregnant patients with sickle cell disease: A randomized cooperative study. *N Engl J Med* 1988; 319:1447–1452.

157. Koskiniemi M, Happonen JM, Jarvenpaa AL Pettay O, Vaheri A: Neonatal herpes simplex virus infection: A report of 43 patients. *Pediatr Infect Dis J* 1989; 8:30–35.

158. Koskiniemi M, Lappalainen M, Hedman K: Toxoplasmosis needs evaluation. *Am J Dis Child* 1989; 143:724–728.

159. Kouyoumdjian A: Velamentous insertion of the umbilical cord. *Obstet Gynecol* 1980; 56:737–742.

160. Labarrere CA, Althabe OH: Chronic villitis of unknown etiology and maternal arterial lesions in preeclamptic pregnancies. *Eur J Obstet Gynecol Reprod Biol* 1985; 20:1–11.

161. Labarrere CA, Althabe OH: Intrauterine growth retardation of unknown letiology. II Serum complement and circulating immune complexes in maternal sera and their relationship with parity and chronic villitis. *Am J Reprod Immunol* 1986; 12:4–6.

162. Labarrere CA, McIntyre JA, Faulk WP: Immunohistologic evidence that villitis in human normal term placentas is an immunologic lesion. *Am J Obstet Gynecol* 1990; 162:515–522.

163. Lauweryns J, Bernat R, Lerut A, Detournay G: Intrauterine pneumonia, an experimental study. *Biol Neonate* 1973; 22:301–318.

164. Leake RD, Stimling B, Emmanouilides GC: Intrauterine cardiac failure with hydrops fetalis; Case report in a twin with the hypoplastic left heart syndrome and review of the literature. *Clin Pediatr* 1973; 12:649–651.

165. Lee MML, Yeh MN: II. Fetal microcirculation of abnormal human placenta. Scanning electron microscopy of placental vascular casts from fetus with severe erythroblastosis fetalis. *Am J Obstet Gynecol* 1986; 154:1139–1146.

166. Lehtovirta T, Forss M: The acute effect of smoking on intervillous blood flow of the placenta. *Br J Obstet Gynaecol* 1978; 85: 729–731.

167. Lemtis H, Hadrich G: Über die Gewichtsabnahme des Mutterkuchens nach des Geburt und die Bedeutung für den Quotienten aus Plazenta- und Kindesgewicht. Geburtshilfe and Frauenheilkunde 1974; 34:618–622.

168. Leung A, Kwok P, Chang A: Association between prostaglandin E2 and placental abruption, *Br J Obstet Gynaecol* 1987; 94: 1001–1002.

169. Levene MI, Fenton AC, Evans DH, Archer LNJ, Shortland DB, Gibson NA: Severe birth asphyxia and abnormal cerebral blood flow velocity. *Dev Med Child Neurol* 1989; 31:427–434.

170. Leviton C, VanMarter L, Kuban KCK: Respiratory distress syndrome and intracranial hemorrhage: Cause or association? Inference from surfactant clinical trials. *Pediatrics* 1989; 84:915–922.

171. Lewis SH, Reynolds-Kohler C, Fox HE, Nelson JA: HIV-1 in trophoblastic and villous Hofbauer cells and haematological precursors in eight-week fetuses. *Lancet* 1990; 335:565–568.

172. Lin C, Evans MI: *Intrauterine Growth Retardation.* New York, McGraw-Hill Book Co, 1984, pp 81–85.

173. Lisboa AC: On congenital Chagas' disease, anatomic-pathological study of six cases. *Rev Inst Med Trop Sao Paulo* 1960; 2:319–334.

174. Lockshin MD, Druzin ML, Goei S, Qamar T, Magid MS, Jovanovic L, Ferenc M: Antibody to cardiolipin as a predictor of fetal distress or death in pregnant patients with systemic lupus erythematosus. *N Engl J Med* 1985; 313:152–156.

175. Lockwood CJ, Romero R, Feinberg RF, Clyne LP, Coster B, Hobbins JC: The prevalence and biologic significance of lupus anticoagulant and anticardiolipin antibodies in a general obstetric population. *Am J Obstet Gynecol* 1989; 161:369–373.

176. Loizou S, Byron MA, Englert HJ, David J, Houghes GRV, Walport MJ: Association of quantitative anticardiolipin antibody levels

with fetal loss and time of loss in systemic lupus erythematosus. *Q J Med* 1988; 68:525–531.

177. Lou HC, Lassen NA, Friis-Hansen B: Impaired autoregulation of cerebral blood flow in the distressed newborn infant. *J Pediatr* 1979; 94:118–121.

178. Low JA, Forese AF, Galbraith RS, Sauerbrei EE, McKinven JP, Karchmar EJ: The association of fetal and newborn metabolic acidosis with severe periventricular leukomalacia in the preterm newborn. *Am J Obstet Gynecol* 1990; 162:977–982.

179. Lubbe WF, Butler WS, Palmer SJ, Liggins GC: Lupus anticoagulant in pregnancy. *Br J Obstet Gynaecol* 1984; 91:357–363.

180. Lubbe WF, Liggins GC: Lupus anticoagulant and pregnancy. *Am J Obstet Gynecol* 1985; 153:322–327.

181. Lunell NO, Nylund LE, Lesander R, Sarby B: Uteroplacental blood flow in pre-eclampsia. Measurements with indium-113m and a computer-linked gamma camera. *Clin Exp Biol* 1982; 1:105–117.

182. Macpherson TA, Szulman AE: The placenta and products of conception, in Silverberg SG (ed): *Principles and Practice of Surgical Pathology*, ed 2. New York, Churchill Livingston Inc, 1990, p 1825.

183. Madan E, Meyer MP, Amortegui AJ: Isolation of genital mycoplasmas and *Chlamydia trachomatis* in stillborn and neonatal autopsy material. *Arch Pathol Lab Med* 1988; 112:749–751.

184. Maeda H, Shimokawa H, Satoh S, Nakano H, Nunoue T: Nonimmunologic hydrops fetalis resulting from intrauterine human parovirus B-19 infection: Report of two cases. *Obstet Gynecol* 1988; 72:482–485.

185. Malan AF: Special infections in the newborn (syphilis, tetanus, tuberculosis), in Stern L, Vert P (eds): *Neonatal Medicine*. New York, Masson Publishing, 1987, pp 622–636.

186. Malan AF, Woods DL, Van Der Elst CW, Meyer MP: Relative placental weight in congenital syphilis. *Placenta* 1990; 11:3–6.

187. Martius J, Krohn MA, Hillier SL, Stamm WE, Holmes KK, Eschenbach DA: Relationships of vaginal lactobacillus species, cervical *Chlamydia trachomatis*, and bacterial vaginosis to preterm birth. *Obstet Gynecol* 1988; 71:89–95.

188. Maury W, Potts BJ, Rabson AB: HIV-1 Infection of first-trimester and term human placental tissue: A possible mode of maternal-fetal transmission. *J Infect Dis* 1989; 160:583–588.

189. McCombs HL, Craig JM: Decidual necrosis in normal pregnancy. *Obstet Gynecol* 1964; 24:436–442.

190. McCown LM, Mullen BM, Ritchie K: Umbilical artery flow velocity waveforms and the placental vascular bed. *Am J Obstet Gynecol* 1987; 157:900–902.

191. McGregor IA. Epidemiology, malaria and pregnancy. *Am J Trop Med Hyg* 1984; 33:517–525.

192. McGregor JA, French JI, Richter R, Franco-Buff A, Johnson A, Hillier S, Judson FN, Todd JK: Antenatal microbiologic and maternal risk factors associated with prematurity. *Am J Obstet Gynecol* 1990; 163:1465–1473.

193. McShane PM, Heyl PS, Epstein MF: Maternal and perinatal morbidity resulting from placenta previa. *Obstet Gynecol* 1985; 65: 176–182.

194. Menon R. Pregnancy and malaria. *Med J Malaysia* 1972; 27:115–119.

195. Mercado A, Johnson G Jr, Calver D, Sokol RJ: Cocaine, pregnancy and postpartum intracerebral hemorrhage. *Obstet Gynecol* 1989; 73:467–468.

196. Miller ME, Higginbottom M, Smith DW: Short umbilical cord, its origin relevance. *Pediatrics* 1981; 67:618–621.

197. Miller ME, Jones MC, Smith DW: Tension, the basis of umbilical cord growth. *J Pediatr* 1982; 101:844.

198. Minkoff HL, Henderson C, Mendez H, Gail MH, Holman S, Willoughby A, Goedett JJ, Rubinstein A, Stratton M, Walsh JH, Landesman SH: Pregnancy outcomes among mothers infected with human immunodeficiency virus and uninfected control subjects. *Am J Obstet Gynecol* 1990; 163:1598–1604.

199. Minkoff HL, Willoughby A, Mendez H, Moroso G, Holman S, Goedert JJ, Landesman SH: Serious infections during pregnancy among women with advanced human immunodeficiency virus infection. *Am J Obstet Gynecol* 1990; 162:30–34.

200. Mitchell APB, Anderson GS, Russell JK: Perinatal death from foetal exsanguination. *Br Med J* 1957: 1:611–614.

201. Moessinger AC, Blanc WA, Marone PA, Polsen DC: Umbilical cord length as an index of fetal activity: Experimental study and clinical implications. *Pediatr Res* 1982; 16:109–112.

202. Morales WJ: The effect of chorioamnionitis on the developmental outcome of preterm infants at one year. *Obstet Gynecol* 1987; 70:183–186.

203. Morales WJ, Angel JL, O'Brien WF, Knuppel RA, Finazzo M: A randomized study of antibiotic therapy in idiopathic preterm labor. *Obstet Gynecol* 1988; 72:829–833.

204. Morrow RJ, Ritchie JWK: Uteroplacental and umbilical artery blood velocity waveforms in placental abruption assessed by doppler ultrasound. Case report. *Br J Obstet Gynaecol* 1988; 95:723–724.

205. Mortimer G, MacDonald DJ, Smeeth A: A pilot study of the frequency and significance of placental villitis. *Br J Obstet Gynaecol* 1985; 92:629–633.

206. Morton NE, Chiu D, Holland C, Jacobs PA, Pettay D: Chromosome anomalies as predictors of recurrence risk for spontaneous abortion. *Am J Med Genet* 1987; 28:353–360.

207. Moscoso G, Guillerot Y: Nonimmune hydrops fetalis associated with genetic disorders. *Obstet Gynecol* 1990; 75:568–572.

208. Mostoufi-Zadeh M, Driscoll SG, Biano SA, Kundsin RB: Placental evidence of cytomegalovirus infection of the fetus and neonate. *Arch Pathol Lab Med* 1984; 108:403–406.

209. Naeye RL: Cytomegalic inclusion disease, the fetal disorder. *Am J Clin Pathol* 1967; 47: 738–744.

210. Naeye RL: New observations in erythroblastosis fetalis. *JAMA* 1967; 200:281–286.

211. Naeye RL: Prenatal organ and cellular growth with various chromosomal disorders. *Biol Neonate* 1967; 11:248–255.

212. Naeye RL: Placental infarction leading to fetal or neonatal death. *Obstet Gynecol* 1977; 50:583–588.

213. Naeye RL: Causes of perinatal mortality excess in prolonged gestations. *Am J Epidemiol* 1978; 108:429–433.

214. Naeye RL: Placenta previa, predisposing factors and effects on the fetus and surviving infants. *Obstet Gynecol* 1978; 52:521–525.

215. Naeye RL: The duration of maternal cigarette smoking, fetal and placental disorders. *Early Hum Dev* 1979; 3:229–243.

216. Naeye RL: Coitus and antepartum haemorrhage. *Br J Obstet Gynaecol* 1981; 88:765–770.

217. Naeye RL: Maternal blood pressure and fetal growth. *Am J Obstet Gynecol* 1981; 141: 780–787.

218. Naeye RL: Teenaged and pre-teenaged pregnancies: Consequences of the fetal-maternal competition for nutrients. *Pediatrics* 1981; 67:146–150.

219. Naeye RL: Maternal use of dextroamphetamine and growth of the fetus. *Pharmacology* 1983; 26:117–120.

220. Naeye RL: Maternal floor infarction. *Hum Pathol* 1985; 16:823–828.

221. Naeye RL: Umbilical cord length: clinical significance. *J Pediatr* 1985; 107:278–281.

222. Naeye RL: Do placental weights have clinical significance? *Hum Pathol* 1987; 18:387–391.

223. Naeye RL: Antenatal malarial infections, in Scarpelli DG, Migaki G (eds): *Transplacental Effects on Fetal Health.* New York, Alan R Liss Inc, 1988, pp 165–173.

224. Naeye RL: Sudden infant death syndrome, is the confusion ending? *Mod Pathol* 1988; 1:169–174.

225. Naeye RL: Pregnancy hypertension, placental evidences of low uteroplacental blood flow and spontaneous preterm delivery. *Hum Pathol* 1989; 20:441–444.

226. Naeye RL: The clinical significance of absent subchorionic fibrin in the placenta. *Am J Clin Pathol* 1990; 94:196–198.

227. Naeye RL: Maternal body weight and pregnancy outcome. *Am J Clin Nutr* 1990; 52:273–279.

228. Naeye RL: Preventing the sudden infant death syndrome. *Paediat Perinat Epidemiol* 1990; 4:12–21.

229. Naeye RL, Blanc W: Pathogenesis of congenital rubella. *JAMA* 1965; 194:1277–1283.

230. Naeye RL, Blanc WA, Leblanc W, Khantamee MA: Fetal complications of maternal heroin addiction: Abnormal growth, infections and episodes of stress. *J Pediatr* 1973; 83: 1055–1061.

231. Naeye RL, Harkness WL, Utts J: Abruptio placentae and perinatal death: A prospective study. *Am J Obstet Gynecol* 1977; 124:740–746.

232. Naeye RL, Kissane JM, Kaufman N (eds): *Perinatal Diseases.* Baltimore, Williams & Wilkins Co, 1981.

233. Naeye RL, Maisels MJ, Lorenz RP, Botti JJ: The clinical significance of placental villous edema. *Pediatrics* 1983; 71:588–594.

234. Naeye RL, Peters EC: Causes and consequences of premature rupture of fetal membranes. *Lancet* 1980; 1:192–194.

235. Naeye RL, Ross SM: Amniotic fluid infection syndrome. *Clin Obstet Gynecol* 1982; 9: 593–607.

236. Naeye RL, Ross SM: Coitus and chorioamnionitis: A prospective study. *Early Hum Dev* 1982; 6:91–97.

237. Naeye RL, Tafari N: *Risk Factors in Pregnancy and Diseases of the Fetus and Newborn.* Baltimore, Williams & Wilkins Co, 1983.

238. Naeye RL, Tafari N, Judge D, Maraboe CC: Twins: Causes of perinatal death in 12 United States cities and one African city. *Am J Obstet Gynecol* 1978; 131:267–272.

239. Naib ZM, Nahmias AJ, Josey WE, Wheeler JH: Association of maternal genital herpetic infection with spontaneous abortion. *Obstet Gynecol* 1970; 35:260–263.

240. Nazir MA, Pankuch GA, Botti JJ, Appelbaum PC: Antibacterial activity of amniotic fluid in the early third trimester. *Am J Perinat* 1987; 4:59–62.

241. Nelson AM, Anderson V, Ryder R et al: Placental pathology as a predictor of perinatal HIV infection in infants born to HIV positive women in Kinshasa, Zaire. Presented at Fourth International Conference on AIDS, Stockholm, June 6, 1988, abst 6585.

242. Newton ER, Prihoda TJ, Gibbs RS: Logistic regression analysis of risk factors for intra-amniotic infection. *Obstet Gynecol* 1989; 73:571–575.

243. Newton ER, Turksoy N, Kaplan M, Reinhold R: Pregnancy and liver transplantation. *Obstet Gynecol* 1988; 71:499–500.

244. Nicholaides KH, Thilaganathan B, Rodeck CH, Mibashan RS: Erythroblastosis and reticulocytosis in anemic fetuses. *Am J Obstet Gynecol* 1988; 159:1063–1065.

245. Nickel RE: Maternal floor infarction: an unusual cause of intrauterine growth retardation. *Am J Dis Child* 1988; 142:1270–1271.

246. Novak RW, Platt MS: Significance of placental findings in early-onset group B streptococcal neonatal sepsis. *Clin Pediatr* 1985; 24: 256–258.

247. Oberweiss D, Gillerot Y, Koulischer L, et al: Le placenta des trisomies dans le dernier trimestre de la gestation. *J Gynecol Obst Biol Reprod* 1983; 12:345–349.

248. Orkin SH, Nathan DG: Current concepts in genetics, the thalassemias. *N Engl J Med* 1976; 295:710–714.

249. Page DV, Brady K, Ward S: The placental pathology of substance abuse. *Lab Invest* 1989; 60:A69.

250. Pankuch GA, Cherouny PH, Botti JJ, Appelbaum PC: Amniotic fluid leukotaxis assay as an early indicator of chorioamnionitis. *Am J Obstet Gynecol* 1989; 161:802–807.

251. Pass RF, Little EA, Stagno S, Britt WJ, Alford CA: Young children as a probable source of maternal and congenital cytomegalovirus infection. *N Engl J Med* 1987; 316:1366–1370.

252. Paterson MEL: The aetiology and outcome of abruptio placentae. *Acta Obst Gynecol Scand* 1979; 58:31–35.

253. Paton GR, Silver MF, Allison AC: Comparison of cell cycle time in normal and trisomic cells. *Hum Genet* 1974; 23:173–182.

254. Peckham CS, Logan S: Cytomegalovirus infection in pregnancy, in Cosmi EV, DiRenzo GC (eds): *Proceedings of the 11th European Congress of Perinatal Medicine.* Chur, Switzerland, Harwood, 1988, pp 255–260.

255. Perrin VDK: *Pathology of the Placenta.* New York, Churchill Livingstone Inc, 1984.

256. Perry EH, Bada HS, Ray JD, Korones SB, Arheart K, Magill HL: Blood pressure increases, birthweight-dependent stability boundary, and intraventricular hemorrhage. *Pediatrics* 1990; 85:727–732.

257. Philip AGS, Allan WC, Tito AM, Wheller LR: Intraventricular hemorrhage in preterm infants: Declining incidence in the 1980s. *Pediatrics* 1989; 84:797–801.

258. Phillip K, Skodler WD, Pateisky N: Uteroplacental blood flow measurement using radioisotopes in small placentas. *Gynecol Obstet Invest* 1986; 21:70–75.

259. Potau N, Riudor E, Ballabriga A: Insulin receptors in human placenta in relation to fetal weight and gestational age. *Pediatr Res* 1981; 15:798–802.

260. Preece PM, Ades A, Thompson RG, Brooks JH: *Chlamydia trachomatis* infection in late pregnancy: A prospective study. *Paediatr Perinat Epidemiol* 1989; 3:268–277.

261. Preece PM, Blount JM, Glover J, Fletcher GM, Peckham CS, Griffiths PD: The consequences of primary cytomegalovirus infection in pregnancy. *Arch Dis child* 1983; 58: 970–975.

262. Preece PM, Pearl KN, Peckham CS: Congenital cytomegalovirus infection. *Arch Dis Child* 1984; 59:1120–1126.

263. Pritchard JA, Macdonald PL, Gant NE: Diseases and abnormalities of the placenta and fetal membranes, in *Williams Obstetrics*, ed 17. New York, Appleton-Century-Crofts, 1985, p 441.

264. Pryse-Davies J, Dewhurst CJ, Campbell S: Placenta membranacea. *J Obstet Gynaecol Br Commonw* 1973; 80:1106–1112.

265. Quinn PA, Butany J, Chipman M, Taylor J, Hannah W: A prospective study of microbial infection in stillbirths and early neonatal death. *Am J Obstet Gynecol* 1985; 151: 238–249.

266. Rappaport VJ, Hirata G, Yap HK, Jordon SC: Anti-vascular endothelial cell antibodies in severe preeclampsia. *Am J Obstet Gynecol* 1990; 162:138–146.

267. Rappaport F, Rabinovitz M, Toaff R, Krochick N: Genital listeriosis as a cause of repeated abortion. *Lancet* 1960; 1:1273–1275.

268. Redline RW, Abramowsky CR: Clinical and pathologic aspects of recurrent placental villitis. *Hum Pathol* 1985; 16:727–731.

269. Reik W, Collick A, Norris ML, Barton SC, Surani MA: Genomic imprinting determines methylation of parental alleles in transgenic mice, *Nature* 1987; 328:248–251.

270. Reiner L, Fries E: Chorangioma associated with arteriovenous aneurysm. *Am J Obstet Gynecol* 1965; 93:58–64.

271. Reinhardt MC: The African newborn in Abidjan, maternal and environmental factors influencing the outcome of pregnancy, in Abei H, Whitehead R (eds): *Maternal Nutrition During Pregnancy and Lactation*. Bern, Hans Huber, 1980, p 132.

272. Rhoads GG, Jackson LG, Schlesselman SE et al: The safety and efficacy of chorionic villus sampling for early prenatal diagnosis of cytogenetic abnormalities. *N Engl J Med* 1989; 320:609–617.

273. Ricci JM, Fojaco RM, O'Sullivan MJ: Congenital syphilis: the University of Miami/Jackson Memorial Medical Center experience, 1986–1988. *Obstet Gynecol* 1989; 74:687–693.

274. Rice JP, Kay HH, Mahony BS: The clinical significance of uterine leiomyomas in pregnancy. *Am J Obstet Gynecol* 1989; 160:1212–1216.

275. Robb JA, Benirschke K, Barmeyer R: Intrauterine latent herpes simplex virus infection. I. Spontaneous abortion. *Hum Pathol* 1986; 17:1196–1209.

276. Robertson WB, Brosens I, Dixon HG: Uteroplacental vascular pathology. *Eur J Obstet Gynecol Reprod Biol* 1975; 5:47–65.

277. Rochelson B, Kaplan C, Guzman E, Arato M, Hansen K, Trunca C: A quantitative analysis of placental vasculature in the third-trimester fetus with autosomal trisomy. *Obstet Gynecol* 1990; 75:59–63.

278. Rodgers GM, Taylor RN, Roberts JM: Preeclampsia is associated with a serum factor cytotoxic to human endothelial cells. *Am J Obstet Gynecol* 1988; 159:908–914.

279. Rodriguez J, Claus D, Verellen G, Lyon G: Periventricular leucomalacia: Ultrasonic and neuropathological correlations. *Dev Med Child Neurol* 1990; 32:347–355.

280. Romero R, Brody DT, Oyarzun E, Mazor M, Wu YK, Hobbins JC, Durum SK: Interleukin-1: A signal for the onset of parturition. *Am J Obstet Gynecol* 1989; 160:1117–1123.

281. Romero R, Emamian M, Quintero R, Wan M, Hobbins JC, Mazor M, Edberg S: The value and limitations of the Gram stain examination in the diagnosis of intraamniotic infection. *Am J Obstet Gynecol* 1988; 159:114–119.

282. Romero R, Emamian M, Quintero R, Wan M, Scioscia AL, Hobbins JC, Edberg S: Diagnosis of intra-amniotic infection: the acridine orange stain. *Am J Perinat* 1989; 6:41–45.

283. Romero R, Kadar N, Hobbins JC, Duff GW: Infection and labor, the detection of endotoxin in amniotic fluid. *Am J Obstet Gynecol* 1987; 157:815–819.

284. Romero R, Mazor M: Infection and preterm labor. *Clin Obstet Gynecol* 1988; 31:553–584.

285. Romero R, Oyarzun E, Mazor M, Sirtori M, Hobbins JC, Bracken M: Meta-analysis of the relationship between asymptomatic bacteriuria and preterm delivery/low birth weight. *Obstet Gynecol* 1989; 73:576–582.

286. Romero R, Scharf K, Mazor M, Emamian M, Hobbins JC, Ryan JL: The clinical value of gas-liquid chromatography in the detection of intra-amniotic microbial invasion. *Obstet Gynecol* 1988; 72:44–50.

287. Romero R, Sirtori M, Oyarzun E, Avila C, Mazor M, Callahan R, Sabo V, Athanassiadis AP, Hobbins JC: Prevalence, microbiology, and clinical significance of intraamniotic infection in women with preterm labor and intact membranes. *Am Obstet Gynecol* 1989; 161:817–824.

288. Rosenbert MJ, Schulz KF, Burton N: Sexually transmitted diseases in sub-saharan Africa. *Lancet* 1986; 2:152–153.

289. Rosove MH, Tabsh K, Wasserstrum N, Howard P, Hahn BH, Kalunian KC: Heparin therapy for pregnant women with lupus anticoagulant or anticardiolipin antibodies. *Obstet Gynecol* 1990; 75:630–634.

290. Rushton DI: Examination of products of conception from previable human pregnancies. *J Clin Pathol* 1981; 34:819–835.

291. Russell P, Inflammatory lesions of the human placenta. III: The histopathology of villitis of unknown aetiology. *Placenta* 1980; 1:227–244.

292. Rutter D, Griffiths P, Trompeter RS: Cytomegalic inclusion disease after recurrent maternal infection. *Lancet* 1985; 2:1182.

293. Ryan GM, Abdella TN, McNeeley SG, Baselski VS, Drummond DE: *Chlamydia trachomatis* infection in pregnancy and effect of treatment on outcome. *Am J Obstet Gynecol* 1990; 162:34–39.

294. Saigal S, Lunyk O, Bryce-Larke RP, Chernesky MA: The outcome in children with con-

genital cytomegalovirus infection: A longitudinal follow-up study. *Am J Dis Child* 1982; 136:896–901.

295. Salafia CM, Mangam HE, Weigl CA, Foye GJ, Silberman L: Abnormal fetal heart rate patterns and placental inflammation. *Am J Obstet Gynecol* 1989; 160:140–147.

296. Salafia CM, Weigl C, Silberman L: The prevalence and distribution of acute placental inflammation in uncomplicated term pregnancies. *Obstet Gynecol* 1989; 73:383–389.

297. Samra JS, Obhrai MS, Constantine G: Parvovirus infection in pregnancy. *Obstet Gynecol* 1989; 73:832–834.

298. Sander CH, Kinnane L, Stevens NG, Echt R: Haemorrhagic endovasculitis of the placenta: A review with clinical correlation. *Placenta* 1986; 7:551–574.

299. Scott JS: Placenta extra-chorialis (placenta marginata and circumvallata): A factor in ante-partum haemorrhage. *J Obstet Gynaecol Br Commonw* 1960; 67:904–918.

300. Scott JR, Branch DW, Kochenour NK, Ward K: Intravenous immunoglobulin treatment of pregnant patients with recurrent pregnancy loss caused by antiphospholipid antibodies and Rh immunization. *Am J Obstet Gynecol* 1988; 159:1055–1056.

301. Screening for congenital CMV. *Lancet* 1989; 2:599–600.

302. Scott GB, Hutto C, Makuch RW, Mastrucci MT, O'Connor T, Mitchell CD, Trapido EJ, Parks WP: Survival in children with perinatally acquired human immunodeficiency virus type 1 infection. *N Engl J Med* 1989; 321: 1791–1796.

303. Shen-Schwarz S, Macpherson TA, Mueller-Heubach E: The clinical significance of hemorrhagic endovasculitis of the placenta. *Am J Obstet Gynecol* 1988; 159:48–51.

304. Shen-Schwarz S, Ruchelli E, Brown D: Villous oedema of the placenta, a clinicopathological study. *Placenta* 1989; 10:297–307.

305. Sibai BM, Taslimi MM, El-Nazer A, Amon E, Mabie BC, Ryan GM: Maternal and perinatal outcome associated with the syndrome of hemolysis, elevated liver enzymes, and low platelets in severe preeclampsia-eclampsia. *Am J Obstet Gynecol* 1986; 155:501–509.

306. Sidiropoulos D, Herrmann U, Morell A, von Muralt G, Barandun S. Transplacental passage of intravenous immunoglobulin in the last trimester of pregnancy. *J Pediatr* 1986; 109:505–508.

307. Silver HM, Sperling RS, St Clair PJ, Gibbs RS: Evidence relating bacterial vaginosis to intraamniotic infection. *Am J Obstet Gynecol* 1989; 161:808–812.

308. Silver MM, Yeger H, Lines LD: Hemorrhagic endovasculitis-like lesion induced in placental organ culture. *Hum Pathol* 1988; 19:251–256.

309. Silver RK, Dooley SL, MacGregor SN, Depp R: Fetal acidosis in prolonged pregnancy cannot be attributed to cord compression alone. *Am J Obstet Gynecol* 1988; 159: 666–669.

310. Silver RK, Gibbs RS, Castillo M: Effect of amniotic fluid bacteria on the course of labor in nulliparous women at term. *Obstet Gynecol* 1986; 68:587–592.

311. Simpson WJ: A preliminary report on cigarette smoking and the incidence of prematurity. *Am J Obstet Gynecol* 1957; 73:808–815.

312. Smith LG, Summers PR, Miles RW, Biswas MK, Pernoll ML: Gonococcal chorioamnionitis associated with sepsis: A case report. *Am J Obstet Gynecol* 1989; 160:573–574.

313. Soyannwo MAO, Armstrong MJ, McGeown MG: Survival of the foetus in a patient in acute renal failure. *Lancet* 1966; 2:1009–1011.

314. Spark RP: Does transplacental spread of coccidioidomycosis occur? Report of a neonatal fatality and review of the literature. *Arch Pathol Lab Med* 1981; 105:347–350.

315. Spencer JAD: Perinatal listeriosis. *Br Med J* 1987; 295:349.

316. Spaun E, Klunder K: *Candida* chorioamnionitis and intrauterine contraceptive device. *Acta Obstet Gynecol Scand* 1986; 65:183–184.

317. Stafford PA, Biddinger PW, Zumwalt RE: Lethal intrauterine fetal trauma. *Am J Obstet Gynecol* 1988; 159:485–489.

318. Stagno S, Pass RF, Cloud G, Britt WJ, Henderson RE, Walton PD, Veren DA, Page F, Alford CA: Primary cytomegalovirus infection in pregnancy. *JAMA* 1986; 256:1904–1908.

319. Stern D, Nawroth P, Handley D, Kisiel W: An endothelial cell-dependent pathway of coagulation. *Proc Natl Acad Sci USA* 1985; 82: 2523–2527.

320. Strauss L, Driscoll SG: Congenital neuroblastoma involving the placenta. Reports of two cases. *Pediatrics* 1964; 34:23–31.

321. Stuart MJ, Clark DA, Sunderji SG, Allen JB, Yambo T, Elrad H, Slott JH: Decreased prostacyclin production: A characteristic of chronic placental insufficiency syndromes. *Lancet* 1981; 1:1126–1128.

322. Sumawong V, Nondasuta A, Thanapath S, Budthimedhee V: Placenta accreta. A review of the literature and a summary of ten cases. *Obstet Gynecol* 1966; 27:511–516.

323. Swartzberg JE, Remington JS: Transmission of *Toxoplasma*. *Am J Dis Child* 1975; 129: 777–779.

324. Sweet RL, Landers DV, Walker C, Schachter J: *Chlamydia trachomatis* infection and pregnancy outcome. *Am J Obstet Gynecol* 1987; 156:824–833.

325. Sweet L, Reid WE, Robertson NRC: Hydrops fetalis in association with chorangioma of the placenta. *J Pediatr* 1973; 82:91–94.

326. Sybulski S, Tremblay PC: Pathways of glucose metabolism in human placentas from normal pregnancies and from pregnancies associated with intrauterine fetal malnutrition. *Am J Obstet Gynecol* 1969; 103: 1148–1153.

327. Symonds EM: Renin and reproduction. *Am J Obstet Gynecol* 1988; 158:754–761.

328. Tafari N, Ross SM, Naeye RL, Galask RP, Zaar B. Failure of bacterial growth inhibition by amniotic fluid. *Am J Obstet Gynecol* 1977; 128:187–189.

329. Taylor RN, Green JR: Abruptio placentae following nipple stimulation. *Am J Perinat* 1987; 4:94–97.

330. Teasdale F: Histomorphometry of the human placenta in pre-eclampsia associated with severe intrauterine growth retardation. *Placenta* 1987; 8:119–128.

331. Teasdale F, Jean-Jacques G: Morphometry of the microvillous membrane of the human placenta in maternal diabetes mellitus. *Placenta* 1986; 7:81–88.

332. Thomas GB, Sbarra AJ, Feingold M, Cetrulo CL, Shakr C, Newton E, Selvaraj RJ: Antimicrobial activity of amniotic fluid against *Chlamydia trachomatis, Mycoplasma hominis*, and *Ureaplasma urealyticum*. *Am J Obstet Gynecol* 1988; 158:16–22.

333. Torpin R, Hart BF: Placenta bilobata. *Am J Obstet Gynecol* 1941; 42:38–49.

334. Toth A, O'Leary WM, Ledger WL: Evidence for microbial transfer by spermatozoa, *Obstet Gynecol* 1982; 59:556–559.

335. Tremblay PC, Sybulski S, Maughan GB: Role of the placenta in fetal malnutrition. *Am J Obstet Gynecol* 1965; 91:597–605.

336. Triplett DA: Antiphospholipid antibodies and recurrent pregnancy loss. *Am J Reprod Immunol* 1989; 20:52–67.

337. Trudinger BJ, Cook CM: Doppler umbilical and uterine flow waveforms in severe pregnancy hypertension. *Br J Obstet Gynaecol* 1990; 97:142–148.

338. Trudinger BJ, Giles WB, Cook CM, Bombardieri J, Collins L: Fetal umbilical artery flow velocity waveforms and placental resistance: clinical significance. *Br J Obstet Gynaecol* 1985; 92:23–30.

339. VanBergen WS, Fleury FJ, Cheatle EL: Fatal maternal disseminated coccidioidomycosis in a non-endemic area. *Am J Obstet Gynecol* 1976; 124:661–664.

340. van de Bor M, Guit GL, Schreuder AM, Wondergem J, Vielvoye GJ: Early detection of delayed myelination in preterm infants. *Pediatrics* 1989; 84:407–411.

341. Van Der Velde WJ, Peereboom-Stegeman JHJC, Treffers PE, James J: Basal lamina thickening in the placentae of smoking mothers. *Placenta* 1985; 6:329–340.

342. Vaughan JE, Ramirez H: Coccidioidomycosis as a complication of pregnancy. *Calif Med* 1975; 74:121–125.

343. Vetter VL, Rashkind WJ: Congenital complete heart block and connective-tissue disease. *N Engl J Med* 1983; 309:236–238.

344. Vintzileos AM, Campbell WA, Nochimson DJ, Weinbaum PJ: Preterm premature rupture of the membranes: A risk factor for the development of abruptio placentae. *Am J Obstet Gynecol* 1987; 156: 1235–1238.

345. Volpe JJ, *Neurology of the Newborn*, ed 2. Philadelphia, WB Saunders Co, 1987.

346. Volpe JJ: Intraventricular hemorrhage in the premature infant, current concepts, Part I. *Ann Neurol* 1989; 25:3–11.

347. Wallenburg HC: Chorangioma of the placenta: 13 new cases and a review of the literature from 1939–1970 with special reference to clinical complications. *Obstet Gynecol Surv* 1971; 26:411–425.

348. Walsh SW: Preeclampsia: An imbalance in placental prostacyclin and thromboxane production. *Am J Obstet Gynecol* 1985; 152: 335–340.

349. Walter PR, Garin Y, Blot P: Placental pathology changes in malaria, a histologic and ultrastructural study. *Am J Pathol* 1982; 109:330–342.

350. Wendel GD, Maberry MC, Christmas JT, Goldberg MS, Norgard MV: Examination of amniotic fluid in diagnosing congenital syphilis with fetal death. *Obstet Gynecol* 1989; 74:967–970.

351. Whyte RK, Hussain Z, deSa D: Antenatal infections with *Candida* species. *Arch Dis Child* 1982; 57:528–535.

352. Wigglesworth JS: Morphological variations of the insufficient placenta. *J Obstet Gynaecol Br Commonw* 1964; 71:87–184.

353. Wisot AL: Silent abruptio placentae with marked hypofibrinogenemia. *JAMA* 1969; 207:557–558.

354. Wittek AE, Yeager AS, Au DS, Hensleigh PA: Asymptomatic shedding of herpes simplex virus from the cervix and lesion site during pregnancy: Correlation of antepartum shedding with shedding at delivery. *Am J Dis Child* 1984; 138:439–442.

355. Woods JR, Plessinger MA, Clark KE: Effect of cocaine on uterine blood flow and fetal oxygenation. *JAMA* 1987; 257:957–961.

356. Yoder PR, Gibbs RS, Blanco JD, Castaneda YS, St. Clair PJ: A prospective controlled study of maternal and perinatal outcome after intra-amniotic infection at term. *Am J Obstet Gynecol* 1983; 145: 695–701.

357. Yow MD: Congenital cytomegalovirus disease: a NOW problem. *J Infect Dis* 1989; 159:163–167.

CHAPTER 8

Disorders of the Fetal Membranes

METHODS OF PREPARING SECTIONS FOR MICROSCOPIC EXAMINATION

Sections should be prepared from the extraplacental membranes. In the case of twins, one or more sections from the dividing membranes are also needed. In addition, sections of all grossly visible abnormalities whose nature and clinical significance are not obvious should be prepared. After inspecting the membranes, cut out a segment that is approximately 10 cm in length and 5 cm in width, starting at the point of rupture and proceeding toward the margin of the pla-

centa. Be very careful not to strip off the amnion during this procedure. Edema of the amnion is common and the amnion is very easily detached when it is edematous. Roll up the excised segment of membranes with forceps and place the roll in buffered formalin. After fixing for at least 24 hours, trim the specimen so the membranes will appear in a rolled-up configuration on the slide for microscopic examination. Figure 8–1 is a cross-sectional photograph of a normal extraplacental membrane.

DISORDERS OF THE FETAL MEMBRANES

Premature Rupture

Premature rupture of the fetal membranes is defined as membrane rupture 2 hours or more before the onset of labor.

Causes of premature rupture. – In the laboratory, membranes that have ruptured prematurely usually resist further rupture by pressures as high as those generated by labor. Most of this strength is in a zone of connective tissue beneath the amnion, and usually little or no abnormality has been found in the collagen and the elastic tissue content of membranes that have ruptured prematurely.[16] A likely explanation is that many premature ruptures start in localized abnormalities.

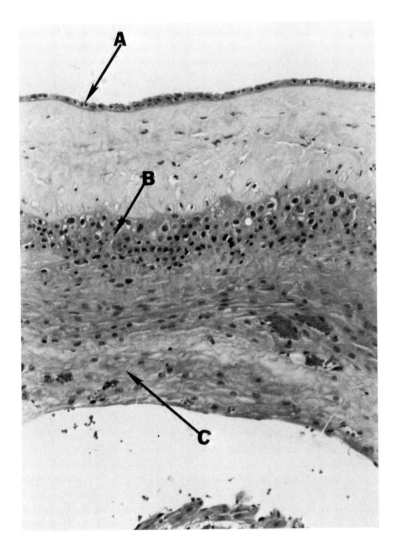

FIG 8–1.
Cross-sectional view of normal fetal membranes. Amnion *(A)*, chorion *(B)*, decidua capsularis *(C)*. Hematoxylin-eosin (HE) stain, ×300.

When the ruptures pass through these local abnormalities, normal or near-normal remnants are left behind for analysis. This possibility is supported by Bourne's finding that lesions are often present at the site of premature rupture but not elsewhere.[7] In my experience the most frequent of these local lesions is acute chorioamnionitis with associated membrane necrosis (Figs 8–2 and 8–3).[3,17,46] In the Collaborative Perinatal Study (CPS) chorioamnionitis was twice as frequent when fetal membranes ruptured 1 to 4 hours before the onset of labor as when the membranes ruptured just after labor began.[46] This is evidence that chorioamnionitis preceded about half of

the premature membrane ruptures because it takes more than 4 hours for the microscopic findings of chorioamnionitis to develop after membrane rupture. In the absence of acute chorioamnionitis premature membrane ruptures occur most often between 2 and 4 A.M. which is the time that normal labor most often begins.[11,12] Cooperstock et al. found that this early morning peak of membrane rupture was absent when acute chorioamnionitis was present.[12] This is additional evidence that acute chorioamnionitis antedates many premature membrane ruptures. In still another study maternal and umbilical cord serum levels of IgM were often elevated when membranes had been rup-

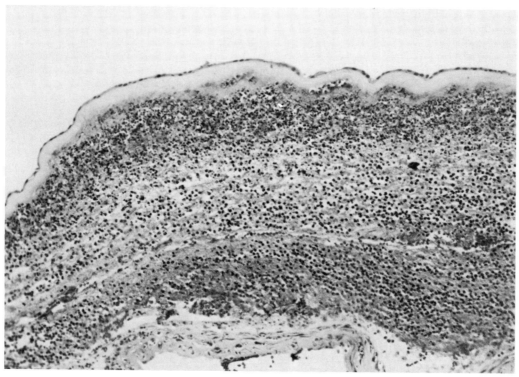

FIG 8–2.
A heavy infiltrate of neutrophils is present in the extraplacental membranes near the site of a spontaneous premature rupture of the fetal membranes. HE stain, ×120.

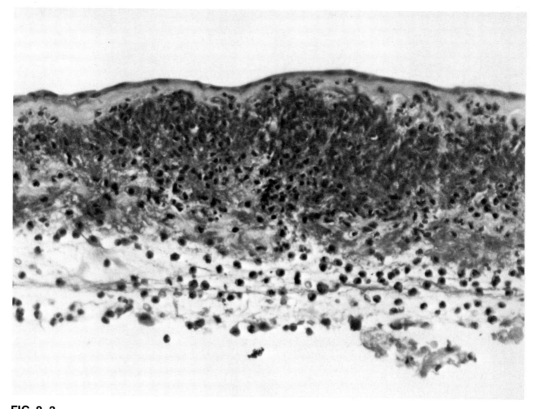

FIG 8–3.
A heavy infiltrate of neutrophils with associated necrosis immediately adjacent to the site of a spontaneous premature rupture of the fetal membranes. HE stain, ×300.

tured for only 12 to 24 hours, suggesting that infection had preceded most of these membrane ruptures.[25]

In our analyses acute chorioamnionitis accounted for 44% of the premature membrane ruptures that took place 1 to 12 hours before the onset of labor in the CPS (Table 8–1), (Fig 8–4). In these analyses the perinatal mortality rate was threefold higher when acute chorioamnionitis was present than when it was absent. This was true for both preterm births (182/1,000 vs. 66/1,000, $P < .001$) and for full-term births (24/1,000 vs. 8/1,000, $P < .001$). When acute chorioamnionitis was taken into consideration, stillbirths and neonatal deaths were less frequent when the membranes ruptured prematurely than when labor preceded membrane rupture (see Table 8–1). Premature membrane rupture was not followed by an increase in the frequency of neurologic abnormalities at 7 years of age when antecedent risk factors were taken into consideration. All of these findings support the view that acute chori-

oamnionitis and preterm delivery are the factors mainly responsible for the poor outcomes associated with premature membrane rupture.

What are the circumstances in which bacteria reach the fetal membranes and initiate acute chorioamnionitis? The vaginal pH usually decreases during pregnancy and this suppresses bacterial growth.[32] When the vaginal pH is high, the frequency of premature membrane rupture is reported to increase severalfold, presumably because the bacteria that initiate acute chorioamnionitis grow more easily.[15] Specifically, larger numbers of anaerobic bacteria, mycoplasmas, *Chlamydia trachomatis* and *Trichomonas vaginalis* are apt to be present when the vaginal pH is high during pregnancy.[15,22,56] Coitus can also temporarily raise vaginal pH.[19]

The microbial products that initiate acute chorioamnionitis appear to activate collagen degradation by recruiting inflammatory cells that both produce and

TABLE 8–1.

Risk Estimates for Antecedents to the Development of Fetal Membrane Rupture 1 to 12 Hours Before Onset of Labor*

Risk Factors	No. of Cases of Premature Membrane Rupture per 1,000 Cases With Risk Factor†	Relative Risks (95% Confidence Intervals)	Attributable Risks (95% Confidence Intervals)
All cases	98 (*5,829*)		
Maternal factors			
Smoked during pregnancy	**117** (*1,325*), $P < .001$	**1.3** (1.2, 1.4)	**.05** (.04, .06)
Age ($\geq$ 35 yr)	**124** (*448*), $P < .001$	**1.3** (1.2, 1.5)	**.02** (.01, .02)
Incompetent cervix	**201** (*48*), $P < .001$	**2.2** (1.2, 4.1)	**.01** (.00, .01)
Placental factor			
Acute chorioamnionitis	**160** (*1,349*), $P < .001$	**1.9** (1.8, 2.1)	**.44** (.41, .47)
Markers for high fetal motor activity			
Diffuse subchorionic fibrin	**109** (*862*), $P < .001$	**1.2** (1.1, 1.3)	**.04** (.03, .05)
Unusually long umbilical cord	**111** (*662*), $P < .01$	**1.1** (1.0, 1.2)	**.02** (.01, .03)
Other indicators			**.02** (.00, .05)
Population attributable risk			***.59*** (*.56, .63*)
Pregnancy Outcomes			
Preterm birth	**113** (*1,380*), $P < .001$	**1.2** (1.1, 1.3)	
Fetal growth retardation	**124** (*560*), $P < .001$	**1.3** (1.2, 1.4)	
Stillbirth	**28** (*62*), $P < .001$	**0.7** (0.5, 1.0)	
Neonatal death	**66** (*71*), $P < .001$	**0.7** (0.5, 1.0)	
Neurologic abnormalities at 7 yrs	**114** (*193*), $P < .02$	1.0 (0.8, 1.2)	

Significant values are in boldface.
†Numbers of cases are in parentheses.

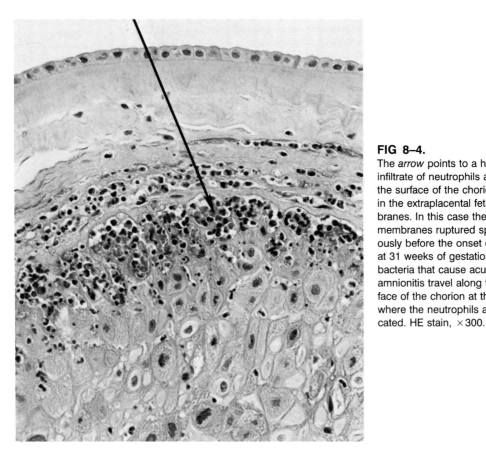

FIG 8–4.
The *arrow* points to a heavy infiltrate of neutrophils along the surface of the chorion in the extraplacental fetal membranes. In this case the fetal membranes ruptured spontaneously before the onset of labor at 31 weeks of gestation. The bacteria that cause acute chorioamnionitis travel along the surface of the chorion at the site where the neutrophils are located. HE stain, ×300.

stimulate the production of collagenase.[53,63,64] It is noteworthy that the presence of *Staphylococcus aureus* and *Escherichia coli* potentiate the in vitro weakening of the fetal membranes, whereas group B streptococci do not.[51,52] This might explain why *E. coli* and *S. aureus* are common isolates from the membranes and placenta in cases of acute chorioamnionitis, whereas group B streptococci have not been shown to cross intact fetal membranes and initiate acute chorioamnionitis.

Local lesions caused by acute chorioamnionitis are not the only explanation for premature membrane ruptures. There are published reports that zinc deficiency is associated with acute chorioamnionitis and that it interferes with protein production.[54] Collagen is both degraded and regenerated at a rate higher than normal in membranes that rupture prematurely.[62] Fetal movements that strike the fetal membranes and coital-induced orgasm appear to be additional mechanisms that prematurely rupture the fetal membranes.[9,45] Two markers for vigorous motor activity by the fetus, namely long umbilical cords (>90th percentile) and diffuse fibrin beneath the chorionic (fetal) plate of the placenta, had positive correlations with premature membrane rupture (see Table 8–1).

It has been known for some years that female orgasm can induce uterine contractions, and we have postulated that fetal membranes locally weakened by infection are more likely to be ruptured by uterine contractions than are undamaged membranes.[18,20] A prospective study which we conducted found a strong, positive correlation between maternal orgasm and premature membrane rupture when acute chorioamnionitis was present (Fig 8–5).[44,45] Other risk factors for premature membrane rupture in the CPS

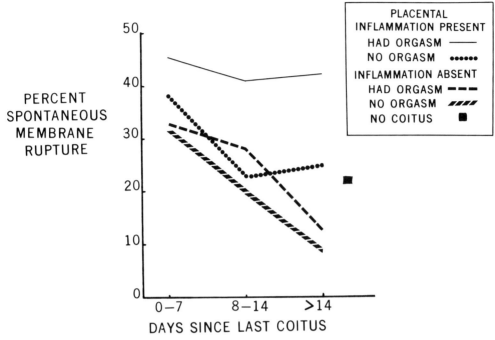

FIG 8–5.
Premature rupture of the fetal membranes was most frequent when acute chorioamnionitis was present and women had coital-induced orgasm.

were maternal cigarette smoking during pregnancy and gravidas being 35 years of age or older (see Table 8–1). A recent study found that cerclage performed for an incompetent cervix did not improve the outcome of preterm premature membrane ruptures.[5]

Prevention of Preterm Labor Following Premature Membrane Rupture. — The labor that follows premature membrane rupture is usually initiated by acute chorioamnionitis, even when the chorioamnionitis follows rather than antedates the membrane rupture. Days or weeks sometimes pass between the time that membranes rupture and delivery takes place. During this interval acute chorioamnionitis usually develops if it did not antedate the rupture.[4] Antibiotics administered prophylactically after preterm membrane rupture reportedly delay the onset of labor and reduce the incidence of infections in neonates.[1,41] It is worth repeating that perinatal mortality rates were much lower in the CPS when premature membrane

rupture was not accompanied by acute chorioamnionitis than when acute chorioamnionitis was present.

Prognosis. — Premature membrane rupture before 27 weeks of gestation had a very poor prognosis in a 1984 study.[59] Only about 25% of the liveborns survived and the majority of the survivors subsequently had psychomotor abnormalities.[59] Outcomes were somewhat better in a 1988 study of children born after premature membrane rupture at this early gestational age.[42] A third survived and only a third of these survivors had a developmental abnormality during the first year of life. Seven of the 12 impaired children had cerebral palsy and three had lesser neurologic abnormalities. It remains to be seen if more subtle psychomotor abnormalities emerge as the initially normally developing children grow older. Severe neonatal respiratory distress, cerebral intraventricular hemorrhage, pneumonia, sepsis, necrotizing enterocolitis, a persistent fetal circulation, and bronchopulmonary dysplasia are common in those who are born after premature membrane rupture at very early gestational ages. Severe antenatal hypoxia caused by severe placental villous edema and the immaturity of the cerebral circulation are the major risk factors for psychomotor impairments after very early premature membrane rupture. In the CPS premature membrane rupture did not increase the frequency of neurologic abnormalities at 7 years of age when gestational age and placental villous edema were taken into consideration (see Table 8–1). It is important to note that very few deliveries can be delayed for more than 2 to 3 weeks after the membranes have ruptured.[42] In one study only 7% of pregnancies had labor delayed more than 48 hours following premature membrane rupture.[13] The presence of group B streptococci in the cervix at the time of rupture increases the risk of maternal endometritis and group B streptococcal infection in the neonate.[47]

Under some circumstances pulmonary hypoplasia can follow premature membrane rupture.[31] When all or most of the amniotic fluid is lost, pressure on the fetal thorax by the uterus can slow lung expansion, maturation, and growth.[48,49] The inhibition of normal breathing movements and an abnormal balance of fluid volume and pressure within the pulmonary alveoli are reportedly responsible for the slow growth and maturation of the fetal lungs.[29,31] The diagnosis of pulmonary hypoplasia following premature membrane rupture is based on clinical, radiologic, and postmortem findings. Suggestive clinical signs include a subnormal chest circumference, neonatal respiratory insufficiency that is severe enough to require high ventilatory pressures, and persistent pulmonary arterial hypertension.[50] Radiologic findings include small, well-aerated lung fields, markedly elevated diaphragms, and downward sloping ribs.[30] The diagnosis is confirmed by finding very small lungs for body size at postmortem examination. Compression deformities of the chest are not always present at birth, and when they are

present they usually disappear as the child grows older.

Oligohydramnios of only a week's duration can lead to pulmonary hypoplasia.[31] In fact, the duration of oligohydramnios has less effect on the development of pulmonary hypoplasia than does the timing of its appearance. More than 80% of neonates will have hypoplastic lungs if oligohydramnios develops and is persistent in the first trimester of pregnancy.[50] The frequency of lung hypoplasia progressively decreases as the onset of oligohydramnios is delayed. Approximately 25% of neonates will have clinically symptomatic lung hypoplasia when oligohydramnios starts at 22 weeks of gestation. The figure drops to 10% when oligohydramnios starts at 25 weeks and to nearly zero when oligohydramnios starts after 28 weeks of gestation. The mortality rate with symptomatic hypoplastic lungs exceeds 60% in most published studies.[50] Mortality is reported to be lowest when the infant was observed to make breathing movements before birth.[6]

Necrosis

Necrosis of the amnion was observed in 14.3% of the extraplacental fetal membranes in the CPS (Fig 8–6). Antecedent risk factors included acute chorioamnionitis, meconium in the fetal membranes, postterm birth, fetal malformations, and markers for vigorous fetal motor activity (Table 8–2). The markers for vigorous movements were unusually long umbilical cords and excessive fibrin beneath the chorionic (fetal) plate of the placenta. Long umbilical cords often appear to be the consequence of vigorous fetal movements that put tension on the umbilical cord, while there is evidence that diffusely distributed subchorionic fibrin is often the result of fetal movements that traumatize the fetal surface of the placenta (see Chapters 6,7).

In preterm born children the frequency of amnion necrosis was 167/1,000 in fetal membranes without chorioamnionitis, 242/1,000 when chorioamnionitis was mi-

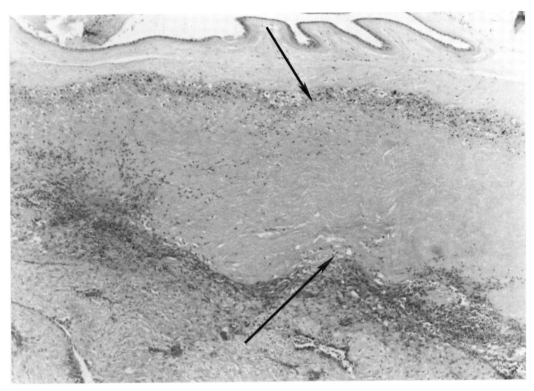

FIG 8–6.
A large area of necrosis is present in the extraplacental membranes between the *arrows*. Inflammation is absent.
HE stain, ×120.

croscopically mild, and 331/1,000 when chorioamnionitis was severe (*P* < .001). The comparable figures for full-term born infants were 58/1,000, 71/1,000, and 97/ 1,000 (*P* < .001). After taking acute chorioamnionitis and the other antenatal risk factors into consideration, amnion necrosis in the fetal membranes was not associated with any unfavorable pregnancy outcome (see Table 8–2).

Gross Edema

Gross edema of the fetal membranes was observed in 5.8% of the births in the CPS. The most frequent antecedent risk factors were preeclampsia, eclampsia, and acute chorioamnionitis (Table 8–3). The frequency of such edema increased in preterm born children from 34/1,000 in those without microscopic chorioamnionitis to 44/1,000 in those with mild chorioamnionitis, and to 64/1,000 in those with severe chorioamnionitis (*P* < .01). The

comparable figures for full-term born infants were 58/1,000, 72/1,000 and 95/ 1,000 (*P* < .001). This edema had prognostic significance for perinatal mortality only when acute chorioamnionitis was present. The perinatal mortality rate was 57/1,000 when acute chorioamnionitis was present vs. 29/1,000 when it was absent (*P* < .001). After taking acute chorioamnionitis, preeclampsia, eclampsia, and major fetal malformations into consideration, gross edema of the fetal membranes was not associated with any unfavorable pregnancy outcome (see Table 8–3).

Microscopic edema of the fetal membranes is many times more frequent than grossly visible edema. It characteristically separates the amnion from the chorion (Fig 8–7). It is so often associated with acute chorioamnionitis that we always make a thorough search for chorioamnionitis when edema is present in the fetal membranes (Fig 8–8).

TABLE 8–2.

Risk Estimates for Antecedents to the Development of Necrosis of the Fetal Membranes (Amnion)*

Risk Factors	No. of Cases of Membrane Necrosis per 1,000 Cases With Risk Factor†	Relative Risks (95% Confidence Intervals)	Attributable Risks (95% Confidence Intervals)
All cases	143 (*6,603*)		
Maternal factor			
Preeclampsia, eclampsia	**293** (1,905), *P* < .001	**1.1** (1.1, 1.2)	**.03** (.01, .04)
Fetal factors			
Postterm birth	**324** (921), *P* < .001	**1.3** (1.1, 1.4)	**.02** (.01, .03)
Minor fetal malformations	**301** (*1,756*), *P* < .001	**1.1** (1.0, 1.2)	**.02** (.01, .03)
Major fetal malformations	**289** (595), *P* < .05	**1.1** (1.0, 1.2)	**.01** (.00, .02)
Placental factors			
Acute chorioamnionitis	**347** (*2,341*), *P* < .001	**1.6** (1.5, 1.7)	**.14** (.12, .16)
Meconium in fetal membranes	**325** (*1,611*), *P* < .001	**1.3** (1.2, 1.4)	**.05** (.04, .07)
Markers for vigorous fetal motor activity			
Diffuse subchorionic fibrin	**304** (*1,756*), *P* < .001	**1.2** (1.1, 1.3)	.04 (.03, .06)
Unusually long umbilical cord	**287** (*1,772*), *P* < .001	**1.1** (1.0, 1.2)	**.02** (.00, .03)
Other indicators			.01 (.00, .03)
Population attributable risk			**.34** (*.31, .37*)
Pregnancy outcomes			
Preterm birth (only full-term births were included in the analyses)			
Fetal growth retardation	270 (*604*), *P* > .1	1.0 (0.8, 1.2)	
Stillbirth	**120** (*21*), *P* < .01	**0.8** (0.6, 1.0)	
Neonatal death	99 (*18*), *P* < .1	**0.7** (0.6, 0.9)	
Neurologic abnormalities at 7 yrs	**264** (*181*), *P* < .001	1.0 (0.7, 1.4)	

*Significant values are in boldface.
†Numbers of cases are in parentheses.

TABLE 8–3.

Risk Estimates for Antecedents to the Development of Gross Edema in the Fetal Membranes*

Risk Factors	No. of Cases of Edema of the Fetal Membranes per 1,000 Cases with Risk Factor†	Relative Risks (95% Confidence Intervals)	Attributable Risks (95% Confidence Intervals)
All cases	58 (*2,857*)		
Maternal factor			
Preeclampsia, eclampsia	**85** (*746*), *P* < .001	**1.4** (1.2, 1.6)	**.09** (.04, .15)
Fetal factor			
Major fetal malformations	**71** (*229*), *P* < .02	**1.2** (1.0, 1.4)	**.01** (.00, .02)
Placental factor			
Acute chorioamnionitis	**72** (*656*), *P* < .001	**1.3** (1.2, 1.5)	**.06** (.05, .07)
Population attributable risk			**.16** (*.11, .21*)
Pregnancy outcomes			
Preterm birth	**42** (*429*), *P* < .001	0.7 (0.4, 1.1)	
Fetal growth retardation	**44** (*178*), *P* < .001	1.3 (0.9, 1.8)	
Stillbirth	**105** (*90*), *P* < .001	0.8 (0.3, 1.6)	
Neonatal death	**55** (*49*), *P* > .1	1.0 (0.5, 1.5)	
Neurologic abnormalities at 7 yrs	**59** (*90*), *P* > .1	0.9 (0.7, 1.2)	

*Significant values are in boldface.
†Numbers of cases are in parentheses.

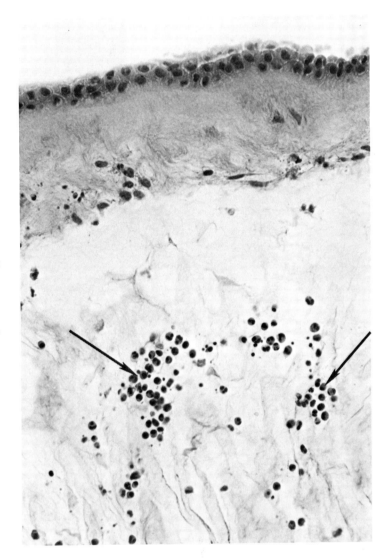

FIG 8–7.
Severe edema has separated the amnion from the chorion in the extraplacental membranes. The *arrows* point to two of the many nests of neutrophils in the wide zone of edema. The chorion is not visible. HE stain, ×600.

Meconium in the Amniotic Fluid

Meconium is the bile-stained contents of the fetal intestine. Its appearance in the amniotic fluid is the result of fetal defecation. It is assumed by most to be the consequence of fetal stress and by some to be specific evidence of fetal hypoxia or asphyxia. The stress that initiates defecation does not need to be severe and stress severe enough to cause stillbirth does not always result in meconium being passed into the amniotic fluid.[4] A hormone in the fetal blood called *motilin* reportedly initiates the intestinal motor activity that leads to the passage of meconium into the amniotic fluid.[35,36] Its low levels in the

blood prior to late gestation is the presumed reason why meconium is rarely present in the amniotic fluid before 34 weeks of gestation. In a recent study, cord blood levels of motilin had a positive correlation with meconium in the amniotic fluid, but had no correlation with antecedent fetal stress.[36]

In the literature, meconium in the amniotic fluid has been associated with premature rupture of the fetal membranes, acute chorioamnionitis, abruptio placentae, and the use of cocaine.[38,46] In the CPS, 64% of the cases of meconium in the amniotic fluid were associated with the presence of acute chorioamnionitis, 6%

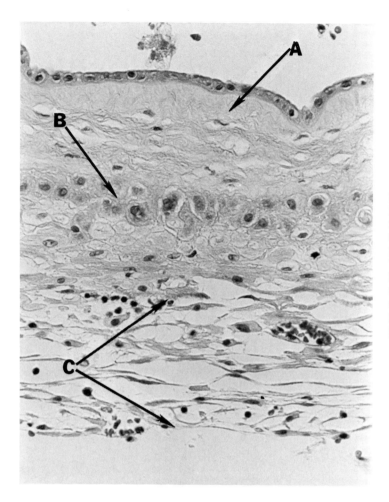

FIG 8–8.
In this case the edema is in the decidua capsularis *(C)* rather than between the amnion *(A)* and the chorion *(B)*. There are many neutrophils infiltrating the edematous decidua. The findings of acute chorioamnionitis were present in the chorionic plate of the placenta. HE stain, × 600.

with postterm birth, 6% with disorders that cause low blood flow from the uterus to the placenta, and smaller percentages with advanced maternal age, maternal cigarette smoking during pregnancy, and major congenital malformations in the fetus (Table 8–4). Only 0.2% of the meconium-stained amniotic fluids were attributable to birth asphyxial disorders. This would explain why correlations have usually been poor between meconium staining of the amniotic fluid, electronically monitored fetal heart rate abnormalities in labor, low umbilical arterial cord blood pH values, and low Apgar scores.[57] In one study only 3 of 323 neonates with meconium-stained amniotic fluid had metabolic acidemia.[66] Meconium in the amniotic fluid should never be interpreted as evidence of intrapartum hypoxia or asphyxia unless there is conclusive evidence of such hypoxemia and acidosis in fetal scalp blood or umbilical arterial blood.

After all of the antecedent risk factors had been taken into account, meconium in the amniotic fluid had only one unfavorable pregnancy outcome, the presence of neurologic abnormalities at 7 years of age (see Table 8–4). These neurologic abnormalities were of three types: quadriplegic cerebral palsy, lesser motor disorders with associated severe mental retardation and chronic seizure disorders. These neurologic abnormalities are likely to be the consequence of vasoconstrictive effects of the meconium (see Chapter 11).

Studies have shown that meconium staining of the placental surface can occur within an hour of the time that meconium

TABLE 8–4.

Risk Estimates for Antecedents to Meconium in the Amniotic Fluid*

Risk Factors	No. of Cases of Meconium in the Amniotic Fluid per 1,000 Cases With Risk Factor†	Relative Risks (95% Confidence Intervals)	Attributable Risks (95% Confidence Intervals)
All cases	191 *(10,401)*		
Maternal factors			
Age ≥ 35 yr	**270** *(879)*, *P* < .001	**1.6** (1.4, 1.8)	**.03** (.02, .04)
Smoked during pregnancy	**208** *(2,218)*, *P* < .001	**1.2** (1.1, 1.3)	**.02** (.01, .03)
Preeclampsia, eclampsia	**267** *(2,087)*, *P* < .001	**1.4** (1.3, 1.5)	**.06** (.05, .07)
Fetal factors			
Postterm birth	**255** *(1,633)*, *P* < .001	**1.2** (1.1, 1.3)	**.06** (.04, .08)
Major fetal malformations	**222** *(1,106)*, *P* < .001	**1.2** (1.1, 1.3)	**.03** (.02, .04)
Birth asphyxial disorder	**454** *(49)*, *P* < .001	**6.4** (2.9, 14.0)	.002
Placental factor			
Acute chorioamnionitis	**567** *(7,371)*, *P* < .001	**2.7** (2.3, 3.0)	**.64** (.62, .67)
Population attributable risk			**.80** (.76, .85)
Pregnancy outcomes			
Preterm birth	**146** *(1,691)*, *P* < .001	0.8 (0.5, 1.3)	
Fetal growth retardation	**201** *(898)*, *P* < .02	1.0 (0.9, 1.1)	
Stillbirth	**427** *(374)*, *P* < .001	0.9 (0.5, 1.4)	
Neonatal death	**232** *(235)*, *P* < .02	0.8 (0.8, 1.2)	
Neurologic abnormalities at 7 yrs	**230** *(381)*, *P* < .001	**1.2** (1.0, 1.4)	
Motor abnormalities + severe mental retardation		**1.5** (1.1, 2.0)	
Hyperactivity		**1.4** (1.0, 1.8)	

*Significant values are in boldface.
†Numbers of cases are in parentheses.

enters the amniotic fluid.[39] The frequency of such staining increases with the length of exposure to meconium and with its concentration in the amniotic fluid. Within 3 hours meconium can be picked up by macrophages and transported into the chorionic plate of the placenta. It appears as faint yellow-green pigment in macrophages (Fig 8–9). Occasionally it appears as amorphous material between the amnion and chorion in the extraplacental membranes. Within 12 to 20 hours the amnion can show signs of pseudostratification, cell degeneration, and even necrosis.[39] Macrophages with meconium can continue to be found in the amnion or chorion for up to a week after meconium is no longer visible in the amniotic fluid. Because of these findings the presence of meconium in the amniotic fluid and membranes usually has little value in establishing the time when the fetus first experi-

enced the event that led to passage of meconium into the amniotic fluid.

The Meconium Aspiration Syndrome

The presence of meconium in the trachea below the vocal cords, accompanied by tachypnea in the newborn period, is widely known as the *meconium aspiration syndrome.* Many of the affected children have a low Apgar score at birth and most are born at or near term. The syndrome had a frequency of 9/1,000 births in the CPS, which was approximately 5% of the cases of meconium-stained amniotic fluid in the study. This is close to the frequencies reported by previous investigators.[65] The syndrome has long been recognized to be associated with a high perinatal mortality.[14] Sixty-three percent of the neonates with the meconium aspiration syndrome in the CPS died, which is a much

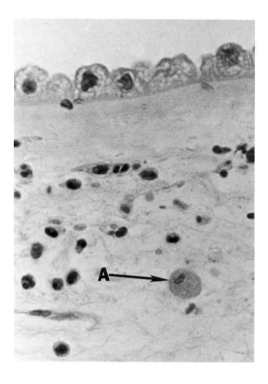

FIG 8–9.
A meconium-filled macrophage *(A)* is in an edematous zone beneath the amnion of the extraplacental membranes in a case of acute chorioamnionitis. There are many neutrophils in this edematous zone in addition to the macrophage with meconium. HE stain, ×1,200.

higher death rate than has been reported with the syndrome during the last few years.[65] Fifty-nine percent of the mortality in CPS children who had the meconium aspiration syndrome was attributable to moderate or severe acute chorioamnionitis. The rest was attributable to major malformations in the child, placental abruptions, or disorders that produce chronic low uteroplacental blood flow. In the CPS there were no neonatal deaths associated with the meconium aspiration syndrome when children with major malformations, children exposed to acute chorioamnionitis, to low uteroplacental blood flow disorders, and to abruptio placentae were excluded from the analysis.

The meconium aspiration syndrome is often assumed to be the result of the fetus being hypoxic during labor, gasping and aspirating meconium which then obstructs airways.[10,61] Such obstruction is very rare at postmortem examination in infants who die with the syndrome, including those who had a documented acute asphyxial event such as abruptio placentae, a tight knot in the umbilical

cord, or umbilical cord prolapse. Any pulmonary inflammation that is present has been in cases in which acute chorioamnionitis was also present, so the pneumonia was presumably the result of the fetus having aspirated infected amniotic fluid. The instillation of meconium into the airways of experimental animals causes no more pulmonary inflammation or necrosis than is produced by the aspiration of clear amniotic fluid.[27] In the CPS aspiration in the presence of acute chorioamnionitis increased the frequency of neonatal respiratory distress tenfold, so in many cases the tachypnea or respiratory distress associated with meconium aspiration is probably due to the aspiration of infected amniotic fluid.

Chronic disorders are often responsible for the meconium aspiration syndrome. In one study 10 of 11 infants who had persistent pulmonary arterial hypertension after aspirating meconium had a marked increase of muscle in their small pulmonary arteries at postmortem examination.[43] In the CPS, 30% of full-term born neonates who had the meconium aspiration syndrome had hemoglobin values of 21 g/dL or greater vs. 19% of age-matched controls ($P < .01$). These high hemoglobin values raise the possibility of protracted antenatal hypoxemia. There are also many reports that major congenital malformations are common with the meconium aspiration syndrome.[65] In the CPS, chronic risk factors were more frequent with the meconium aspiration syndrome than with meconium in the amniotic fluid without aspiration. Of the meconium aspiration cases, 19% were associated with major fetal malformations vs. 3% for cases of meconium in the amniotic fluid without aspiration. Of the children with the meconium aspiration syndrome, 10% were born postterm vs. 6% of the children in whom meconium was present in the amniotic fluid but not aspirated. Of the meconium aspiration syndrome cases, 7% were attributable to maternal cigarette smoking vs. 2% of cases in which meconium was in the amniotic fluid but not aspirated. This indicates that chronic fetal disorders and conditions had a much larger role in the genesis of the meconium aspiration syndrome than in the passage of meconium into the amniotic fluid without aspiration. Birth asphyxial disorders were associated with 3.0% of the cases in which meconium was aspirated vs. 0.2% of the cases in which meconium was present in the amniotic fluid but not aspirated. Thus, the meconium aspiration syndrome should never be automatically assumed to be the consequence of antenatal hypoxia or asphyxia.

Both the frequency and the case fatality rate of the meconium aspiration syndrome appear to have markedly decreased in the last two decades.[65] Some might attribute this to the introduction of routine intubation and suctioning of the oropharynx and trachea, but the many other changes in perinatal care could also have contributed to this improvement. This includes the current frequent administration of antibiotics in neonates with respiratory distress and the other managements of the neonatal respiratory distress syndrome. Survivors of the meconium aspiration syndrome are reported often to have long-term pulmonary sequelae, including evidence of chronic airway obstruction, hyperinflation, elevated airway closing volumes, and airway hyperactivity.[58] These abnormalities are usually much less severe than the pulmonary abnormalities that are associated with bronchopulmonary dysplasia.

Hemosiderin in the Fetal Membranes

Hemosiderin is a breakdown product of hemolyzed red cells. It can be easily identified by iron stains. It was identified in the fetal membranes of 1.9% of the births in the CPS (Table 8–5). Its presence is a marker for antecedent hemorrhage. Identified risk factors for hemosiderin in the fetal membranes were unevenly accelerated placental maturation, acute chorioamnionitis, abruptio placentae, circumvallate placenta, and various markers for vigorous fetal motor activity (see Table 8–5). Taken together, these risk factors accounted for 42% of the deliveries in the CPS in which the fetal membranes had macrophages with hemosiderin. Each of the risk factors for hemosiderin in the fetal membranes has an easily explained relationship to the finding. Unevenly accelerated placental maturation is a marker for chronic low uteroplacental blood flow. This is a disorder that is also associated with placental infarcts, which are a frequent source of hemosiderin. Hemorrhage at the edge of the placenta is a postulated cause of circumvallate placenta, so such a hemorrhage may be the connection of circumvallate placentas with hemosiderin in the fetal membranes. Trauma to the fetal membranes by vigorous fetal movements is the presumed reason why markers of vigorous fetal activity were associated with hemosiderin in the fetal membranes (see Chapter 7). Hemosiderin in the fetal membranes was associated with a high rate of stillbirths, but most of this high rate disap-

TABLE 8–5.

Risk Estimates for Antecedents to the Development of Hemosiderin in the Fetal Membranes*

Risk Factors	No. of Cases of Hemosiderin in the Fetal Membranes per 1,000 Cases With Risk Factor†	Relative Risks (95% Confidence Intervals)	Attributable Risks (95% Confidence Intervals)
All cases	19 *(991)*		
Placental factors			
Unevenly accelerated maturation	**69** *(355)*, *P* < .001	**1.8** (1.5, 2.0)	**.16** (.14, .19)
Acute chorioamnionitis	**72** *(356)*, *P* < .001	**1.7** (1.5, 2.0)	**.15** (.12, .17)
Abruptio placentae	**31** *(29)*, *P* < .01	**1.6** (1.1, 2.3)	**.01** (.00, .02)
Circumvallate placenta	**29** *(34)*, *P* < .02	**1.5** (1.1, 2.2)	**.01** (.01, .02)
Markers for vigorous fetal motor activity			
Unusually long umbilical cord	**59** *(298)*, *P* < .001	**1.3** (1.1, 1.5)	**.06** (.04, .08)
Other indicators			**.05** (.03, .07)
Population attributable risk			**.42** *(.39, .45)*
Pregnancy Outcomes			
Preterm birth	45 *(190)*, *P* > .1	0.9 (0.5, 1.2)	
Fetal growth retardation	53 *(91)*, *P* > .1	0.9 (0.7, 1.1)	
Stillbirth	**119** *(32)*, *P* < .001	**1.4** (1.1, 1.9)	
Neonatal death	53 *(18)*, *P* > .1	1.1 (0.8, 1.5)	
Neurologic abnormalities at 7 yrs	53 *(30)*, *P* > .1	1.1 (0.6, 1.7)	

Significant values are in boldface.
†*Numbers of cases are in parentheses.*

peared when confounding risk factors were taken into consideration (see Table 8–5).

Squamous Metaplasia of the Amnion

Squamous metaplasia is focal keratinization of the amnion (Fig 8–10). Grossly it appears as small pale plaques on the fetal surface of the placenta. Unlike the plaques of amnion nodosum, the plaques of squamous metaplasia are difficult to rub off the placenta. Grossly visible squamous metaplasia had a frequency of 0.9% in the CPS. Microscopic plaques of squamous metaplasia are present in up to 60% of placentas.[4] The plaques are most frequent near the insertion of the umbilical cord. In the CPS the antecedents of squamous metaplasia of the fetal membranes were being black, preeclampsia, eclampsia, and full-term birth (Table 8–6). These findings support the thesis that such plaques are a normal maturational finding. There were no unfavorable pregnancy outcomes associated with squamous metaplasia of the amnion (see Table 8–6).

Amnion Nodosum

Amnion nodosum manifests as nodular elevations or plaques of debris and cells on the fetal surface of the placenta. The underlying disorder is oligohydramnios. When amniotic fluid is absent, exfoliated cells from the fetal skin and amnion are not washed off the surface of the placenta.[42] On gross inspection the plaques are 1 to 5 mm in diameter, round or ovoid, yellow-gray, shiny, waxy to the touch, and easily detached, sometimes leaving a small depression on the surface of the placenta at the site of removal (Fig 8–11). The ease with which the nodules of amnion nodosum are detached from the surface of the placenta helps distinguish it from the plaques of squamous metaplasia, which do not readily detach from the placental surface. Microscopically, amnion nodosum appears as granular or

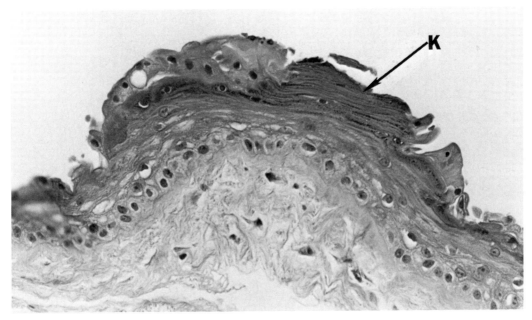

FIG 8–10.
Focal keratinization *(K)* of the amnion, known as *squamous metaplasia.* HE stain, ×600.

amorphous, eosin-staining material that is sometimes fibrillar in appearance with embedded cells and fragments of cells (Fig 8–12). The lesions stain positively with periodic acid-Schiff and Alcian blue stains. They do not elicit an inflammatory reaction.

Amnionic Band Syndrome

The amnionic band syndrome is the triad of an amnion-denuded placenta, a fetus entangled in remnants of the amnion, and fetal deformities, malformations, or disruption. Some prefer to call this the *early amnion rupture sequence* and

TABLE 8–6.
Risk Estimates for Antecedents to the Development of Squamous Metaplasia of the Amnion*

Risk Factors	No. of Cases With Squamous Metaplasia of the Amnion per 1,000 Cases with Risk Factor†	Relative Risks (95% Confidence Intervals)	Attributable Risks (95% Confidence Intervals)
All cases	8 (452)		
Maternal factors			
Race: black	**12** (317), P<.001	**2.8** (2.8, 3.4)	**.45** (.42, .48)
Full term birth	9 (397), P<.02	**1.7** (1.3, 2.2)	**.08** (.06, .10)
Preeclampsia, eclampsia	**11** (122), P<.02	**1.3** (1.0, 1.6)	**.06** (.05, .07)
Population attributable risk			*.58 (.56, .61)*
Pregnancy outcomes			
Preterm birth	8 (80), P>1	0.9 (0.2, 1.7)	
Fetal growth retardation	**6** (24), P<.02	**0.6** (0.3, 1.0)	
Stillbirth	8 (7), P>1<.001	0.9 (0.2, 1.8)	
Neonatal death	14 (13), P>1	1.5 (0.8, 2.3)	
Neurologic abnormalities at 7 yrs	11 (17), P>.1	1.2 (0.6, 1.9)	

*Significant values are in boldface.
†Numbers of cases are in parentheses.

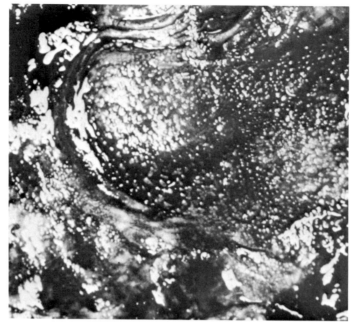

FIG 8–11.
The waxy plaques on the surface of the placenta are characteristic of amnion nodosum.

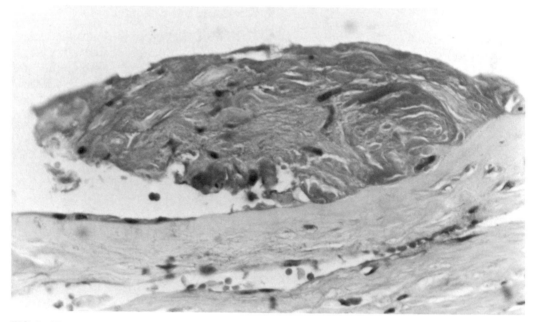

FIG 8–12.
The plaques of amnion nodosum are comprised of fibrillar debris with embedded cells and fragments of cells. HE stain, ×600.

define it as a spectrum of fetal anomalies and malformations resulting from one of the following: (a) constriction by amniotic bands, (b) constriction by aberrant amniotic sheets, (c) deformity that is the result of swallowing the loose end of an amniotic membrane string, or (d) the mechanical effects of fetal containment.[24,26,40] Whichever of the two terms is used to identify the disorder, its most common clinical fea-

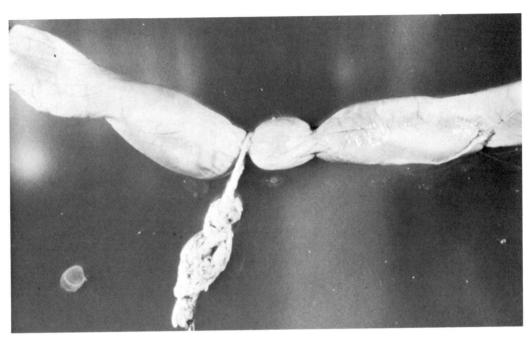

FIG 8–13.
An amnionic band constricts the umbilical cord. The result was stillbirth.

tures include syndactyly and acrosyndac-tyly (fused digits); craniofacial defects such as cleft palate and cleft lip, clubfoot, and visceral and cranial anomalies; con-striction of the umbilical cord; and fetal or neonatal death (Fig 8–13). Transverse amputations of body parts are presumed to be the result of mechanical constriction by an amniotic band.[60] Acrosyndactyly is claimed to be the result of digits being tied together by amniotic bands. Abdominal wall and visceral abnormalities are pos-tulated often to be the consequence of truncal bands. The time at which the amnion is torn could explain the character of many of the malformations. Anenceph-aly could date back to as early as the third week of gestation, limb reduction anoma-lies and body wall defects to the fifth week, and omphalocele and amputations from 7 weeks onward.[55]

Hypotheses not related to amniotic bands have been suggested to explain the genesis of many of the aforementioned malformations and deformations. How-ever, the asymmetric distribution of the abnormalities, their frequent peripheral location, and the fact that no two victims have exactly the same malformations have convinced most observers that the amni-otic band theory best explains their origin. The frequency of the disorder has been estimated to be about 1 in 10,000 births. It is most frequent in males, the offspring of young mothers, and in blacks.[21] Chil-dren with epidermolysis bullosa are par-ticularly prone to develop the syndrome because they have abnormally fragile amnions.[37]

Those who dissent from the constrict-ing band hypothesis to explain the syn-drome cite the fact that affected twins are predominantly monozygous, and monozy-gous twinning has a teratogenic ori-gin.[33,34] Other arguments against a purely amniotic band origin of the syndrome cite features of the syndrome that have been produced in experimental animals by re-moving part of the amniotic fluid at mid-gestation and by the intraamniotic in-jection of a variety of vasoactive sub-stances.[23,28] In this last model the devel-opment of amnionic bands appears to be a secondary event, analogous to adhesion formation.[34] From this multitude of evi-dence some investigators have concluded that the amniotic band syndrome is the result of many different processes that are responsible for developmental malformations, and fetal ectodermal and mesenchymal disruption. Based on this pathogenesis Lockwood et al. have proposed renaming the syndrome the "fetal disruption complex."[34]

REFERENCES

1. Amon E, Lewis SV, Sibai BM, Villar MA, Arheart KL: Ampicillin prophylaxis in preterm premature rupture of the membranes: A prospective randomized study. *Am J Obstet Gynecol* 1988; 159:539–543.

2. Appelbaum PC, Holloway Y, Ross SM, Dhupelia I. The effect of amniotic fluid on bacterial growth in three population groups. *Am J Obstet Gynecol* 1977; 128:868–871.

3. Benirschke K, Altschuler G: The future of perinatal physiopathology, in Abramson H (ed): *Symposium on the Functional Physiopathology of the Fetus and Neonate.* CV Mosby Co, St Louis, 1971, pp 158–168.

4. Benirschke K, Kaufmann P: *Pathology of the Human Placenta.* New York, Springer-Verlag, 1990.

5. Blickstein I, Katz Z, Lancet M, Molgilner BM: The outcome of pregnancies complicated by preterm rupture of the membranes with and without cerclage. *Int J Gynecol Obstet* 1989; 28:237–242.

6. Blott M, Greenough A, Nicolaides KH, Moscoso G, Gibb D, Campbell S: Fetal breathing movements as predictor of favourable pregnancy outcome after oligohydramnios due to membrane rupture in second trimester. *Lancet* 1987; 2:129–131.

7. Bourne G: *The Human Amnion and Chorion.* London, Lloyd-Luke, 1962, p 175.

8. Boyd PA: Placenta and umbilical cord, in Keeling JW (ed): *Fetal and Neonatal Pathology.* London, Springer Verlag, 1987, pp 45–76.

9. Buchsbaum HJ: *Trauma in Pregnancy.* Philadelphia, WB Saunders Co, 1979.

10. Coltart TM, Bryne DL, Bates SA: Meconium aspiration syndrome: A 6-year retrospective study. *Br J Obstet Gynaecol* 1989; 96:411–414.

11. Cooperstock M, England JE, Wolfe RA: Circadian incidence of premature rupture of the membranes in term and preterm births. *Obstet Gynecol* 1987; 69:936–941.

12. Cooperstock M, England JE, Wolfe RA: Circadian incidence of labor onset hour in preterm

birth and chorioamnionitis. *Obstet Gynecol* 1987; 70:852–855.

13. Cox SM, Williams ML, Leveno KJ: The natural history of preterm ruptured membranes: What to expect of expectant management. *Obstet Gynecol* 1988; 71:558–562.

14. Dooley SL, Pesavento DJ, Depp R, Socol ML, Tamura RK, Wiringa KS: Meconium below the vocal cords at delivery: Correlation with intrapartum events. *Am J Obstet Gynecol* 1985; 153:767–770.

15. Ernest JM, Meis PJ, Moore ML, Swain M: Vaginal pH: A marker of preterm premature rupture of the membranes. *Obstet Gynecol* 1989; 74:734–738.

16. Evaldson GR, Larsson B, Jiborn H: Is the collagen content reduced when the fetal membranes rupture? *Gynecol Obstet Invest* 1987; 24:92–94.

17. Evaldson GR, Malmborg AS, Nord CE. Premature rupture of the membranes and ascending infection. *Br J Obstet Gynaecol* 1982; 89:793–801.

18. Flood B, Naeye RL: Factors that predispose to premature rupture of the fetal membranes. *JOGN Nurs* 1984; 13:119–122.

19. Fox CA, Meldrum SJ, Watson BW: Continuous measurement by radio-telemetry of vaginal pH during human coitus. *J Reprod Fertil* 1973; 33:69–75.

20. Goodlin RC, Schmidt W, Creevy DC: Uterine tension and fetal heart rate during maternal orgasm. *Obstet Gynecol* 1972; 39:125–127.

21. Garza A, Cordero JF, Mulinare J: Epidemiology of the early amnion rupture spectrum of defects. *Am J Dis Child* 1988; 142:541–544.

22. Hanna NF, Taylor-Robinson D, Kalodiki-Karamanoli M, Harris JRW, McFadyen IR: The relation between vaginal pH and the microbiological status in vaginitis. *Br J Obstet Gynecol* 1985; 92:1267–1271.

23. Herva R, Karkinen-Jaaskelainen M: Amniotic adhesion malformation syndrome: Fetal and placental pathology. *Teratology* 1984; 29:11–19.

24. Higginbottom MC, Jones KL, Hall BD, Smith DW: The amniotic band disruption complex: Timing of amniotic rupture and variable spectra of consequent defects. *J Pediatr* 1979; 95:544–549.

25. Ismail MA, Yang SL, Abusharif AN, Moawad AH: Immunoglobulins in prolonged ruptured membranes. *Am J Obstet Gynecol* 1985; 153:390–393.

26. Jones KL, Miscellaneous sequences: Early amnion rupture sequence, in Jones KL (ed): *Smith's Recognizable Patterns of Human Mal-*

formations. Philadelphia, WB Saunders Co, 1988, pp 576–583.

27. Jovanovic R, Nguyen HT: Experimental meconium aspiration in guinea pigs. *Obstet Gynecol* 1989; 73:652–656.

28. Kino Y: Clinical and experimental studies of the congenital constriction band syndrome, with an emphasis on its etiology. *J Bone Joint Surg [AM]* 1975; 57:636–643.

29. Lawrence S, Rosenfeld CR: Fetal pulmonary development and abnormalities of amniotic fluid volume. *Semin Perinatol* 1986; 10:142–153.

30. Leonidas JC, Bhan I, Beatty EC: Radiographic chest contour and pulmonary air leaks in oligohydramnios-related pulmonary hypoplasia (Potter's syndrome). *Invest Radiol* 1982; 17:6–10.

31. Liggins D, Thurlbeck WM: Conditions altering normal lung growth and development, in Thibeault DW, Gregory GA (eds): *Neonatal Pulmonary Care*, ed 2. Norwalk, Conn, Appleton-Century-Crofts, 1986; p 3.

32. Lindner JGEM, Plantema FHF, Hoogkamp-Korstanje JAA: Quantitative studies of the vaginal flora of healthy women and of obstetric and gynaecological patients. *J Med Microbiol* 1978; 11:233–241.

33. Lockwood C, Ghidini A, Romero R: Amniotic band syndrome in monozygotic twins: Prenatal diagnosis and pathogenesis. *Obstet Gynecol* 1988; 71:1012–1016.

34. Lockwood C, Ghidini A, Romero R, Hobbins JC: Amniotic band syndrome: Reevaluation of its pathogenesis. *Am J Obstet Gynecol* 1989; 160:1030–1033.

35. Lucas A, Christofides ND, Adrian TE, Bloom SR, Aynsley-Green A: Fetal distress, meconium, and motilin. *Lancet* 1979; 1:718.

36. Mahmoud EL, Benirschke K, Vaucher YE, Poitras P: Motilin levels in term neonates who have passed meconium prior to birth. *J Pediatr Gastroenterol Nutr* 1988; 7:95–99.

37. Marras A, Dessi C, Macciotta A: Epidermolysis bullosa and amniotic bands. *Am J Med Genet* 1984; 19:815–817.

38. Mastrogiannis DS, Decavalas GO, Verma U, Tejani N: Perinatal outcome after recent cocaine usage. *Obstet Gynecol* 1990; 76:8–11.

39. Miller PW, Coen RW, Benirschke K: Dating the time interval from meconium passage to birth. *Obstet Gynecol* 1985; 66:459–462.

40. Miller ME, Graham JM Jr, Higginbottom MC, Smith DW: Compression-related defects from early amnion rupture: Evidence for mechanical teratogenesis. *J Pediatr* 1981; 98:292–297.

41. Morales WJ, Angel JL, O'Brien WF, Knuppel RA: Use of ampicillin and corticosteroids in premature rupture of membranes: A randomized study. *Obstet Gynecol* 1989; 73:721–726.

42. Moretti M, Sibai BM: Maternal and perinatal outcome of expectant management of premature rupture of membranes in the midtrimester. *Am J Obstet Gynecol* 1988; 159:390–396.

43. Murphy JD, Vawter GF, Reid LM: Pulmonary vascular disease in fatal meconium aspiration. *J Pediatr* 1984; 104:758–762.

44. Naeye RL, Ross SM: Amniotic fluid infection syndrome. *Clin Obstet Gynecol* 1982; 9:593–607.

45. Naeye RL, Ross SM: Coitus and chorioamnionitis: A prospective study. *Early Hum Dev* 1982; 6:91–97.

46. Naeye RL, Tafari N: *Risk Factors in Pregnancy and Diseases of the Fetus and Newborn.* Baltimore, Williams & Wilkins Co, 1983.

47. Newton ER, Clark M: Group B streptococcus and preterm rupture of membranes. *Obstet Gynecol* 1988, 71:198–202.

48. Nimrod C, Varela-Gittings F, Machin G, Campbell D, Wesenberg R: The effect of very prolonged membrane rupture on fetal development. *Am J Obstet Gynecol* 1984; 148:540–543.

49. Perlman M, Williams J, Hirsch M: Neonatal pulmonary hypoplasia after prolonged leakage of amniotic fluid. *Arch Dis Child* 1976; 51:349–353.

50. Rotschild A, Ling EW, Puterman ML, Farquharson D: Neonatal outcome after prolonged preterm rupture of the membranes. *Am J Obstet Gynecol* 1990; 162:46–52.

51. Sbarra AJ, Thomas GB, Cetrulo CL, Shakr C, Chaudhury A, Paul B: Effect of bacterial growth on the bursting pressure of fetal membranes in vitro. *Obstet Gynecol* 1987; 70:107–110.

52. Schoonmaker JN, Lawellin DW, Lunt B, McGregor JA: Bacteria and inflammatory cells reduce chorioamniotic membrane integrity and tensile strength. *Obstet Gynecol* 1989; 74:590–596.

53. Sibille Y, Lwebuga-Mukasa JS, Polomski L, Merrill WW, Ingbar DH, Gee JBL: An in vitro model for polymorphonuclear-leukocyte-induced injury to an extracellular matrix. *Am Rev Respir Dis* 1986; 134:134–140.

54. Sikorski R, Juszkiewicz T, Paszkowski T: Zinc status in women with premature rupture of membranes at term. *Obstet Gynecol* 1990; 76:675–677.

55. Smith DW. Early amnion rupture spectrum, in Smith DW (ed): *Recognizable Patterns of Human Malformations*. London, WB Saunders Co, 1982, pp 488–489.

56. Spiegel CA, Amsel R, Eschenbach D, Schoenknecht F, Holmes KK: Anaerobic bacteria in nonspecific vaginitis. *N Engl J Med* 1980; 303:601–607.

57. Steer PJ, Eigbe F, Lissauer TJ, Beard RW: Interrelationships among abnormal cardiotocograms in labor, meconium staining of the amniotic fluid, arterial cord blood pH, and apgar scores. *Obstet Gynecol* 1989; 74:715–721.

58. Swaminathan S, Quinn J, Stabile MW, Bader D, Platzker ACG, Keens TG: Long-term pulmonary sequelae of meconium aspiration syndrome. *J Pediatr* 1989; 114:356–361.

59. Taylor J, Garite TJ: Premature rupture of membranes before fetal viability. *Obstet Gynecol* 1984; 64:615–620.

60. Torpin R: *Fetal Malformations Caused by Amnion Rupture During Pregnancy*. Springfield, Ill, Charles C Thomas, Publisher, 1968.

61. Tyler DC, Murphy J, Cheney FW: Mechanical and chemical damage to lung tissue caused by meconium aspiration. *Pediatrics* 1978; 62:454–459.

62. Vadillo-Ortega F, Gonzalez-Avila G, Karchmer S, Cruz NM, Ayala-Ruiz A, Lama MS: Collagen metabolism in premature rupture of amniotic membranes. *Obstet Gynecol* 1990; 75:84–88.

63. Vaes G: Cell-to-cell interactions in the secretion of enzymes of connective tissue breakdown, collagenase and proteoglycan-degrading neutral proteases. A review. *Agents Actions* 1980; 10:474–485.

64. Wahl LM, Wahl SM, Mergenhagen SE, Martin GR: Collagenase production by endotoxin-activated macrophages. *Proc Natl Acad Sci USA* 1974; 71:3598–3601.

65. Wiswell TE, Tuggle JM, Turner BS: Meconium aspiration syndrome: Have we made a difference? *Pediatrics* 1990; 85:715–721.

66. Yeomans ER, Gilstrap LC, Leveno KJ, Burris JS: Meconium in the amniotic fluid and fetal acid-base status. *Obstet Gynecol* 1989; 73:175–178.

CHAPTER 9

Preterm Birth

Birth before 37 weeks of gestation is a major cause of fetal and neonatal morbidity and mortality in every population in the world where it has been studied. It has been estimated that about $5 billion are spent each year in the United States for the newborn care of preterm born infants and that another $45 billion will be required for their lifelong care. Many contemporary authors still report that most such preterm births are unexplained.[11] This is true in the sense that the biochemical mechanisms that initiate most preterm births have not been identified. However,

in a clinical sense the possibility of preventing preterm labors rests far more on finding ways to prevent the disorders that initiate the biochemical mechanisms than on knowledge of the biochemical mechanisms. This chapter shows that knowledge of the biochemical mechanisms might have very limited clinical value because most of the initiating disorders would be a serious threat to fetal survival if the pregnancies continued. The chapter focuses on the identity of the disorders that initiate most preterm births and on the possibilities of their prevention.

It has long been known that many preterm births are related to premature rupture of the fetal membranes, abruptio placentae, overdistention of the uterus, uterine cervical incompetence, major malformations in the fetus, and other disorders that severely stress gravidas and uterine anomalies. In recent years several additional disorders have been identified as causes of preterm birth. Acute chorioamnionitis appears to initiate as many as a third of preterm births. This is a disorder in which the fetal membranes and the amniotic fluid are invaded by bacteria or mycoplasmas.[23,25,29] Acute chorioamnionitis also appears to be responsible for about half of the premature fetal membrane ruptures that lead to preterm birth.[23,29] Very recently it has been determined that low blood flow from the uterus to the placenta is another likely cause of many preterm births.[24]

DATA BASE FOR THE ANALYSES

The large data base of the Collaborative Perinatal Study (CPS) affords a unique opportunity to analyze the disorders that initiate preterm birth. Most of the findings in this chapter are the product of analyses of the CPS data.[9,29,31] The CPS was set up to identify antepartum and subsequent events that affect children's morbidity, mortality, and long-term development. Details of the study are found in the introduction to this book. The CPS data are 25 years old but they are worth analyzing because the frequency of preterm births in the United States has not decreased since the data were collected, and nearly all of the disorders that cause preterm delivery are still uncontrolled today.

The disorders that caused most of the preterm births in the CPS were acute chorioamnionitis, chronically low uteroplacental blood flow, abruptio placentae, premature rupture of the fetal membranes, placenta previa, multiple fetuses, major fetal malformations, incompetent cervix, hydramnios, malformations of the uterus, and serious maternal illnesses during pregnancy (Table 9–1).[23–25,29] Placentas were available for more than half of the births in the study.

We made the diagnosis of acute chorioamnionitis when acute inflammatory cells were found in the chorionic plate of the placenta or were present in large numbers in the blood clot beneath the chorionic plate.[23,25] Acute inflammatory cells are attracted to these sites by the presence of bacteria or mycoplasmas in the amniotic fluid.[16,32] Chronically low uteroplacental blood flow was identified by the finding of unevenly accelerated placental villous maturation. In some cases this accelerated maturation was accompanied by an abnormally small placenta and placental infarcts. The accelerated maturation was identified by finding abnormally small placental villi and both more and larger syncytiotrophoblastic knots in the placenta than was normal for gestational age.[23,24,29] When present throughout the placenta, these findings are characteristic evidence of chronic low blood flow from the uterus to the placenta.[8,24] Such findings, sometimes without hypertension, were common in women who were having repeat spontaneous preterm deliveries, making it likely that chronic low uteroplacental blood flow is an important cause of preterm birth.[24] The diagnosis of premature rupture of the fetal membranes was made when the membranes ruptured preterm 2 or more hours before the onset of labor. Abruptio placentae was diagnosed when a blood clot was found in a depression on the maternal surface of the placenta. Finding an infarct or other evidence of ischemia in the placenta beneath the blood clot confirmed that the abruption had been present for some time. We also made the diagnosis of abruptio placentae when obstetricians observed a prematurely separated placenta with evidence of bleeding into the uterine cavity.[23,29] Additional details on the criteria used to make these diagnoses can be found in Chapters 7 and 8.

Incompetent cervix, hydramnios, malformations of the uterus, and serious maternal disorders are among the less common causes of preterm delivery. For purposes of the current analyses these less common anomalies and disorders were placed in a single consolidated category termed "other identified disorders" (Table 9–1). Anomalies of the uterus included malformations and benign neoplasms. Serious maternal disorders during pregnancy included organic heart disease that limited physical activity, pneumonia, burns, shock, status asthmaticus, major surgery, glomerulonephritis, hepatitis, and urinary tract infections that produced a temperature greater than 39° C. It would be of interest to quantitate individually the roles of each of these maternal disorders in preterm births, but there were not enough cases in most of these diagnostic categories to do so.

TABLE 9–1.

Risk Estimates for Factors Associated With Premature Birth

Risk Factors	Attributable Risks (95% Confidence Intervals)
Gestational Age 13–23 wk	
Acute chorioamnionitis	**.67** (.60, .76)
Abruptio placentae	**.16** (.10, .23)
Twins	**.04** (.01, .07)
Unevenly accelerated placental maturation	**.02** (.00, .04)
Premature membrane rupture	**.02** (.00, .04)
Major fetal malformations	**.02** (.00, .04)
Other identified disorders	**.07** (.06, .09)
Population attributable risk	***.98*** *(.96, 1.00)*
Gestational age 24–30 wk	
Acute chorioamnionitis	**.41** (.38, .44)
Abruptio placentae	**.07** (.05, .09)
Twins	**.07** (.05, .09)
Major fetal malformations	**.07** (.05, .08)
Premature membrane rupture	**.06** (.04, .08)
Unevenly accelerated placental maturation	**.03** (.01, .07)
Other identfied disorders	**.11** (.10, .12)
Population attributable risk	***.80*** *(.78, .82)*
Gestational Age 31–34 wk	
Acute chorioamnionitis	**.37** (.35, .40)
Unevenly accelerated placental maturation	**.12** (.10, .13)
Premature membrane rupture	**.08** (.07, .09)
Twins	**.03** (.02, .04)
Major fetal malformations	**.03** (0.2, .04)
Abruptio placentae	**.02** (.00, .04)
Other identified disorders	**.06** (0.5, .07)
Population attributable risk	***.67*** *(.65, .69)*
Gestational age 35–37 wk	
Acute chorioamnionitis	**.23** (.22, .25)
Unevenly accelerated placental maturation	**.17** (.16, .18)
Premature membrane rupture	**.09** (.08, .11)
Twins	**.03** (.02, .04)
Abruptio placentae	**.01** (.00, .02)
Major fetal malformations	**.01** (.00, .02)
Other identified disorders	**.08** (.07, .09)
Population attributable risk	***.60*** *(.58, .62)*

We included each risk factor for preterm birth as an independent variable in a logistic regression model that enabled us to estimate attributable risks for each risk factor (see Table 9–1).[3,5,15,27] This method made it possible to estimate the relative contribution of each risk factor to preterm delivery when adjusted for all of the other risk factors in the model. For example, acute chorioamnionitis at 13 to 23 weeks of gestation had an attributable risk estimate of .67 for preterm labor and delivery (see Table 9–1). This indicates that 67% of the spontaneous preterm births in this gestational period could be attributed to acute chorioamnionitis, given adjustments for all of the other risk factors in the analysis.

DISORDERS ASSOCIATED WITH PRETERM BIRTH

Of the 1,129 deliveries that took place between 13 and 23 weeks of gestation, 98% were explained by findings of the study (see Table 9–1). Acute chorioamnionitis accounted for 67%, abruptio placentae for 16%, twins for 4%, and other disorders for the rest of these deliveries (see Table 9–1). Acute chorioamnionitis and major congenital malformations accounted for a progressively smaller proportion of preterm deliveries as pregnancy advanced, but the actual number of weekly preterm deliveries attributable to these two risk factors increased because the frequency of deliveries increased week by week as gestation advanced. Presumed low uteroplacental blood flow and premature rupture of the fetal membranes were responsible for an increasing proportion of total preterm deliveries as pregnancy advanced, and the number of weekly births due to these disorders increased very rapidly with gestational age. The only risk factor not associated with an increasing number of births as pregnancy advanced was abruptio placentae (see Table 9–1).

INDIVIDUAL DISORDERS ASSOCIATED WITH PRETERM BIRTH

Acute Chorioamnionitis

Acute chorioamnionitis was the most frequent cause of preterm delivery in the study. Only about 1 in 10 of these infections can be recognized prior to delivery by clinical and laboratory signs of infection in the gravida, so microscopic examination of the placenta is usually needed to make the diagnosis. Most of the bacteria and mycoplasmas that are present in the vagina and cervix can cause acute chorioamnionitis, and an abnormal flora at these sites increases the risk for preterm birth.[16,20,29,32] This is discussed in detail in Chapter 7.

Plausible mechanisms have been proposed for how acute chorioamnionitis initiates preterm labor. Bejar et al. reported in 1981 that many of the microorganisms that cause chorioamnionitis produce phospholipase A_2 which can cleave arachidonic acid from the fetal membranes, thereby making arachidonic acid available to start the prostaglandin cascade and initiate labor.[2] Recently Cox et al. claimed that bacterial endotoxin initiates chorioamnionitis-induced labors by stimulating decidual cells to produce cytokines and prostaglandins.[10] Mitchell has found increased levels of several cytokines in the amniotic fluid of women with acute chorioamnionitis who delivered preterm.[21] These women also had increased levels of specific hydroxyeicosatetraenoic acids, leukotriene B_4, and prostaglandins, indicating that activation had taken place of both the lipoxygenase and cyclooxygenase pathways of arachidonic acid metabolism. Once started, rarely, if ever, can the labors initiated by acute chorioamnionitis be stopped by tocolytic agents, rest, and hydration.[30]

Chronic Low Uteroplacental Blood Flow

Chronic low uteroplacental blood flow appeared to be the second most frequent cause of spontaneous preterm delivery in the CPS. As previously explained, the surrogate we used for low uteroplacental blood flow was unevenly accelerated placental villous maturation. In our analyses this surrogate was associated with a 2.5-fold greater-than-expected frequency of

spontaneous preterm deliveries.[5] Furthermore, when a woman had a preterm delivery with these placental findings, her next pregnancy had a 64% frequency of terminating preterm with the same placental findings.[24]

The preterm labors and births associated with presumed low uteroplacental blood flow could be due to an excess of thromboxane or a paucity of the prostacyclin that is produced by the placenta because prostacyclin inhibits and thromboxane stimulates uterine activity.[35] This possibility is supported by evidence that preeclampsia can sometimes be prevented by the prophylactic administration of small doses of aspirin.[1] Aspirin maintains or restores the normal balance between the placental productions of prostacyclin and thromboxane.[1] Low uteroplacental blood flow will often not be recognized as the presumed cause of preterm birth if the placentas from preterm births are not routinely examined for evidence of uneven maturation. This is particularly true in cases where gravidas were normotensive throughout their pregnancies.

Preterm Rupture of the Fetal Membranes

Spontaneous premature rupture of the fetal membranes before term was the third most frequent cause of spontaneous preterm delivery in the CPS. In the laboratory, membranes that spontaneously ruptured preterm have usually resisted rupture by pressures as high as those generated by labor.[33] This does not mean that these membranes were normal at the time they ruptured. The tissue damage responsible for many such ruptures is present only at the site of rupture, so the rupture when it takes place tends to destroy the evidence of its origin.[4] The identification of this localized damage sometimes requires the microscopic examination of hundreds of tissue samples from the margins of the rupture site, an impractical procedure for routine case investigation. In other cases acute chorioamnionitis is present in the membranes and this disorder is a well-documented cause of premature membrane rupture.

Collagenase and elastase released by acute inflammatory cells are major suspects for weakening the membranes in many cases of premature membrane rupture in which acute chorioamnionitis is present.[19] Acute chorioamnionitis and cervical instrumentation before pregnancy appear to predispose to at least half of premature membrane ruptures.[13,23] In the CPS chorioamnionitis was twice as frequent when fetal membranes ruptured during the 4 hours before the onset of preterm labor as when labor preceded preterm membrane ruptures.[23,29] Four hours is too short a time for bacteria to invade the fetal membranes and initiate the microscopic findings of acute chorioamnionitis, so this finding suggests that chorioamnionitis antedated as many as half of the preterm membrane ruptures in the CPS (see Chapter 8).

Coital-induced orgasm appears to be an important cofactor with chorioamnionitis in some premature membrane ruptures.[28] It has been known for some years that orgasm can induce uterine contractions during pregnancy, and a prospective study found that inflamed fetal membranes were much more prone to rupture after coital-induced orgasm than were uninflamed, presumably undamaged membranes.[28]

Twins and Triplets

The next most frequent cause of spontaneous preterm delivery in the CPS was twins or triplets. The assumption is often made that preterm labor in such cases is due to overdistention of the uterus by the multiple fetuses or by hydramnios.[11] We have found that the placental findings of acute chorioamnionitis are present in about two-thirds of the twins who deliver spontaneously before 30 weeks of gestation. Between 30 weeks and term more than two-thirds of twin placentas either have acute chorioamnionitis or display unevenly accelerated placental villous maturation, which is suggestive evidence that uteroplacental blood flow was low. It can therefore be argued that infection and low uteroplacental blood flow, rather than an overdistended uterus, are the most frequent causes of preterm birth when twins or triplets are present.

Abruptio Placentae

Abruptio placentae was another frequent cause of preterm birth in the CPS. The retroplacental hemorrhages that start most placental abruptions presumably originate in the rupture of an arteriole or artery in the decidua basalis. This can occur when the vessel is torn or its wall weakened by necrosis or infection. Abdominal trauma, uterine tumors, uterine malformations, hydramnios, maternal gestational hypertension, a short umbilical cord, sudden decompression of the uterus, occlusion or compression of the inferior vena cava, lupus erythematosus, and the use of anticoagulants are the causes of abruptio placentae that are usually mentioned.[11] However, taken as a group, all of these risk factors explained less than 1 in 4 of the placental abruptions in the CPS. Maternal cigarette smoking, presumed chronically low uteroplacental blood flow, acute chorioamnionitis, and advanced maternal age appeared to explain nearly half of placental abruptions in the CPS (see Chapter 7).[22,29]

A placental examination is needed to identify the presence of many of these risk factors. Cigarette smoking damages the decidua, which may explain its association with placental abruptions. Evidence of this damage is the decidual necrosis that is often present at the edge of the placenta in cigarette smokers.[29] Uterine arterial and arteriolar damage, particularly in the spiral arteries, is frequent in hypertensive gravidas, in older gravidas, and in those with lupus erythematosus antibodies, which may explain the increased frequency of abruptio placentae in mothers with these risk factors. A placental infarct caused by hypertensive damage to spiral arteries can be a nidus for starting an abruption. In the case of acute chorioamnionitis, the infection often invades the decidua where blood vessel damage may lead to the hemorrhages which initiate some abruptions.[22,23,29] Abruptions are reported to be increased in frequency in cocaine users, perhaps because cocaine induces sharp increases in maternal blood pressure and decreases in uteroplacental blood flow.[6]

Major Congenital Malformations

It is not known why spontaneous preterm delivery is more frequent when a fetus has major congenital malformations, but this finding strengthens the possibility that preterm labor is sometimes initiated by the fetus. The initiating factor could be related to fetal stress because many children with major malformations are stressed before birth by the dysfunctions produced by their malformations. For example, in the CPS children with cyanotic types of congenital heart disease had twice the frequency of spontaneous preterm births as children with noncyanotic types of congenital heart disease. With the cyanotic types of heart disease the fetal heart and brain are perfused with blood having lower-than-normal levels of oxygen, which may be stressful to the fetus. Other evidences of fetal stress or fetal brain dysfunction include abnormalities in fetal heart rate, low Apgar scores at birth, neonatal seizures, and neurologic abnormalities in the early neonatal period.

Other Risk Factors for Preterm Delivery

There are many other claimed causes of preterm delivery. Vigorous physical exertion has been claimed to shorten the length of gestation, but none of the studies that make this claim have taken into consideration most of the disorders just discussed that appear to cause preterm birth.[7,17] In the CPS, maternal work outside of the home that required standing all day did not increase the frequency of preterm births.[26]

CONSEQUENCES OF PRETERM BIRTH

There has been a progressive decrease in the neonatal mortality of preterm born infants during the last two decades. This improvement has been particularly great for infants with birth weights of less than 1.0 kg. However, about two-thirds of the infants weighing less than 750 g still die and some institutions have reported no significant improvement in recent survival rates.[12,14] Within individual preterm birth weight categories the proportion of survivors who have serious neurosensory handicaps 1 to 2 years after birth has reportedly not changed with the introduction of neonatal intensive care and other recently introduced therapies.[12,14] A recent compilation of outcomes from many perinatal care centers disclosed that between 1975 and 1985 major developmental handicaps at 1 to 2 years of age were present in 26% of surviving infants who had birth weights of less than 800 g, 17% who had birth weights of 750 to 1,000 g, and 11% who had birth weights of 1,000 to 1,500 g.[12] Despite this generally discouraging report, some individual centers have reported significantly improved outcomes in recent years.[34]

This failure to reduce the frequency of long-term handicaps, particularly neurodevelopmental impairments, is mainly due to the fact that many of the impairments have their origins in antenatal disorders that are outside of the control of the health care system. Intracranial hemorrhage has been the greatest risk for such impairments and its most frequent initiating event, severe placental villous edema, produces severe fetal hypoxia which usually starts several days before delivery. The details can be found in Chapter 11. Severe chronic lung disease does not seem to affect the psychomotor development of very low-birth-weight infants, but the way in which such infants are parented has been reported to have a large effect on their psychomotor outcome.[18]

CONCLUSIONS

A gross and microscopic examination of the placenta was required to make a presumptive diagnosis of the cause of preterm birth in more than half of such births in the CPS. The following cannot be identified without such a placental examination: nine out of ten cases of acute chorioamnionitis, the cause of about half of premature fetal membrane ruptures, the cause of many placental abruptions, the reason why many twins are born preterm, and the cause of some preterm births associated with presumed chronically low uteroplacental blood flow.

REFERENCES

1. Beaufils M, Uzam S, Donsiomoni R, Colau JC: Prevention of preeclampsia by early antiplatelet therapy. *Lancet* 1985; 1:840–842.

2. Bejar R, Curbelo V, Davis C, Gluck L: Premature labor, II. Bacterial sources of phospholipase. *Obstet Gynecol* 1981; 57:479–482.

3. Benichou J, Gail MH: Variance calculations and confidence intervals for estimates of the attributable risk based on logistic models. *Biometrics* 1990; 46:991–1003.

4. Bourne G: *The Human Amnion and Chorion.* London, Lloyd-Luke, 1962, p 175.

5. Bruzzi P, Green SB, Byar DP, Brinton LA, Schairer C: Estimating the population attributable risk for multiple risk factors using case-control data. *Am J Epidemiol* 1985; 122:904–914.

6. Chasnoff IJ, Burns WJ, Scholl SH, Burns KA: Cocaine use in pregnancy. *N Engl J Med* 1985; 313:666–669.

7. Clapp JF, Dickstein S: Endurance exercise and pregnancy outcome. *Med Sci Sports Exerc* 1984; 16:556–562.

8. Clavero-Nunez JA, Negrueruela J, Botella-Llusia J. Placental morphometry and placental circulometry. *J Reprod Med* 1971; 6:209–217.

9. *The Collaborative Study on Cerebral Palsy, Mental Retardation and Other Neurological and Sensory Disorders of Infancy and Childhood Manual.* Bethesda, Md, US Department of Health, Education and Welfare, 1966.

10. Cox SM, McDonald PC, Casey ML: Cytokines and prostaglandins in amniotic fluid of preterm labor pregnancies: Decidual origin in response to bacterial toxins. Presented at the 36th Annual Meeting of the Society of Gynecological Investigation. March 1989, San Diego.

11. Cunningham FG, MacDonald PC, Gant NF: *William's Obstetrics.* Norwalk, Conn, Appleton & Lange, 1989, pp 702, 748.

12. Ehrenhaft PM, Wagner JL, Herdman RC: Changing prognosis for very low birth weight infants. *Obstet Gynecol* 1989; 74:528–535.

13. Flood B, Naeye RL: Factors that predispose to premature rupture of the fetal membranes. *JOGN Nurs* 1984; 13:119–122.

14. Hack M, Fanaroff AA: Outcomes of extremely-low-birth-weight infants between 1982 and 1988. *N Engl J Med* 1989; 321:1642–1647.

15. Hastings RP (ed): *SUGI: Supplemental Library User's Guide*, ed 5. Cary, NC, SAS Institute, 1986.

16. Hiller SL, Martius J, Krohn M, Kiviat N, Holmes KK, Eschenback DA: A case controlled study of chorioamnionic infection and histologic chorioamnionitis in prematurity. *N Engl J Med* 1988; 319:972–978.

17. Homer CJ, Beresford SAA, James SA, Siegel E, Wilcon S: Work-related physical exertion and risk of preterm, low birthweight delivery. *Pediatr Perinat Epidemiol* 1990; 4:161–174.

18. Leonard CH, Clyman RI, Piecuch RE, Juster RP, Ballard RA, Behle MB: Effect of medical and social risk factors on outcome of prematurity and very low birth weight. *J Pediatr* 1990; 116:620–626.

19. McGregor JA, French JI, Lawellin D, Franco-Buff A, Smith C, Todd JK: Bacterial protease induced reduction of chorioamniotic membrane strength and elasticity. *Obstet Gynecol* 1987; 69:167–174.

20. McGregor JA, French JI, Richter R, Franco-Buff A, Johnson A, Hillier S, Judson FN, Todd JK: Antenatal microbiologic and maternal risk factors associated with prematurity. *Am J Obstet Gynecol* 1990; 163:1465–1473.

21. Mitchell M: Causes of preterm labour, in *International Symposium in Honour of Professor Sir Alexander Turnbull, CBE*, 30 June 1990, Oxford, p 4.

22. Naeye RL: Coitus and antepartum hemorrhage. *Br J Obstet Gynecol* 1981; 88:765–770.

23. Naeye RL: Functionally important disorders of the placenta, umbilical cord and fetal membranes. *Hum Pathol* 1987; 7:680–691.

24. Naeye RL: Pregnancy hypertension, placental evidences of low uteroplacental blood flow and spontaneous preterm delivery. *Hum Pathol* 1989; 20:441–444.

25. Naeye RL: Acute chorioamnionitis, its origins and its clinical consequences, in Bellisario R, Mizejewski GJ (eds): *Transplacental Disorders.* New York, Alan R Liss Inc, 1990, pp 3–15.

26. Naeye RL, Peters EC: Working during pregnancy: Effects on the fetus. *Pediatrics* 1982; 69:724–727.

27. Naeye RL, Peters EC, Bartholomew M, Landis R: Origins of cerebral palsy. *Am J Dis Child* 1989; 143:1154–1161.

28. Naeye RL, Ross SM: Coitus and chorioamnionitis, a prospective study. *Early Hum Dev* 1982; 6:91–97.

29. Naeye RL, Tafari N: *Risk Factors in Pregnancy and Diseases of the Fetus and Newborn.* Baltimore, Williams & Wilkins Co, 1983.

30. Nazir MA, Pankuch GA, Botti JJ, Appelbaum PC: Antibacterial activity of amniotic fluid in early third trimester: Its association with preterm labor and delivery. *Am J Perinat* 1987; 4:59–62.

31. Niswander KR, Gordon M. *The Women and Their Pregnancies,* Philadelphia, WB Saunders Co, 1972.

32. Pankuch GA, Appelbaum PC, Lorenz RP, Botti JJ, Schachter J, Naeye RL: Placental microbiology and histology and the pathogenesis of chorioamnionitis. *Obstet Gynecol* 1984; 64:802–806.

33. Polishuk WZ, Kohane S, Harar A: Fetal weight and membrane tensile strength. *Am J Obstet Gynecol* 1964; 88:248–250.

34. Saigal S, Rosenbaum P, Hattersley B, Milner R: Decreased disability rate among 3-year-old survivors weighing 501–1000 grams at birth and born to residents of a geographically defined region from 1981 to 1984 compared with 1977 to 1980. *J Pediatr* 1989; 114:839–846.

35. Walsh SW: Preeclampsia: An imbalance in placental prostacyclin and thromboxane production. *Am J Obstet Gynecol* 1985; 152:335–340.

CHAPTER 10

Disorders of Twins

FREQUENCY OF TWINS

The frequency of twin births varies greatly from one population to another, being high in many African groups and low in the Orient. Almost all of this variation is in dizygous twinning, so it is presumably related to differences in the frequency of multiple ovulation.[10] One cause of this difference among populations is in the frequency and skill with which fertility drugs are used to induce multiple ovulation. Maternal fatness at the time of conception exerts an even greater influence on the frequency of dizygous twinning. The fatter the gravida, the higher the frequency of dizygous twins (see Chapter 3).[38] In this regard humans are like other mammals. The best-nourished conceive and deliver the most offspring with each pregnancy. The positive correlation of dizygous twinning with maternal weight for height is one reason why maternal hypertension is more frequent in gestations with twins.[24] There is a strong, positive association between maternal pregravid weight for height and gestational hypertension.[38]

Benirschke and Kaufmann have attributed the differences of dizygous twinning between populations to the genes that regulate follicle-stimulating (FSH) and luteinizing hormone (LH) secretions.[6] They point out that both twinning and the FSH/LH ratio in maternal blood increase with age. They note that the Japanese, who have low blood ratios of FSH/LH, have a low rate of twinning. Fatness increases with maternal age and this explains most of the increase of twins with increasing maternal age.[38]

ZYGOSITY

Fetal and neonatal death are several times more frequent in twins and triplets than in single-born infants. Mortality and preterm birth are more frequent in monozygous than in dizygous twins (Table 10–1, Fig 10–1). Twins of different sex are always dizygous. An examination of the

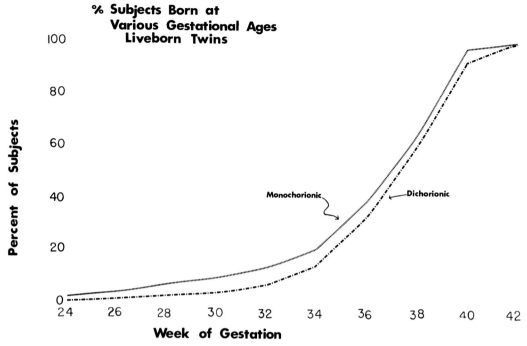

FIG 10–1.
In the CPS, a higher proportion of monochorionic than dichorionic twins were born preterm.

TABLE 10–1.

Type of Twin and Pregnancy Outcome*

	Frequency of Types of Twins	Perinatal Mortality Rate	Fetal Growth Retardation	Neurologic Abnormalities at 7 Years	Preterm Birth
All births in study		41 (2,281)	81 (4,528)	30 (1,684)	161 (8,976)
Monochorionic, monoamnionic	0.3 (15)	200 (3), $P<.01$	267 (4), $P<.001$	67 (1)	467 (7), $P<.001$
Relative risks		5.1, $P<.001$	3.6, $P<.05$	1.6	4.4, $P<.01$
Monochorionic, diamnionic	3 (167)	156 (26), $P<.001$	407 (68), $P<.001$	66 (11)	413 (69), $P<.001$
Relative risks		3.3, $P<.001$	7.3, $P<.001$	2.9, $P<.001$	2.6, $P<.001$
Dichorionic, diamnionic	8 (454)	59 (27), $P<.05$	295 (134), $P<.001$	48 (22)	441 (200), $P<.001$
Relative risks		7.2, $P<.001$	5.9, $P<.001$	1.4	4.6, $P<.001$

*Frequencies per 1,000 births. Numbers of cases are in parentheses. Relative risk values have been calculated to take the following possible confounding variables into consideration: major congenital malformations, acute chorioamnionitis, disorders of low uteroplacental blood flow, and, when appropriate, gestational age at birth.

membranes between the two fetal sacs usually establishes the zygosity of same-sex twins. If chorionic cells are absent in the middle of this dividing membrane, the twins are monochorionic and all monochorionic twins are monozygous (Fig 10–2). If chorionic cells are present in the middle of the dividing membrane, the twins are dichorionic (Fig 10–3). Approximately 18% of same-sex dichorionic twins are monozygous, the rest dizygous. Blood group identification, enzyme markers, HLA, and genetic typing are occasionally required to determine the zygosity of

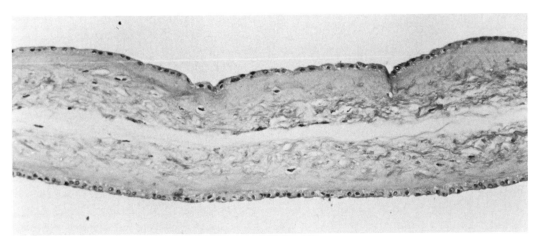

FIG 10–2.
No chorionic cells are present within this fused membrane that separates the two sacs of a twin placenta, indicating that this is a monochorionic placenta. Hematoxylin-eosin (HE) stain, ×134.

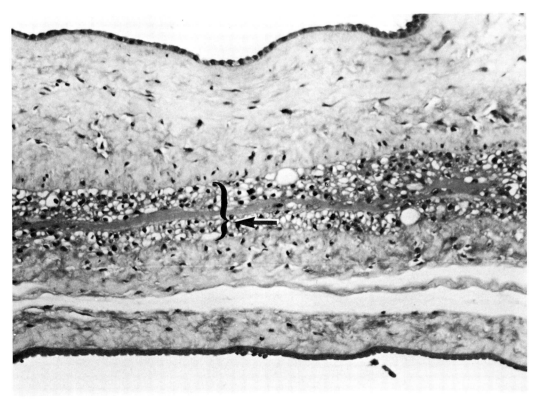

FIG 10–3.
A layer *(arrow)* of chorionic cells in the center of this fused membrane that separates the two sacs of a twin placenta indicates that this is a dichorionic placenta. HE stain, ×134.

phenotypically similar, same-sex dichorionic twins. Sometimes this typing is not definitive because the parents have a similar distribution of antigens.[43] For the same reason, an analysis of multiple-restriction enzyme site polymorphisms with DNA probes can produce a false-positive diagnosis of monozygosity.[17] Chromosome marking is the most definitive method for establishing zygosity.[32]

FETAL GROWTH

On the average, twins weigh about 800 g less at birth than single-born infants. Twins are more often born preterm than singletons, and when this is taken into consideration twins weigh 400 to 500 g less than singletons at birth (Fig 10–4).[39] This difference would probably be even greater if a disproportionate number of dizygous twins were not the offspring of overweight mothers.[38] The overweight mothers of dizygous twins as a group also are taller and have higher levels of several growth-affecting hormones than the mothers of single-born infants.[29] Genetic influences are not the dominant factor that is responsible for the slow growth of twins before birth because this slowing only

becomes striking after the 30th week of gestation, which is a pattern that is characteristic of fetal undernutrition (see Chapter 4).[13,39,41] There are several reasons for such undernutrition. First, uteroplacental blood flow on a per fetus basis is lower in twin than in singleton gestations and this flow is the main determinant of the rate at which nutrients are delivered to the fetus.[18,41] Second, 1 in 4 twin pairs share a common circulation in the placenta, and sometimes shunts between the two sides of the placenta lead large amounts of blood and nutrients to pass from one twin to the other.[5,6,33,39] The donor twin that loses the blood also loses its nutrients, which can markedly retard its growth.[33,39] The donor is probably also deprived of some oxygen, but this is almost

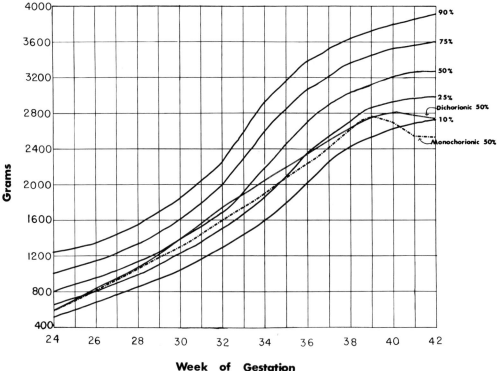

FIG 10–4.
The mean birth weights of monochorionic and dichorionic twins born at various gestational ages compared with the birth weights of single-born infants.

certainly less important than low supply of nutrients in the retarded growth of the donor.[35]

There are still other mechanisms that slow the fetal growth of twins more than the growth of single-born infants. Although most of the growth retardation in twins occurs after 30 weeks of gestation, more twins than single-born infants are growth-retarded early in gestation (see Fig 10–4).[8] One reason is that congenital malformations, which are often associated with growth retardation, are more frequent in twins than in the single-born.[34,36]

CAUSES OF FETAL AND NEONATAL DEATH IN TWINS

In the Collaborative Perinatal Study (CPS) twins were more often stillborn or died in the neonatal period than single-born infants (see Table 10–1).[41,42] This was particularly true when maternal net pregnancy weight gain was low (Fig 10–5). Maternal net pregnancy weight gain is the total maternal weight gain during pregnancy minus the weight of the fetus and placenta. It is mainly a measure of nutrients incorporated into maternal tissues, the weight of the amniotic fluid, and the size of maternal blood volume increase (see Chapter 4). Two of these factors, nutrients incorporated into maternal tissue and the size of maternal blood volume increase, affect both fetal growth and fetal survival. Maternal net pregnancy weight gains of less than 2 kg were associated with perinatal mortality rates that exceeded 100/1,000 in twin gestations (see Fig 10–5).

The following disorders were responsible for the higher perinatal mortality rate of twins than of single-born infants: acute chorioamnionitis, premature rupture of

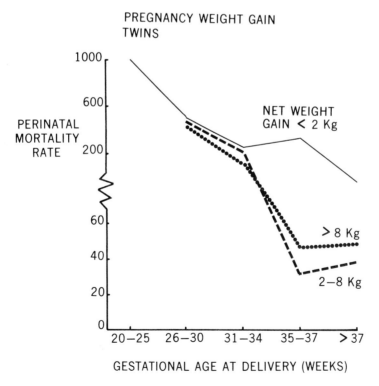

FIG 10–5.
The perinatal mortality rates for twins exceeded 100/1,000 when their mothers had very low net pregnancy weight gains.

the fetal membranes, the transplacental twin-to-twin transfusion syndrome, and congenital fetal malformations (Table 10–2).[41,42] Identifying most of these disorders or their cause requires a gross and microscopic examination of the placenta, umbilical cord, and extraplacental fetal membranes.

Acute Chorioamnionitis

The higher frequency of acute chorioamnionitis in twin than in singleton gestations may be the result of premature opening of the cervix when twins overdistend the uterus and shorten the cervical canal. This would expose the fetal membranes to the bacterial flora of the cervix. Such exposure leads to a high frequency of acute chorioamnionitis when it occurs with an incompetent cervix.[41] This is an attractive hypothesis for the high rate of acute chorioamnionitis with twins in the third trimester, but it is less credible for the high rate of acute chorioamnionitis with twins in earlier gestation. Perhaps the high rate of acute chorioamnionitis in earlier gestation is a secondary phenomenon to some other mechanism that in preparation for labor causes the cervical canal to shorten and thereby predisposes to acute chorioamnionitis.

Premature Rupture of the Fetal Membranes

Premature rupture of the fetal membranes was the second most frequent initiating event that led to the fetal or neonatal death of twins. Acute chorioamnionitis is almost always present, so the mechanisms that are responsible for acute chorioamnionitis may also be responsible for the high rate of premature membrane rupture. The twins may overdistend the uterus and thereby expose the fetal membranes at the cervical os to the bacterial flora of the cervix and vagina. Resulting acute chorioamnionitis weakens the membranes. There is strong evidence that at least half of premature membrane ruptures are secondary to such infections weakening the membranes (see Chapter 8).[41]

Placental Infarctions, Abruptio Placentae, Neonatal Respiratory Distress Syndrome

On a per capita basis uteroplacental blood flow is lower in twin than in singleton gestations.[18] This presumably explains why placental infarcts and abruptions are more frequent in twin than in singleton gestations. A much higher proportion of twin than of singleton placentas have abnormally small villi and excessive syn-

TABLE 10–2.

Initiating Disorders That Led to the Death of Twins (Collaborative Perinatal Study.)

	Singletons	Monozygotic Twins	Dizygotic Twins
Acute chorioamnionitis	3	34	6, $P < .005$
Premature rupture of membranes	3	20	10, $P < .1$
Twin-to-twin transfusion syndrome	0	28	0
Large placental infarcts	2	11	6, $P > .1$
Congenital malformations	10	23	2, $P < .005$
Hydramnios, preterm delivery	0.1	14	5, $P > .1$
Abruptio placentae	4	6	8, $P > .1$
Umbilical cord compression	1	6	2, $P > .1$
Birth trauma	1	3	3, $P > .1$
Incompetent cervix	0.2	0	3
Placenta previa	1	0	3
Other disorders	8	46	27, $P > .005$
Totals	33	191	75, $P < .001$

*Adapted from Naeye RL, Tafari N, Judge D, Marboe CC: Am J Obstet Gynecol 1978; 131:267–272.
†Perinatal deaths per 1,000 births. P values compare perinatal mortality rates in monozygous and dizygous twins.

cytial knots for gestational age. These are the characteristic consequences of subnormal uteroplacental blood flow.[41] Low uteroplacental blood flow appears to be a major cause of spontaneous preterm birth.[37] It is also the underlying cause of most placental infarcts and a frequent underlying cause of abruptio placentae.[41] Bed rest sometimes increases uteroplacental blood flow, but in the case of twins it has not prolonged gestation.[31]

The low uteroplacental blood flow to individual members of twin pairs often accelerates fetal lung and liver maturation. One result was that at every week after 30 weeks of gestation newborn twins had only one-third the frequency of the neonatal respiratory distress syndrome as did single-born infants in the CPS. It has often been observed that the second-born of twins has a higher perinatal mortality rate than the first-born. This difference reportedly disappears when the two twins are of similar birth weight, so it is probably not due to more frequent hypoxia in the second-born as has often been claimed.[52]

Congenital Malformations

Congenital malformations are more frequent in twins than in single-born infants. More of this increase is in monozygous than in dizygous twins (Fig 10–6).[9] This may be because monozygous twinning can be compared to a teratogenic event in that the division of a fertilized egg to form two zygotes is an abnormal event. The better perfusion of one side of the placenta than the other when the two embryos share a single placental circulation might also at times be teratogenic. Polar body fertilization is another mechanism that might help explain why malformations in monozygotic twins are often limited to one member of a pair.[6] Malformations that are particularly frequent in twins include a single umbilical artery and esophageal atresia. Monochorionic, monoamnionic twins reportedly have a high frequency of anencephaly, sirenomelia, and the holoprosencephaly constellation of malformations.[51] Benirschke and Kaufmann have provided a detailed discussion of malformations in twins.[6]

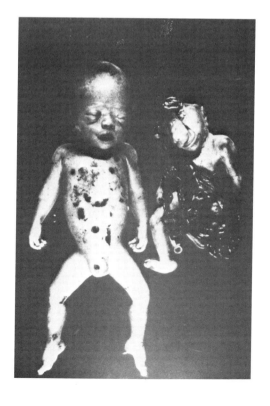

FIG 10–6.
These monozygous twins are markedly discordant in size. The smaller twin has multiple congenital malformations. (From Altshuler G: The placenta, how to examine it, its normal growth and development, in Naeye R, Kissane J, Kaufman N: *Perinatal Diseases.* Baltimore, Williams & Wilkins Co, 1982, pp 21. Used by permission.)

Umbilical Cord Compression

Up to 50% of monochorionic, monoamnionic twins are stillborn because the absence of a membrane between the two fetal sacs permits the two umbilical cords to intertwine and thereby obstruct blood flow in one or both cords (see Table 10–1, Fig 10–7).

Twin-to-Twin Transfusion Syndrome

The perinatal mortality rate for monozygous twins in the CPS was 191/1,000 births compared to 75/1,000 for dizygous twins (see Table 10–2). More frequent major fetal malformations, the twin-to-twin transplacental transfusion syndrome, acute chorioamnionitis, premature rupture of the fetal membranes, and hydramnios explained more than 80% of the higher perinatal mortality rate in the monozygous twins.[41,42] The incidence of the twin-to-twin transfusion syndrome ranges from 5% to 15% in twin pregnancies. It is caused by an unequal shunting of blood from one twin to the other through artery-to-vein, artery-to-artery, and perhaps vein-to-vein anastomoses between the two sides of the placenta (Fig 10–8).[6] Most such shunts are balanced. It is the unbalanced minority that produces the twin-to-twin transfusion syndrome. Injection with colored saline or another contrast material is usually needed to identify these shunts, most of which are deep in the parenchyma of the placenta.[5,6,45] The shunts can sometimes be identified by finding that one side of the placenta is more congested (recipient side) than the other side (donor) (Fig 10–9). Characteristically, the donor twin is anemic, growth-retarded, and associated with oligohydramnios. The recipient is usually plethoric, relatively larger, and develops polyhydramnios in its amniotic sac because of high urine production (Figs 10–10, 10–11).[23,40] The large blood volume in the recipient leads to much larger renal glomerular size, bladder size, and heart weights in the recipient than in the donor twin (see Figs 10–11, 10–12).[33] When the twin-to-twin transplacental

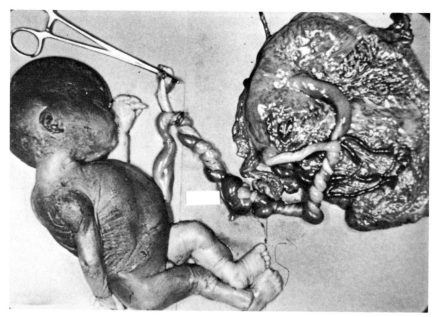

FIG 10–7.
There was no dividing membrane between these two monochorionic, monoamnionic twins. This absence permitted the two umbilical cords to intertwine and thereby obstruct blood flow in one of the cords. The affected twin was stillborn.

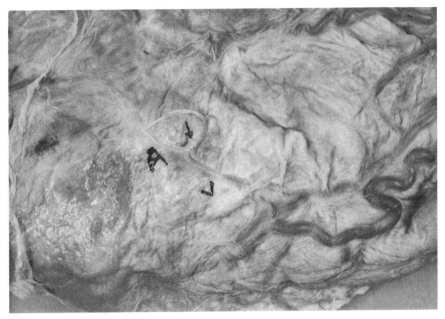

FIG 10–8.
An artery-to-vein anastomosis is shown on the surface of a monochorionic twin placenta. Most such anastomoses are far below the surface of the placenta.

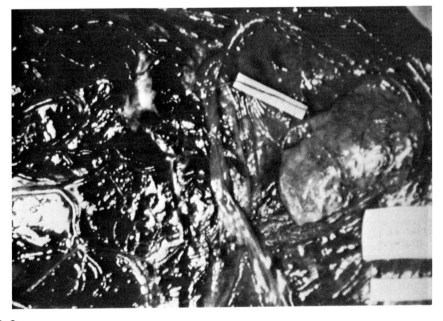

FIG 10–9.
The recipient side is much more congested than the donor side in this placenta from a case of the twin-to-twin transfusion syndrome.

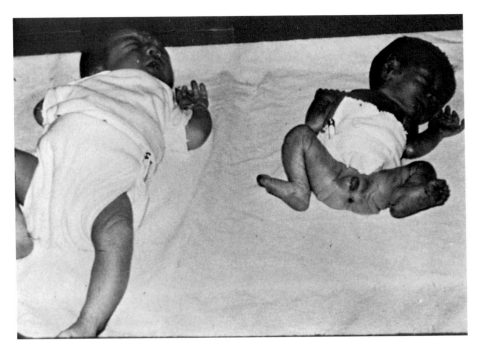

FIG 10–10.
The donor twin is much smaller than the recipient twin in this case of the twin-to-twin transfusion syndrome.

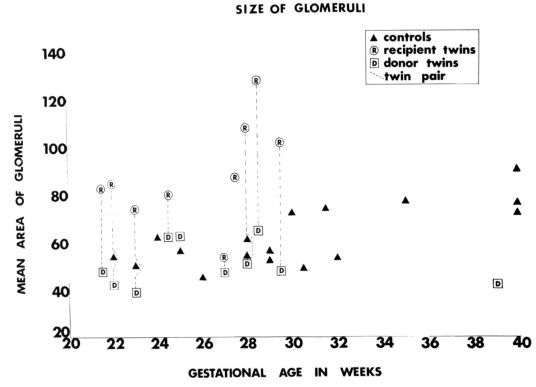

FIG 10–11.
Renal glomerular size is much larger in recipient than in donor members of twin pairs in the twin-to-twin transfusion syndrome. Glomerular size correlates with bladder size and the volume of early neonatal urine output in these twins.

WEIGHT OF HEARTS

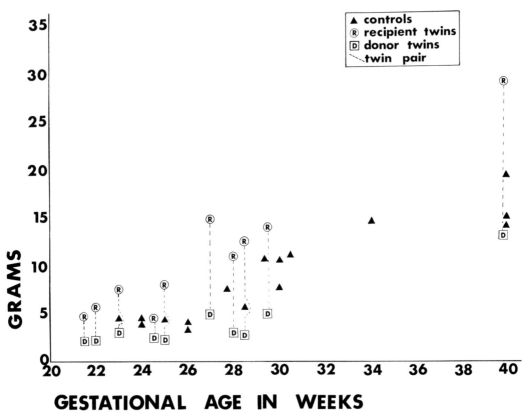

GESTATIONAL AGE IN WEEKS

FIG 10–12.
The weights of hearts are plotted against gestational age for twins with the twin-to-twin transfusion syndrome and for controls. The hearts of recipient twins are abnormally enlarged, whereas those of their donor partners are subnormal in weight.

transfusion syndrome develops in the second trimester of pregnancy, it is usually associated with preterm labor and as many as 80% of the twins die.[21]

Acardia, the absence of a functioning heart, is a rare anomaly that is found only in monochorionic twin gestations.[54] Large artery-to-artery anastomoses in the placenta allow the normal twin to perfuse the entire body of its acardiac partner. This results in a reversal of normal blood flow through the body of the acardiac twin.[7] Organs in the acardiac twin are usually hypoplastic or aplastic. For example, renal hypoplasia or agenesis has been reported in all cases.[54] It is uncertain whether these other organ abnormalities originate independently or are the result of the reversal in blood flow.

Treatments recommended over the years for serious cases of the twin-to-twin transfusion syndrome have included bed rest, serial amniocenteses to decompress the polyhydramnios, digoxin, and tocolytic agents for the mother to try to prevent preterm labor and delivery. There is no convincing evidence that any of these measures have improved survival.[21] The appearance of hydrops in one fetus of a twin pair is a particularly poor prognostic sign. More radical undertakings have included the intrauterine ligation of one umbilical cord and selective feticide.[5,55] Selective feticide has also been tried to salvage one twin from a transplacental twin-to-twin transfusion syndrome that seemed destined to kill both twins.[2] In three such interventions only one came out as planned. Both members of the second pair died and in the third intervention the fetus selected to survive died and the twin who was selected to die survived. The transplacental shunts probably played a role in the two unplanned outcomes. Recently DeLia et al. successfully terminated three cases of the disorder by coagulating the transplacental shunts in utero with a neodynium–yttrium-aluminum-garnet (Nd:YAG) laser beam.[16] Four of the six twins survived.

Transplacental vascular anastomoses are present on rare occasions in fused, dichorionic twin placentas.[5,44,48] This produces chimeras, individuals who possess hematologic tissues derived from two nonidentical individuals. This presumably results from the transplacental passage of hematologic precursors via vascular anastomoses. Such individuals have cross-immunologic tolerance and often more than one blood type. There is one well-documented instance in which artery-to-vein shunts produced a typical twin-to-twin transfusion syndrome in a dichorionic twin pair.[25] Even rarer are dispermic or tetragametic chimeras, who are thought to arise from the early fusion of two separate and genetically distinct zygotes, which then form a single conceptus.

THE INTRAUTERINE DEATH OF ONE TWIN

Twinning is a much more frequent phenomenon than is recognized. Before 8 weeks of gestation the incidence of a lost twin was once thought to be as high as 71%.[11,26] These estimates were based on early ultrasound diagnoses of two gestational sacs and the subsequent disappearance of one of these sacs. More recently it has been concluded that some of these diagnoses were in error and that the frequency of vanishing twins is about 1 in 5, which is close to the first-trimester spontaneous abortion rate for singleton pregnancies.[27] However, it must be emphasized that the true early gestational loss rate of twins is unknown.

The timing, clinical manifestations, placental abnormalities, and long-term consequences of vanishing twins has generated considerable clinical interest. When the loss occurs during the first, or early second trimester, the prognosis for the surviving twin is good.[22] When delivery finally takes place, the part of the placenta that served the dead twin usually appears as a firm, white or yellow plaque that involves the whole thickness of the placenta and is usually less than 3 × 3 cm in size. Microscopically, the lesion is comprised of fibrotic villi that have lost their trophoblastic covering and are surrounded by old fibrin. Occasionally the remnants of the embryo will be present.[22] Most often the gestational sac is resorbed or a blighted ovum is present. The formation of a fetus papyraceous is the least frequent outcome of a twin gestation (Fig 10–13). It has been estimated to occur in about 1 in 184 twin births.[30] After such an occurrence, pregnancy characteristically proceeds without complications for the surviving twin.

Death in the third trimester with one twin surviving is an infrequent event. Three out of four such late deaths involve one member of a monochorionic twin pair.[12] When it occurs, there is a risk of morbidity and death for the gravida as well as for the surviving fetus. The primary threat to the mother is disseminated intravascular coagulation (DIC). The development of DIC with a retained dead fetus is well documented in twin and triplet gestations.[49] Whether or not maternal DIC is detected and treated, the surviving twin is sometimes affected by its dead co-twin. Four case reports have described recent or old necrotic lesions in the surviving twin in the absence of clinically identified maternal DIC.[4,12,15,57] The passage of thromboplastic material from the dead to the surviving twin via transplacental shunts was long assumed to be the explanation for these lesions. A wide range of other abnormalities in the survivors have been attributed to this transplacental transfer of thromboplastin, including a variety of cerebral anomalies, aplasia cutis, and

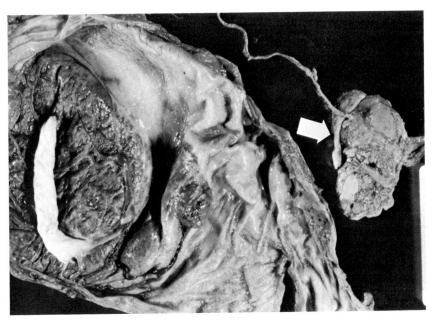

FIG 10–13.
Fetus papyraceus.

intestinal atresia.[50,53] Recently, Benir-schke and Kaufmann have pointed out that sudden bleeding by the survivor, rather than the transfer of thromboplastic material from its dead mate, is the most likely mechanism that damages the surviving twin.[6] This occurs because the death of one twin lowers the blood pressure in its circulation to zero. This is postulated to allow blood to pass rapidly from the surviving twin into the dead co-twin through transplacental shunts until thrombi close these transplacental channels.

Taking all of these factors into consideration, the early delivery of a twin after its partner dies will not necessarily improve the outcome for its partner. In some instances brain damage or maldevelopment is likely to have taken place before a decision can be made to deliver, and deliveries at early gestational ages pose all of the risks associated with immaturity if the surviving twin is still very immature.[12,14] Remaining in utero often benefits the survivor because the competition for oxygen and nutrients has been eliminated.

BRAIN DYSFUNCTION IN TWINS

Nearly 30 years ago Babson et al. found that when twins were greatly dissimilar in size at birth, the smaller member of the pair often had poorer cognitive skills in later years than the larger member.[1] This has been confirmed by several subsequent studies and is most obvious when the intrapair birth weight difference exceeds 25%. The most frequent abnormalities are reportedly in fine motor skills, coordination, and visual-motor perception.[56] There are reportedly few differences between the twin partners in gross motor skills and school grades.[56] We included twins as a risk factor for cognitive, behavioral, sensory, and motor abnormalities in all of our analyses of the CPS data (see Chapter 11). Being a twin proved not to be a risk for any cognitive, motor, or sensory abnormality independent of gestational age at birth, birth weight, head circumference, and all of the other risk factors that applied to psychomotor development in single-born infants. The only abnormalities for which being a twin was an independent risk were having a flat emotional affect and displaying impulsive behavior (see Chapter 11). Perhaps these last two findings are the result of social interactions between the twins, with members of the family, and with others, which is somewhat different for twins than for single-born children. As explained in Chapter 11, early childhood social interactions have a large role in molding behavioral traits.[46,47]

Although twins have the same risk factors as single-born infants for most cognitive, motor, behavioral, and sensory disorders, twins have a higher frequency of many of these disorders because they are more often born preterm, are growth-retarded at birth, and more often have major malformations than do single-born infants. Malformations of the heart and brain are associated with a particularly high frequency of brain malfunction.[19,20] Monozygous partners in the twin-to-twin transfusion syndrome have an increased frequency of antenatal brain damage.[3,25,28,30] The damage is most frequent in donor twins. The lesions are characteristically in the white matter, are hypoxic-ischemic in type, and often cavitate.[3,28,50,57] Such lesions are reportedly most often associated with vein-to-vein transplacental anastomoses and with the intrauterine fetal death of a co-twin.[3] These transplacental shunts have occasionally been reported in fused dichorionic twin placentas.[25] The brain lesions occasionally occur without the fetal death of a co-twin, and without the clinical manifestations of the twin-to-twin transfusion syndrome.[3] Bejar et al. postulate that the mechanism of this latter brain damage are transitory episodes of cardiovascular compromise that decrease blood flow through the fetal brain without causing the death of a co-twin or the full-blown twin-to-twin transfusion syndrome.[3] Larroche et al. postulate that fetal blood pressure instability or episodes of severe hypotension may be responsible for these brain lesions.[28]

I can suggest still another mechanism for this brain damage. In normal pregnancies maternal blood pressure decreases during the first trimester, remains low in the second trimester, and then slowly increases toward the prepregnancy level in the third trimester. In about 10% of gravidas this third-trimester blood pressure rise will be interrupted by episodes of blood pressure decreases to levels that are common in the second trimester. We identified such women in the CPS when they had one or more diastolic blood pressure decreases of more than 20 mm Hg to values below 60 mm Hg. There were 19 surviving twin pairs in the CPS whose mothers had one or more recorded episodes of such blood pressure decrease. There were motor impairments, including cerebral palsy in several instances, in one or both members of seven of the pairs. This raises the possibility that decreases in uteroplacental blood flow, caused by drops in maternal blood pressure, sometimes cause severe enough hemodynamic disturbances in twins to produce serious brain damage.

The donor twin is probably most often affected by these maternal blood pressure drops because its low blood volume and low hepatic glycogen stores make it more susceptible to hypoxemic brain damage than its recipient partner. The fact that brain lesions are in white matter explains how they occur without killing the fetus. White matter lesions point to damage before 32 weeks of gestation. Before about 32 weeks of gestation, there are large amounts of glycogen in the fetal heart. When severe hypoxemia develops, the heart can keep functioning by using this glycogen for a period of up to half an hour. During this time the brain may be severely damaged and the fetus may survive if the hypoxemia is relieved before the cardiac glycogen is exhausted. As term approaches, cardiac glycogen stores markedly decrease, so that the fetus can tolerate severe hypoxemia for only a very short period without dying. As a result, the chance of surviving severe hypoxemia with brain damage is probably less in late than in earlier gestation.

REFERENCES

1. Babson SG, Kangas J, Young N, Bramhall JL: Growth and development of twins of dissimilar size at birth. *Pediatrics* 1964; 33:327–333.

2. Baldwin VJ, Wittmann BK: Pathology of intragestational intervention in twin-to-twin transfusion syndrome. *Pediatr Pathol* 1990; 10:79–93.

3. Bejar R, Vigliocco G, Gramajo H, Solana C, Benirschke K, Berry C, Coen R, Resnik R: Antenatal origin of neurologic damage in newborn infants. *Am J Obstet Gynecol* 1990; 162:1230–1236.

4. Benirschke K: Twin placenta in perinatal mortality. *NY State J Med* 1961; 61:1499–1508.

5. Benirschke K, Driscoll SG: *The Pathology of the Human Placenta*. New York, Springer-Verlag, 1967, pp 205, 232–236.

6. Benirschke K, Kaufmann P: *Pathology of the Human Placenta*. New York, Springer-Verlag, 1990, pp 636–732.

7. Benson CB, Bieber FR, Genest DR, Doubilet PM: Doppler demonstration of reversed umbilical blood flow in an acardiac twin. *J Clin Ultrasound* 1989; 17:291–295.

8. Blickstein I, Shoham-Schwartz Z, Lancet M, Borenstein DR: Characterization of the growth discordant twin. *Obstet Gynecol* 1987; 70:11–15.

9. Bouchard C, Tremblay A, Despres JP, Nadeau A, Lupien PJ, Theriault G, Dussault J, Moorjani S, Pinault S, Fournier G: The response to long-term overfeeding in identical twins. *N Engl J Med* 1990; 322:1477–1482.

10. Boyd PA: Placenta and umbilical cord, in Keeling JW (ed): *Fetal and Neonatal Pathology*. London, Springer-Verlag, 1987, pp 45–76.

11. Bryan EM. The intrauterine hazards of twins. *Arch Dis Child* 1986; 61:1044–1045.

12. Cherouny PH, Hoskins IA, Johnson TRB, Niebyl JR: Multiple pregnancy with late death of one fetus. *Obstet Gynecol* 1989; 74:318–320.

13. Corney G, Robson EB, Strong SJ: The effect of zygosity on the birth weight of twins. *Ann Hum Genet* 1972; 36:45–59.

14. D'Alton ME, Newton ER, Cetrulo CL: Intrauterine fetal demise in multiple gestation. *Acta Genet Med Gemellol (Roma)* 1984; 33:43–49.

15. David TJ: Vascular basis for malformations in a twin. *Arch Dis Child* 1985; 60:166–167.

16. De Lia JE, Cruikshank DP, Keye WR Jr. Fetoscopic neodymium:YAG laser occlusion of placental vessels in severe twin-twin transfusion syndrome. *Obstet Gynecol* 1990; 75:1046–1053.

17. Derom C, Bakker E, Vlietinck R, Derom R, Van Den Berghe H, Thiery M, Pearson P: Zygosity determination in newborn twins using DNA variants. *J Med Genet* 1985; 22:279–282.

18. Dixon HG, Browne JCM, Davey DA: Choriodecidual and myometrial blood-flow. *Lancet* 1963; 2:369.

19. Glauser TA, Rorke LB, Weinberg PM, Clancy RR: Congenital brain anomalies associated with the hypoplastic left heart syndrome. *Pediatrics* 1990; 85:984–990.

20. Glauser TA, Rorke LB, Weinberg PM, Clancy RR: Acquired neuropathologic lesions associated with hypoplastic left heart syndrome. *Pediatrics* 1990; 85:991–1000.

21. Gonsoulin W, Moise KJ Jr, Kirshon B, Cotton DB, Wheeler JM, Carpenter RJ Jr: Outcome of twin-twin transfusion diagnosed before 28 weeks' gestation. *Obstet Gynecol* 1990; 75:214–216.

22. Jauniaux E, Elkazen N, Leroy F, Wilkin P, Rodesch F, Hustin J: Clinical and morphologic aspects of the vanishing twin phenomenon. *Obstet Gynecol* 1988; 72:577–581.

23. Kirshon B: Fetal urine output in hydramnios. *Obstet Gynecol* 1989; 73:240–242.

24. Kovacs BW, Kirschbaum TH, Paul RH: Twin gestations: I. Antenatal care and complications. *Obstet Gynecol* 1989; 74:313–317.

25. Lage JM, Vanmarter LJ, Mikhail E: Vascular anastomoses in fused, dichorionic twin placentas resulting in twin transfusion syndrome. *Placenta* 1989; 10:55–59.

26. Landy HJ, Keith L, Keith D: The vanishing twin. *Acta Genet Med Gemellol (Roma)* 1982; 31:179–194.

27. Landy HJ, Weiner S, Corson SL, Batzer FR, Bolognese RJ: The "vanishing twin": Ultrasonographic assessment of fetal disappearance in the first trimester. *Am J Obstet Gynecol* 1986; 155:14–19.

28. Larroche JC, Droulle P, Delezoide AL, Narcy F, Nessmann C: Brain damage in monozygous twins. *Biol Neonate* 1990; 57:261–278.

29. Little J, Bryan E: Congenital anomalies in twins. *Semin Perinatol* 1986; 10:50–64.

30. Livnat EJ, Burd L, Cadkin A, Keh P, Ward AP: Fetus papyraceus in twin pregnancy. *Obstet Gynecol* 1978; 5(suppl):41S.

31. MacLennan AH, Green RC, O'Shea R, Brookes C, Morris D: Routine hospital admission in twin pregnancy between 26 and 30 weeks of gestation. *Lancet* 1990; 335:267–269.

32. McCracken AA, Daly PA, Zolnick MR, Clark AM: Twins and Q-banded chromosome polymorphisms. *Hum Genet* 1978; 45:253–258.

33. Naeye RL: Human intrauterine parabiotic syndrome and its complications. *N Engl J Med* 1963; 268:804–809.

34. Naeye RL: Transposition of the great arteries and prenatal growth. *Arch Pathol* 1966; 82:412–418.

35. Naeye RL: New observations in erythroblastosis fetalis. *JAMA* 1967; 20:281–286.

36. Naeye RL: Prenatal abnormal organ and cellular growth with various chromosomal disorders. *Biol Neonate* 1967; 11:248–255.

37. Naeye RL: Pregnancy hypertension, placental evidences of low uteroplacental blood flow and spontaneous preterm delivery. *Hum Pathol* 1989; 20:441–444.

38. Naeye RL: Maternal body weight and pregnancy outcome. *Am J Clin Nutr* 1990; 52:273–279.

39. Naeye RL, Benirschke K, Hagstrom JWC, Marcus CC: Intrauterine growth in twins as estimated from liveborn birth weight data. *Pediatrics* 1966; 37:409–416.

40. Naeye RL, Blanc WA: Fetal renal structure and the genesis of amniotic fluid disorders. *Am J Pathol* 1972; 67:95–108.

41. Naeye RL, Tafari N: *Risk Factors in Pregnancy and Diseases of the Fetus and Newborn.* Baltimore, Williams & Wilkins Co, 1983.

42. Naeye RL, Tafari N, Judge D, Marboe CC: Twins: causes of perinatal death in 12 United States cities and one African city. *Am J Obstet Gynecol* 1978; 131:267–272.

43. Nylander PPS: The determination of zygosity, a study of 608 pairs of twins born in Aberdeen. *J Obstet Gynaecol Br Commonw* 1970; 77:506–510.

44. Nylander PPS, Osunkoya BO: Unusual monochorionic placentation with heterosexual twins. *Obstet Gynecol* 1970; 36:621–625.

45. Perrin VDK: *Pathology of the Placenta.* New York, Churchill Livingstone Inc, 1984.

46. Plomin R, Chipuer HM, Loehlin JC: Behavior genetics and personality, in Pervin LA (ed): *Handbook of Personality, Theory and Research.* New York, Guilford Press, 1990, pp 225–243.

47. Plomin R, DeFries JC, McClearn GE: *Behavioral Genetics: A Primer,* ed 2. New York, WH Freeman, 1990.

48. Robertson EG, Neer KJ: Placental injection studies in twin gestation. *Am J Obstet Gynecol* 1983; 147:170–174.

49. Romero R, Duffy TP, Berkowitz RL, Chang E, Hobbins JC: Prolongation of a preterm pregnancy complicated by death of a single twin in utero and disseminated intravascular coagulation. *N Engl J Med* 1984; 310:772–774.

50. Schinzel AAGL, Smith DW, Miller JR: Monozygotic twinning and structural defects. *J Pediatr* 1979; 95:921–930.

51. Smith DW: Recognizable patterns of human malformation, in Smith DW (ed): *Major Problems in Clinical Paediatrics,* vol 7. WB Saunders, London, 1982, p 506.

52. Spellacy WN, Handler A, Ferre CD: A case-control study of 1253 twin pregnancies from a 1982–1987 perinatal data base. *Obstet Gynecol* 1990; 75:168–171.

53. Szymonowicz W, Preston H, Yu VH: The surviving monozygotic twin. *Arch Dis Child* 1986; 61:454–458.

54. Van Allen MI, Smith DW, Shepard JH: Twin reversed arterial perfusion (TRAP) sequence: A study of 14 twin pregnancies with acardia. *Semin Perinatol* 1983; 7:285–293.

55. Wittmann BK, Farquharson DF, Thomas WDS, Baldwin VJ, Wadsworth LD. The role of feticide in the management of severe twin transfusion syndrome. *Am J Obstet Gynecol* 1986; 155:1023–1026.

56. Ylitalo V, Kero P, Erkkola R: Neurological outcome of twins dissimilar in size at birth. *Early Hum Dev* 1988; 17:245–255.

57. Yoshioka H, Kadomoto Y, Mino M, Morikawa Y, Kasubuchi Y, Kusunoki T: Multicystic encephalomalacia in liveborn twin with a stillborn macerated co-twin. *J Pediatr* 1979; 95:798–800.

CHAPTER 11

Disorders of the Central Nervous System

This chapter includes many findings derived from the Collaborative Perinatal Study (CPS), which collected information to look for the origins of central nervous system (CNS) disorders.[28,115,125] It followed prospectively the course of over 56,000 pregnancies in 12 medical school–affiliated hospitals in different regions of the United States between 1959 and 1966. Events of gestation, labor, delivery, and the neonatal period were recorded as well as children's mental, motor, sensory, and physical development to 7 years of age. Sociocultural, lifestyle, and hereditary data were also collected. Placentas were routinely examined and their findings recorded. We used data from all of these sources to identify risk factors for motor, cognitive, and behavioral disorders. All of the diagnoses of these disorders are based on the results of neurologic and psychological examinations undertaken on the children at 7 years of age. This age was selected because abnormalities diagnosed at this age are more often permanent than abnormalities that are present at earlier ages. More details about the CPS can be found in the introduction to this book.

RISK FACTORS

The risk factors that we selected to screen for their roles in the genesis of cognitive, motor, and behavioral disorders fall into three broad categories: (1) familial, (2) antenatal maldevelopment or damage, and (3) damage during labor, delivery, the neonatal period, or later. We placed each risk factor in the category that seems to reflect its dominant character, recognizing that some of the risk factors could have been placed in more than one category. For example, mothers who smoke cigarettes differ in their lifestyles and personalities in some respects from nonsmokers.[158] All of the risk factors were used as independent variables.

Familial Factors

Familial risk factors are divided into two subcategories. The first contains factors that have mainly a *genetic* component (Table 11–1). Individuals with IQ scores between 60 and 79 were considered to have mild mental retardation. IQ values in this range often have a genetic component, as evidenced by the fact that siblings of children with these low scores have an increased frequency of low values.

The second category, entitled *environmental*, contains a potpourri of factors that reflect child-raising practices based in part on culture and custom, factors that sometimes deprive children of stimulation because one or both parents are absent or are culturally deprived. It also includes factors that are markers for both nourishing and destructive interactions with near-of-age siblings and parents, and specific adverse conditions in the home. These interactions and experiences are highly individual and often have different effects on different children in the same family. Adverse social conditions included having a high level of conflict in the home, losing or living away from one or both parents, and being chronically ill. It has long been known that children with chronic illnesses are at an increased risk for social, educational, and emotional difficulties.[137,139] Socioeconomic scores of 0 to 30 were considered to be low. This score is based on values given to family income, maternal

TABLE 11–1.

Risk Factors by Categories

Familial factors	
Mainly genetic (one or more family members)	*Environmental*
Mild mental retardation	Low socioeconomic status
Mental illness	Race: black
Motor disorders	Father living apart from family
Congenital syndromes	Mother: blue collar worker outside of home
Sex: male	Adverse social conditions in home
	Near-of-age older siblings
Antenatal brain maldevelopment or damage	
Placental and umbilical cord abnormalities	*Subnormal fetal motor activity*
Unevenly accelerated placental maturation	Abnormally short umbilical cord
Retarded placental maturation	Absent subchorionic fibrin, placenta
Maternal floor infarction, placenta	
Bipartite or tripartite placenta	*Fetal abnormalities*
Succenturiate lobe, placenta	Birth weight, percentiles 1–10
Circumvallate placenta	Head circumference, percentiles 1–10
Single umbilical artery	Major malformations
Velamentous insertion of umbilical cord	Multiple births
Umbilical cord meconium-stained	*No intrapartum or postnatal explanations for brain dysfunctions*
Maternal pregnancy factors	
Cigarette smoking	Cerebral palsy
Diabetes mellitus	Other poor motor coordination
Seizure disorder	Severe mental retardation
Severe anemia	Other neurologic abnormalities
Low pregnancy weight gain	
Damage during labor, delivery, the neonatal period, or later	
Birth asphyxia	CNS infections
Preterm birth	Neonatal serum bilirubin >18 mg/dL
Meconium in the amniotic fluid	
Severe neonatal respiratory distress	

education, and the type of job held by the head of household.

Antenatal Maldevelopment or Damage

Antenatal brain maldevelopment or damage was divided into several subcategories (see Table 11–1). The first of these subcategories is *placental and umbilical cord abnormalities*. Some of these disorders impair placental or umbilical function and thereby indirectly affect the fetal brain. Others are markers for early gestational events that also lead to maldevelopment of the CNS. Details on the origins and clinical significance of these placental and umbilical cord disorders can be found in Chapters 6 and 7.

The second subcategory is *maternal pregnancy factors*. Included are maternal cigarette smoking during pregnancy, severe gestational anemia, diabetes mellitus,

and a chronic seizure disorder without reference to whether the seizures were under control or out of control during pregnancy. Smoking reduces uteroplacental blood flow.[76] Children of mothers who smoked during pregnancy had increased frequencies of hyperactive behavior and mild cognitive impairments.[112] Maternal diabetes mellitus and seizure disorders were included as risk factors because both are sometimes teratogenic (see Chapter 2). Maternal gestational anemia was included as an antenatal risk factor because it increases fetal and neonatal mortality.[115]

The third subcategory consists of markers for *subnormal fetal motor activity*. This topic is covered in detail in Chapter 7. A number of placental, umbilical cord, and fetal membrane abnormalities appear to be the consequence of trauma administered by vigorous movements of the fetus. Their absence is sometimes a manifestation of low fetal motor activity and also has a positive correlation with both cognitive and motor impairments in older children. We postulate that factors that adversely affect motor areas of the brain sometimes also affect cognitive areas as well.

The fourth subcategory is *fetal abnormalities*. It includes fetal growth retardation, congenital malformations, and multiple births. The first two are either markers or consequences of influences that lead to brain maldevelopment or damage. For example, congenital malformations can be markers for brain maldevelopment or they can damage brains because they cause organ malfunction. An example of the latter are the brain lesions sometimes associated with congenital heart disease.[58,59,64,128] Twins have a much higher frequency of CNS malfunctions than single-born infants. The reasons for this finding can be found in Chapter 10.

The fifth subcategory, *no intrapartum or postnatal explanations for brain dysfunction,* includes well-known motor and cognitive disorders which have no intrapartum or postnatal explanation and are therefore assumed to originate before birth. The category includes children who had an IQ score of less than 60 at 7 years of age. This is presumably not usually a genetic disorder because the siblings of children with these very low IQ scores have a normal distribution of IQ values.[122,140] In the absence of an intrapartum or postnatal explanation, this finding suggests that scores less than 60 usually reflect antenatal brain damage or maldevelopment.

Brain Damage During Labor, Delivery, the Neonatal Period, or Later

This category includes birth asphyxial disorders, meconium in the amniotic fluid preterm birth, CNS infections, and neonatal serum bilirubin values greater than 18 mg/dL. *Preterm birth* was included as a risk factor because the disorders that cause preterm birth sometimes damage

the fetal brain. In addition, the brains of preterm born infants are sometimes damaged as the result of their immaturity, particularly the immaturity of the mechanisms that control blood flow through their brains.[177] Meconium can reportedly damage fetuses by enducing vasoconstriction in the placenta and umbilical cord.[3] The other risk factor in the category that needs definition is *birth asphyxia*. This is a composite category that includes several disorders that cause acute intrapartum fetal hypoxia or asphyxia. The identity of these disorders and how we decided that they cause hypoxia or asphyxia is explained in the introduction. Disorders and conditions that can cause antenatal hypoxia or ischemia for several days or longer were consolidated into a category which we termed *chronic antenatal hypoxia disorders*. The details of this category are also in the introduction.

Methods of Analysis

Multiple logistic regression was the method used to identify risk factors that were significantly associated with individual cognitive, motor, and behavioral disorders.[70] To make the tables in this chapter easy to understand, risk factors that were not significantly associated with the cognitive, motor, and behavioral disorders analyzed are excluded from the tables.

A method for estimating population attributable risk from logistic regression models, described by Bruzzi et al., was utilized to estimate the relative contribution of each risk factor for a neurologic or behavioral disorder when adjusted for all of the other risk factors in the model.[18,114] For example, an attributable risk of 0.02 for congenital malformations in Table 11–2 indicates that 2% of the mild mental retardation in the analysis was estimated to be attributable to congenital malformations, given adjustments for all of the other risk factors in the model. The recently developed methods of Benichou and Gail were employed to construct 95% confidence intervals for the relative risk and attributable risk estimates.[6] A relative risk of 2.4 for parental mental retardation in Table 11–2 indicates that mental retardation in one or both parents was associated with a 2.4-fold increase in the risk for long-term mild mental retardation in their children.

COGNITIVE DISORDERS

Mental Retardation

We analyzed data from the CPS to try to determine the relative roles of organic, genetic, and sociocultural influences on the genesis of mental retardation. Starting 25 years ago, Drillien et al.,[39] Penrose,[133] Zigler,[190] and others developed the two-population model to explain the causes of mental retardation. In this model sociocultural deprivation and heredity are the main factors responsible for mild mental retardation, whereas brain damage and maldevelopment cause most severe mental retardation. This two-population model has been challenged in recent years by reports that potentially damaging disorders sometimes antedate mild as well as severe mental retardation.[16,29,30,38,67] No disorder that might damage brains has been identified for most published cases of mild mental retardation, but a few instances of maternal bleeding or hypertension during pregnancy; placental infarcts; asphyxia at birth; kernicterus; and neonatal cyanosis have been described.[15,16,30,38,39,67]

Other reported antenatal risk factors for mental retardation include maternal seizure disorders, maternal cigarette smoking during pregnancy, maternal alcoholism, severe maternal gestational anemia, fetal growth retardation, congenital cytomegalovirus infection, congenital syndromes, minor and major congenital malformations, a high hemoglobin value in the neonate, congenital hypothyroidism, the neonatal respiratory distress syndrome, dietary deficiencies of iron, chloride, and other nutrients during early infancy, an abnormal distribution of blood flow within the brain, and a host of sociocultural and polygenic influences.*

Seven percent of the children in the CPS had IQ scores between 60 and 79 on the Wechsler Intelligence Scale, which identified them as mildly retarded, while 2% had IQ scores of less than 60, which classified them as severely retarded (see Tables 11–2, 11–3).[182] Children in the two categories were further classified by whether or not they had associated neurologic abnormalities (see Tables 11–2 through 11–5).[28]

Mild Mental Retardation Without Accompanying Neurologic Abnormalities

Risk factors were identified for 91% of the IQ scores between 60 and 79 in the CPS (Table 11–2). Seventy percent of this risk was familial. Race and low socioeconomic status were the dominant risk factors in this category. Sixteen percent of the risk was in the antenatal maldevelopment or damage category and the major risk factors were congenital malformations, fetal growth retardation, and unevenly accelerated maturation of the placenta.

It is noteworthy that only 2% of the mild mental retardation in CPS children was attributable to mental retardation in either parent (see Table 11–2). Does this mean that there is less influence of inheritance on IQ values than is usually assumed, or is the inheritance somehow included as part of other risk factors that seem to have a much greater influence on low IQ values, such as low socioeconomic status and race? The cultural bias in the IQ test is widely accepted to be the reason why blacks have lower IQ values than whites. Cultural bias probably also accounts for some of the association between low IQ scores and low socioeconomic status.

One can speculate on the meaning of the other risk factors for mild mental retardation. Unevenly accelerated placen-

* References 29, 33, 53, 75, 82–84, 86, 88, 112, 113, 120, 132, 180, and 185.

TABLE 11–2.

Risk Factors for Mild Mental Retardation Without Accompanying Neurologic Abnormalities at 7 Years of Age*

Risk Factors	No. of Mildly Retarded Children per 1,000 Children With Risk Factor†	Relative Risks (95% Confidence Intervals)	Attributable Risks (95% Confidence Intervals)
All cases	70 (4,053)		
Familial			
Race: black	**196** (1,908), *P* < .001	**2.5** (2.1, 2.8)	**.37** (.36, .39)
Low family socioeconomic status	**150** (3,042), *P* < .001	**2.0** (1.8, 2.1)	**.20** (.19, .22)
Mother employed outside home	**92** (1,154), *P* < .001	**1.2** (1.1, 1.4)	**.07** (.05, .09)
Sex: male	**77** (1,285), *P* < .001	**1.2** (1.1, 1.3)	**.05** (.03, .07)
Parental mental retardation	**250** (35), *P* < .001	**2.4** (1.7, 3.4)	**.02** (.01, .03)
Antenatal maldevelopment or damage			
Fetal abnormalities			
Congenital malformations	**92** (422), *P* < .001	**1.1** (1.0, 1.3)	**.02** (.01, .03)
Birth weight, percentiles 1–10	**120** (242), *P* < .001	**1.4** (1.2, 1.6)	**.02** (.01, .03)
Placental, umbilical cord abnormalities			
Unevenly accelerated maturation	**80** (918), *P* < .001	**1.2** (1.1, 1.3)	**.05** (.03, .07)
Subchorionic fibrin absent	**98** (622), *P* < .001	**1.3** (1.0, 1.6)	**.03** (.01, .05)
Succenturiate lobe present	**102** (75), *P* < .001	**1.4** (1.0, 1.8)	**.01** (.00, .01)
Opaque fetal surface	**91** (335), *P* < .001	**1.1** (1.0, 1.2)	**.01** (.00, .01)
Retarded maturation	**86** (256), *P* < .01	**1.1** (1.0, 1.2)	**.01** (.00, .02)
Unusually short umbilical cord	**100** (162), *P* < .001	**1.3** (1.0, 1.6)	**.01** (.00, .01)
Labor and delivery			
Preterm birth	**93** (715), *P* < .001	**1.2** (1.1, 1.4)	**.04** (.03, .06)
Population attributable risk			**.91** (.89, .93)

*Significant values are in boldface.
†Number of children with mental retardation are in parentheses. P values compared with value in all cases in study.

tal maturation is a manifestation of chronic low blood flow from the uterus to the placenta (see Chapter 7). This low blood flow sometimes restricts the delivery of oxygen and nutrients to the fetus to a degree that retards fetal growth, and based on the current findings may also adversely affect brain development. A short umbilical cord and absent fibrin beneath the chorionic plate of the placenta are often evidence of weak or infrequent fetal movements, which in turn are sometimes manifestations of fetal brain dysfunction.[105,108] Preterm birth has long been known to be a risk factor for mild mental retardation, in part because immaturity of the cerebral circulation sometimes predisposes to brain damage during the neonatal period.[85,106,107] Fetal growth retardation and congenital malformations are presumably surrogates for antenatal disorders that damage or retard brain development before birth.[58,59,115]

Severe Mental Retardation Without Accompanying Neurologic Abnormalities

An IQ score of less than 60 placed a child in the severely mentally retarded category (Table 11–3). This category comprised 0.2% of the children without accompanying motor or other neurologic abnormalities. Risk factors were identified for 88% of this retardation. Forty-six percent of this risk was in the familial category and involved the same risk factors as were present in the familial category for mild mental retardation (see Table 11–2). Thirty-one percent of the risk was in the antenatal maldevelopment or damage category. Fetal growth retardation accounted for most of this risk. Preterm birth accounted for the final 11% of the identified risk.

Familial factors had a relatively larger role in mild than in severe mental retardation, but such factors were very impor-

TABLE 11–3.

Risk Factors for Severe Mental Retardation Unaccompanied by Neurologic Abnormalities at 7 Years of Age*

Risk Factors	No. of Severely Retarded Children per 1,000 Children With Risk Factor†	Relative Risks (95% Confidence Intervals)	Attributable Risks (95% Confidence Intervals)
All cases	2 (114)		
Familial			
Low family socioeconomic status	**5** (46), *P* < .001	**2.0** (1.2, 3.2)	**.18** (.13, .24)
Race: black	**4** (49), *P* < .001	**1.7** (1.0, 2.7)	**.15** (.11, .20)
Sex: male	**4** (47), *P* < .001	**1.5** (1.0, 2.4)	**.13** (.09, .17)
Antenatal maldevelopment or damage			
Fetal abnormalities			
Birth weight, percentiles 1–10	**6** (23), *P* < .001	**3.0** (1.6, 5.7)	**.13** (.06, .19)
Head circumference at birth, percentiles 1–10	**8** (20), *P* < .001	**3.7** (1.9, 7.0)	**.11** (.04, .18)
Placental abnormalities			
Unevenly accelerated maturation	**4** (34), *P* < .02	**1.2** (1.1, 1.3)	**.03** (.00, .06)
Subchorionic fibrin absent	**4** (17), *P* < .05	**1.2** (1.1, 1.3)	**.04** (.01, .07)
Neonatal period			
Preterm birth	**4** (26), *P* < .001	**1.9** (1.2, 3.1)	**.11** (.06, .16)
Population attributable risk			***.88*** (.85, .91)

*Significant values are in boldface.
†Numbers of children with mental retardation are in parentheses. P values compared with value in all cases in category.

tant with both degrees of mental retardation. Antenatal maldevelopment and damage factors were more important antecedents of severe than of mild retardation, but these risk factors were also important with both degrees of retardation (see Tables 11–2, 11–3). Fetal growth retardation, often a manifestation of antenatal maldevelopment or damage, was 12 times more frequent among the severely retarded than among the mildly retarded (see Tables 11–2, 11–3). Preterm birth was three times more frequent among the severely retarded than among the mildly retarded. Severe mental retardation in the prematurely born was not just a reflection of the disorders that caused the preterm births because these latter disorders were among the risk factors included as independent variables in our analyses (see Chapter 9). Absent fibrin beneath the chorionic (fetal) plate of the placenta, which is sometimes the consequence of subnormal fetal motor activity, had about the same frequency in the placentas of mildly and severely mentally retarded children.[108] Unevenly accelerated placen-

tal maturation, a manifestation of low uteroplacental blood flow, was slightly more frequent in the placentas of the mildly retarded (5%) than in the placentas of the severely retarded (3%).

It is noteworthy that no association was found between congenital malformations and severe mental retardation, between meconium in the amniotic fluid and severe mental retardation or between disorders that cause acute fetal hypoxia or asphyxia and severe mental retardation. The reason is that cerebral malformations and meconium and hypoxic brain damage rarely affect cognitive skills without also impairing motor functions. Our analyses found no association between severe mental retardation in children and mental retardation in their parents.

Mild Mental Retardation With Accompanying Neurologic Abnormalities

Of the children in the CPS, 2.1% were placed in this category because they had IQ scores between 60 and 79 and a specific neurologic disorder at 7 years of age

(Table 11–4). One out of every four children with mild mental retardation in the CPS also had neurologic abnormalities. Antecedent risk factors were identified for 84% of this mild retardation that was accompanied by neurologic abnormalities (see Table 11–4). Fifty-six percent of the risk was in the familial category and 25% in the antenatal maldevelopment or damage category. Familial factors were only a slightly less important risk for mild mental retardation with neurologic abnormalities than for mild retardation without neurologic abnormalities (see Tables 11–2, 11–4).

Race and low socioeconomic status were major risks for mild mental retardation with and without accompanying neurologic abnormalities (see Tables 11–2, 11–4). Being a male was a greater risk factor for mild mental retardation accompanied by neurologic abnormalities than for such retardation without neurologic abnormalities. Preterm birth, manifestations of weak fetal motor activity, and parental mental retardation accounted for about the same percentages of mild mental retardation with and without neurologic abnormalities (see Tables 11–2, 11–4). Maternal floor infarction, a disorder in which fibrin fills the intervillous space of the placenta, was associated with mild mental retardation only when neurologic abnormalities were present (see Table 11–4).

Many of the children who had both neurologic abnormalities and mild mental retardation at 7 years of age had neurologic abnormalities persisting through the newborn period (see Table 11–7). Such early persisting neurologic abnormalities were absent in children who had mild mental retardation without long-term neurologic abnormalities.

Severe Mental Retardation With Accompanying Neurologic Abnormalities

Neurologic abnormalities were present in three out of four children who had

TABLE 11–4.

Risk Factors for Mild Mental Retardation Accompanied by Neurologic Abnormalities at 7 Years of Age*

Risk Factors	No. of Mildly Retarded Children per 1,000 Children With Risk Factor†	Relative Risks (95% Confidence Intervals)	Attributable Risks (95% Confidence Intervals)
All cases	21 (1,247)		
Familial			
Race: black	**50** (855), *P* < .001	**2.0** (1.8, 2.2)	**.23** (.21, .25)
Low socioeconomic status	**50** (726), *P* < .001	**1.9** (1.7, 2.1)	**.17** (.16, .19)
Sex: male	**36** (731), *P* < .001	**1.4** (1.2, 1.6)	**.11** (.09, .13)
Mother employed outside home	**37** (568), *P* < .001	**1.3** (1.1, 1.5)	**.05** (.04, .07)
Parental mental retardation	**102** (33), *P* < .001	**3.1** (2.1, 4.4)	**.01** (.01, .02)
Antenatal maldevelopment or damage			
Fetal abnormalities			
Congenital malformations	**80** (287), *P* < .001	**1.5** (1.3, 1.7)	**.05** (.04, .07)
Birth weight, percentiles 1–10	**48** (173), *P* < .001	**1.6** (1.3, 2.0)	**.04** (.03, .05)
Head circumference at birth, percentile 1–10	**42** (129), *P* < .001	**2.1** (1.7, 2.5)	**.04** (.03, .05)
Placental, umbilical cord abnormalities			
Abnormally short umbilical cord	**48** (47), *P* < .001	**1.8** (1.3, 1.7)	**.05** (.04, .07)
Maternal floor infarction	**68** (10), *P* < .005	**2.2** (1.1, 3.4)	**.04** (.00, .09)
Retarded placental maturation	**39** (94), *P* < .001	**1.3** (1.0, 1.6)	**.03** (.00, .06)
Neonatal period			
Preterm birth	**46** (361), *P* < .001	**1.3** (1.1, 1.5)	**.04** (.03, .05)
CNS infections	**99** (15), *P* < .001	**2.8** (1.7, 4.8)	**.01** (.00, .01)
Population attributable risk			**.84** (.83, .86)

*Significant values are in boldface.
†Numbers of children with mental retardation are in parentheses. P values compared with value in all cases category.

severe mental retardation compared with only one of four children who had mild mental retardation (see Tables 11–2 through 11–5). This suggests that brain damage or maldevelopment that is severe enough to cause severe mental retardation usually also affects motor control areas of the brain.

In the CPS, risk factors were identified for 93% of the severe mental retardation that was accompanied by neurologic abnormalities (Table 11–5). Most of the risk factors for severe mental retardation without accompanying neurologic abnormalities were also risk factors for severe mental retardation with neurologic abnormalities. However, the list was longer when neurologic abnormalities were present. The additional risk factors included parental mental retardation and multiple markers for antenatal brain damage or maldevelopment. These latter markers included congenital malforma-

tions, meconium in the amniotic fluid, retarded placental maturation, an unusually short umbilical cord, maternal placental floor infarction, a single umbilical artery, birth asphyxial disorders and central nervous system infections (Tables 11–3, 11–5). The association with congenital malformations could be the consequence of a teratogenic influence that also affected the brain, or it could be the result of damage to the brain caused by malfunction of another malformed organ, particularly the heart.[58,59] Altshuler and Hyde have found evidence that meconium causes vasoconstriction in the placenta and umbilical cord which is a plausible explanation for some of the excessive perinatal mortality and psychomotor impairments associated with its presence in the amniotic fluid (Tables 11–5, and 11–6).[3]

As noted in Chapter 8, meconium in the amniotic fluid is a marker for disorders

TABLE 11–5.

Risk Factors for Severe Mental Retardation Accompanied by Neurologic Abnormalities at 7 Years of Age*

Risk Factors	No. of Severely Retarded Children per 1,000 Children With Risk Factor†	Relative Risks (95% Confidence Intervals)	Attributable Risks (95% Confidence Intervals)
All cases	6 (330)		
Familial			
Race: black	**13** (218), *P*<.001	**2.0** (1.6, 2.5)	**.22** (.20, .25)
Low socioeconomic status	**12** (178), *P*<.001	**1.6** (1.3, 2.0)	**.13** (.11, .16)
Parental mental retardation	**33** (11), *P*<.001	**4.0** (2.1, 7.4)	**.02** (.01, .04)
Antenatal maldevelopment or damage			
Fetal abnormalities			
Congenital malformations	**34** (122), *P*<.001	**3.0** (2.4, 3.8)	**.17** (.14, .22)
Birth weight, percentiles 1–10	**20** (68), *P*<.001	**2.8** (2.1, 3.7)	**.09** (.07, .12)
Head circumference at birth, percentiles 1–10	**13** (53), *P*<.001	**3.4** (2.5, 4.5)	**.07** (.05, .09)
Meconium in amniotic fluid	**8** (103)	**3.1** (2.3, 4.5)	**.05** (.04, .06)
Placental, umbilical cord abnormalities			
Unevenly accelerated maturation	**34** (144), *P*<.001	**1.3** (1.1, 1.7)	**.07** (.05, .09)
Retarded maturation	**11** (26), *P*<.02	**1.4** (1.0, 1.9)	**.02** (.00, .03)
Unusually short umbilical cord	**14** (18), *P*<.01	**1.5** (1.0, 2.1)	**.02** (.00, .05)
Maternal floor infarction	**27** (4), *P*<.01	**3.4** (1.4, 5.6)	**.01** (.00, .01)
Single umbilical artery	**26** (6), *P*<.02	**2.5** (1.2, 4.1)	**.01** (.00, .01)
Labor, delivery, neonatal period			
Preterm birth	**12** (97), *P*<.001	**1.5** (1.1, 1.9)	**.06** (.04, .08)
Birth asphyxia	**99** (4), *P*<.001	**10.1** (3.7, 27.9)	**.01** (.00, .02)
CNS infections	**26** (4), *P*<.001	**2.4** (1.0, 6.3)	**.01** (.00, .03)
Population attributable risk			**.93** (.91, .95)

*Significant values are in boldface.
†Numbers of children with mental retardation are in parentheses. P values compared with value in all cases category.

that stress the fetus, particularly acute chorioamnionitis and developmental disorders. Low Apgar scores and neonatal seizures increased the risk for severe but not for mild mental retardation (see Tables 11–6, 11–7). Neurologic abnormalities persisting through the neonatal period were a risk for long-term motor abnormalities in both the mildly and the severely mentally retarded (Table 11–7).

TABLE 11–6.

The Rates of Various Cognitive Disorders per 1,000 Children at 7 Years of Age in Full-Term Born Children Who Had Meconium in Their Amniotic Fluid at Birth or Abnormal Apgar Scores*

	Meconium in Amniotic Fluid	
	Absent	*Present*
No motor abnormalities		
Mild mental retardation	69 (2,523)	63 (572), $P<.05$
Severe mental retardation	4 (156)	6 (53), $P>.05$
Motor abnormalities present		
Mild mental retardation	5 (167)	5 (45), $P>.1$
Severe mental retardation	3 (110)	5 (45), $P<.001$

	Apgar Scores at 1 and 10 Minutes		
	0–3, 0–5	*0–3, 7–10*	*7–10, 7–10*
No motor abnormalities			
Mild mental retardation	81 (18)	75 (72)	67 (2,191)
Severe mental retardation	5 (2)	9 (9), $P<.02$	4 (139)
Motor abnormalities present			
Mild mental retardation	13 (3)	4 (4)	4 (132)
Severe mental retardation	22 (5), $P<.001$	6 (6)†	3 (96)

*Number of children with brain malfunction are in parentheses.
†$P<.05$ compared with value in 7–10, 7–10 category.

TABLE 11–7.

The Rates of Various Brain Malfunctions per 1,000 Children at 7 Years of Age in Full-Term Born Children Who Had Neonatal Seizures or Persistent Neurologic Abnormalities in the Neonatal Period*

	Absent	Present
Neonatal seizures		
No motor abnormalities		
Mild mental retardation	69 (3,134)	68 (8)
Severe mental retardation	5 (212)	26 (3), $P<.001$
Motor abnormalities present		
Mild mental retardation	5 (210)	17 (2)
Severe mental retardation	3 (150)	42 (5), $P<.001$
Persistent neurologic abnormalities in neonatal period		
No motor abnormalities		
Mild mental retardation	73 (2,456)	80 (231), $P>.1$
Severe mental retardation	4 (136)	5 (15), $P>.1$
Motor abnormalities present		
Mild mental retardation	3 (113)	8 (23), $P<.001$
Severe mental retardation	2 (52)	9 (26), $P<.001$

*Numbers of children with brain malfunction are in parentheses

Learning Disorders Not Associated With Low IQ Values or Visual or Hearing Impairments

Seven-year-old children who were two or more grades below their expected levels in reading and spelling were placed in this category if the results of IQ, visual, and hearing tests did not provide an explanation for their learning problem. Falling into this category were 1.6% of the children in the CPS (Table 11–8). Antecedents were found for 70% of these learning disorders. Sixty percent of these antecedents were in the familial category. The major factors were being male and low family socioeconomic status. Overall, there was a large similarity between the risk factors for mild mental retardation and for learning disorders with normal IQ values. The one major difference was being a male, which had a sixfold greater influence on the frequency of learning disorders than on mild mental retardation (see Tables 11–2, 11–8). Race had a much smaller influence on learning disorders than it had on low IQ values.

Only 11% of the risk was in the antenatal maldevelopment or damage category.

The two risk factors in this category were maternal smoking during pregnancy and unevenly accelerated placental maturation (see Table 11–8). As previously mentioned, unevenly accelerated placental maturation is caused by chronic low blood flow from the uterus to the placenta, which sometimes restricts the delivery of oxygen and nutrients to the fetus.[115] Its association with learning disorders is still further evidence that such low blood flow may adversely affect fetal brain development.

Children with learning disorders also often exhibit hyperactive behavior, a short attention span, and a poor memory. Lou et al. have reported that a number of children with learning disorders and behavioral abnormalities have low blood flow through the head of the caudate nucleus and the posterior periventricular regions of their brains.[83]

HIGH IQ VALUES

Children who had an IQ value above 120 at 7 years of age were placed in this

TABLE 11–8.

Risk Factors for a Learning Disorder Not Associated With a Low IQ Value (<80) at 7 Years of Age*

Risk Factors	Number of Children With a Learning Disorder per 1,000 Children With Risk Factor†	Relative Risks (95% Confidence Intervals)	Attributable Risks (95% Confidence Intervals)
All cases	16 (780)		
Familial			
Sex: male	**26** (529), *P* < .001	**2.1** (1.8, 2.5)	**.30** (.28, .32)
Low socioeconomic status	**27** (393), *P* < .001	**1.6** (1.4, 1.9)	**.16** (.14, .18)
Race: black	**25** (425), *P* < .001	**1.3** (1.1, 1.5)	**.09** (0.7, .12)
Familial disorders	**29** (25), *P* < .001	**1.9** (1.3, 2.8)	**.03** (.02, .04)
Low maternal IQ value			**.02** (.01, .04)
Antenatal maldevelopment or damage			
Placental abnormality			
Unevenly accelerated maturation	**21** (176), *P* < .001	**1.2** (1.0, 1.4)	**.05** (.04, .07)
Maternal pregnancy factor			
Cigarette smoking	**25** (390), *P* < .001	**1.2** (1.0, 1.4)	**.06** (.05, .08)
Brain damage during pregnancy or neonatal period			
Preterm birth	**23** (176)	**1.1** (.00, 1.2)	**.01** (.00, .02)
Population attributable risk			**.70** (.68, .72)

*Significant values are in boldface.
†Numbers of children with learning disorders are in parentheses. P values compared with value in all cases category.

category. Antecedents were identified for 92% of these high IQ scores (Table 11–9). Forty percent of the antecedents were familial factors, most of which were just the reverse of the antecedents of mild mental retardation (see Table 11–2). The familial factors that had a strong positive correlation with high IQ values were race, high familial socioeconomic status, a mother who had many years of education, and a father who lived with the family. The sex of the child and a high maternal IQ value had only a very weak positive correlation with high IQ values in CPS children. High IQ values in children were not associated with the number of years of the father's education. First-born children more often had IQ scores above 120 than their subsequently born siblings, but this first-born advantage disappeared when the confounding factors in Table 11–9 were taken into consideration.

Nearly half (48%) of the antecedents for high IQ values were antenatal, presumably biologic factors. These were full-term birth, normal fetal growth, the presence of markers of vigorous fetal motor activity, and being single-born.

ABNORMAL SPEECH OR LANGUAGE WITHOUT ABNORMAL HEARING, A LOW IQ VALUE, OR CEREBRAL PALSY

Children were placed in this category when testing at 7 years of age demonstrated a speech or language abnormality without cerebral palsy (CP) or abnormalities in hearing, vision, or an IQ score less than 80. Of the children in the CPS, 0.8% fell into this category (Table 11–10). Risk factors were identified for 65% of these speech and language disorders.

TABLE 11–9.

Risk Factors for Children Having a High IQ Value (> 120) at 7 Years of Age*

Risk Factors	No. of Children With High IQ Values per 1,000 Children With Risk Factor†	Relative Risks (95% Confidence Intervals)	Attributable Risks (95% Confidence Intervals)
All cases	61 (2,293)		
Familial			**.40** (.27, .43)
Race: white	**111** (2,035), *P* < .001	**3.8** (3.3, 4.3)	
Mother of child had high IQ value	**165** (579), *P* < .001	**2.3** (2.0, 2.6)	
High socioeconomic status	**164** (1,405), *P* < .001	**2.0** (1.8, 2.2)	
Sex: female	**72** (1,337), *P* < .001	**1.6** (1.4, 1.7)	
Mother: education beyond high school	**233** (819), *P* < .001	**1.5** (1.3, 1.7)	
Mother of child ≥ 25 yr	**71** (1,116), *P* < .001	**1.4** (1.2, 1.5)	
Father of child living in the home	**74** (2,119), *P* < .001	**1.8** (1.5, 2.1)	
Father: education beyond high school	**215** (731), *P* < .001	1.0 (0.9, 1.1)	
Father of child: professional occupation	**115** (366), *P* < .001	1.0 (0.9, 1.2)	
First-born in family	**75** (751), *P* < .001	1.1 (0.8, 1.3)	
Developmental			
Fetus			
Full-term birth	**68** (2,051), *P* < .001	**1.4** (1.3, 1.7)	**.24** (.22, .25)
Birth weight, > 10th percentile	**64** (2,058), *P* < .001	**1.4** (1.2, 1.7)	**.04** (.03, .06)
Head circumference > 10th percentile	**64** (2,102), *P* < .001	**1.4** (1.2, 1.7)	**.20** (.18, .22)
Single-born	**62** (2,277), *P* < .001	**2.5** (1.5, 4.1)	**.01** (.00, .01)
Placenta, umbilical cord			
Unusually long umbilical cord	**78** (294), *P* < .05	**1.3** (1.2, 1.5)	**.01** (.00, .02)
Excessive subchorionic fibrin	**72** (641), *P* < .001	**1.2** (1.1, 1.3)	**.03** (.01, .04)
Population attributable risk			**.92** (.91, .94)

*Significant values are in boldface.
†Numbers of children are in parentheses. P values compared with value in all cases category.

Sixty-one percent of the risk was in the familial category. All of this risk was related to being male, black, and the family having a low socioeconomic status, which raises the possibility that sociocultural factors had a major role in the genesis of the abnormal speech and language.

Only 5% of the risk was in the antenatal maldevelopment or damage category. The two identified risk factors in this category were microcephaly and an opaque fetal surface of the placenta (see Table 11–10). Lou et al. have reported that seven language-impaired children had abnormally low blood flows in the left prefrontal and central perisylvian regions of their brains.[84] In another study nine children with expressive language dysfunction had low blood flow through their left cerebral hemispheres.[145]

BEHAVIORAL DISORDERS

It has long been recognized that organic brain dysfunction, genetic influences, interactions with family members, and with persons outside of the family circle affect an individual's behavior.[142] It has been difficult to separate the roles of these influences on specific behavioral disorders for several reasons. First most of these influences are difficult to quantitate. Genetic influences on behavior are particularly difficult to quantitate because many genes are involved. Individually, each of these genes has a small effect and their interactive effects on behavior are for the most part nonadditive.[95,141] This nonadditive nature of their interactions is one reason why extreme behavior in a child is usually attenuated or absent in a child's siblings. Studies suggest that overall genetic factors account for only about 29% of the difference in personality traits between monozygous twins who are reared apart and monozygous twins who are reared together.[95,141] There are some exceptions. Hostility, assertiveness, and agreeableness are characteristics that twin studies show are little influenced by genetic factors.[141]

Interacting genes do more than just affect intrinsic behavior. They also appear to mediate the effects of social interactions

TABLE 11–10.
Risk Factors for Children Having Abnormal Speech or Language Not Associated With a Low IQ Value at 7 Years of Age*

Risk Factors	No. of Children With Abnormal Speech or Language per 1,000 Children With Risk Factor†	Relative Risks (95% Confidence Intervals)	Attributable Risks (95% Confidence Intervals)
All cases	8 (469)		
Familial			
Sex: male	17 (333), *P* < .001	**2.5** (2.0, 3.0)	**.24** (.21, .27)
Race: black	17 (321), *P* < .001	**2.1** (1.7, 2.6)	**.20** (.17, .23)
Low socioeconomic status	18 (256), *P* < .001	**1.6** (1.3, 1.9)	**.17** (.15, .20)
Antenatal maldevelopment or damage			
Fetal abnormalities			
Head circumference at birth, percentiles 1–10	14 (42), *P* < .001	**1.8** (1.3, 2.5)	**.03** (.02, .04)
Placental abnormalities			
Opaque fetal surface	16 (47), *P* < .05	**1.2** (1.0, 1.5)	**.02** (.00, .05)
Population attributable risk			**.65** (.63, .67)

*Significant values are in boldface.
†Numbers of children with abnormal speech or language are in parentheses. P values compared with value in all cases category.

and organic brain disorders on children's behavior. Familial and community influences are particularly difficult to untangle because they are very complex and the value of the raw data used to analyze them is often suspect. For example, many behavioral studies have relied on parents' descriptions of their children's behavior or on assessments by adolescents and young adults of their own behavior. Both parents' assessments of their children's behavior and individuals' assessments of their own behavior are subject to distortion. The strong bias in parents' ratings of their children's behavior is well documented in a study in which parents scored much smaller behavioral differences between twins that they mistakenly thought were monozygous than between twins that they correctly identified as dizygous.[62]

Thomas and Chess have advanced the thesis that the emotional and behavioral development of a child is greatly influenced by how well a child and its family are temperamentally suited to each other.[172] The psychological world in which a child develops is also strongly influenced by schoolmates and playmates. Psychological mismatches in the home and in the wider community can make children outcasts with attendant ill effects on their personalities and behavior. All of this can lead to widely differing psychological environments for siblings being reared in the same household. The results of twin studies reveal that most such environmental influences are not shared. Plomin et al. have summarized the results of many of these studies as showing that shared environments account for only about 9% of the variance of 19 personality traits.[141] The only traits on which shared environment has a substantial impact are hostility (20%), assertiveness (31%), and agreeableness (21%). These are the personality traits on which genetic factors reportedly have only a very limited influence.

Analyses of adoptive siblings suggest that family influences account for only about 5% of the variance of personality traits.[31,141] The unshared experiences include different interactions with siblings and parents. Brazelton and colleagues have emphasized that whether or not a child progresses from a limited behavioral problem to a more severe and persistent disorder often depends on how effectively the parent-child relationship and other home and community interactions support the child's coping skills.[14]

Another problem with published studies on children's behavioral disorders is that they have often not included evidence of organic brain dysfunction, or the analyses have been limited to children with such organic dysfunctions.[24] When risk factors for brain damage or maldevelopment have been included in the analyses, the information on these risk factors has usually been retrospective. At best such retrospective information is unsystematic in its collection, unquantitated, and frequently unreliable because of the varying skills and interests of the observers and the distortions in memory that develop with the passage of time.

Data in the CPS avoid some of the aforementioned problems. The volume of the data is large and it was prospectively collected. It starts with pregnancy and follows the physical, mental, motor, and sensory development of children to 7 years of age. Its biggest limitation is that most of the behavioral data originates from a single testing session conducted by specially selected teams of psychologists when the children were 7 years of age.[16] Normal as well as abnormal behavior was systematically sought and recorded during this seventh-year examination.[28] Our analyses of these data took into consideration a large number of genetic, pregnancy, intrapartum, neonatal, and subsequent environmental influences (see Table 11–1). Well-known markers for brain damage and maldevelopment were included as risk factors in the analyses. The methods of analysis were described early in this chapter and in Chapter 1.

Hyperactivity

Hyperactivity Without Accompanying Neurologic Abnormalities

Hyperactivity is a disorder character-ized by motor restlessness, short attention span, easy distractibility, and impulsive-ness.[3,4] This behavior frequently places children in trouble with their parents, teachers, and other children. The behavior also makes many of them underachievers in school even when they are intelligent and have no specific learning disorder. Forty percent to 60% of hyperactive be-havior in children is reported to still be present in adult life.[57,183] In recent years a strong heritability has been identified and an association has been shown with ma-ternal gestational alcohol consumption, parents who have psychiatric disorders, and parents who display antisocial behav-ior.[31,123,143,153,166] Zametkin et al. have demonstrated a subnormal glucose me-tabolism in the premotor cortex, the supe-rior prefrontal cortex, and the brain as a whole in hyperactive adults who were hyperactive as children and had at least one hyperactive child of their own.[189] The prefrontal cortex has an important influ-ence on attention span and the premotor cortex affects voluntary movements that depend on external cues.[96,186,189] For ex-ample, the premotor cortex suppresses relatively automatic responses to some sensory stimuli and could thereby produce motor restlessness.[146,189] Low blood flows through the head of the caudate nucleus and posterior periventricular regions of the brain have been demonstrated in several hyperactive children.[83]

In the CPS each child's activity level was judged on a five-point scale as fol-lows: 1 = extreme inactivity and passiv-ity; 2 = little activity; the child was con-tent to sit still most of the time; 3 = nor-mal amount of activity; the child sat quietly when interested but at times fidg-eted and became restless; 4 = unusual amount of activity and restlessness; the child very seldom sat quietly; 5 = extreme overactivity and restlessness, inability to sit still, constant motion, and activ-ities often not in response to external stimuli.[28]

In our analyses antecedent risk factors were identified for 33% of the extremely overactive behavior in CPS children who did not have neurologic abnormalities (category 5). Familial factors accounted for 19% of the risk (Table 11–11). Being male was the dominant factor in this category. Fifteen percent of the risk was in the antenatal maldevelopment or damage category. Maternal cigarette smoking dur-ing pregnancy was the major risk factor in this category. There is other evidence that smoking had a causal relationship to hyperactive behavior in the CPS children. First, the smoking had a dose relationship with hyperactivity; the more cigarettes a woman smoked during pregnancy, the higher the frequency of hyperactivity in her children.[113] Second, mothers who had two pregnancies in the CPS and who smoked in only one of them had a higher frequency of hyperactive children follow-ing the pregnancy in which they smoked than following the pregnancy in which they did not smoke.[112]

There were no findings that suggested an intrapartum or late gestational origin for the hyperactive behavior. For example, children who were hyperactive had no more frequent meconium in their amni-otic fluid, low Apgar scores, neonatal seizures, persistent neonatal neurologic abnormalities, or placental evidence of low uteroplacental blood flow than non-hyperactive children.

Hyperactivity With Accompanying Neurologic Abnormalities

Risk factors were found for 52% of the hyperactivity in the CPS that was accompanied by neurologic abnormal-ities (Table 11–12). With a few exceptions these risk factors were the same as those associated with hyperactivity without neurologic abnormalities. The most im-portant exception was a meconium-stained umbilical cord, which was a risk factor for hyperactive behavior only when it was accompanied by neuro-

TABLE 11–11.

Risk Factors for Hyperactive Behavior Without Accompanying Neurologic Abnormalities in Children at 7 Years of Age*

Risk Factors	No. of Hyperactive Children per 1,000 Children With Risk Factor†	Relative Risks (95% Confidence Intervals)	Attributable Risks (95% Confidence Intervals)
All cases	15 (727)		
Familial			
Sex: male	**19** (456), *P* < .001	**1.7** (1.4, 2.0)	**.14** (.12, .17)
Race: white	**20** (415), *P* < .001	**1.1** (0.0, 1.3)	**.03** (.02, .06)
Mother employed outside home	**20** (256), *P* < .001	**1.1** (1.0, 1.3)	**.02** (.01, .04)
Antenatal maldevelopment or damage			
Fetal abnormalities			
Birth weight, percentiles 1–10	**18** (71), *P* < .005	**1.2** (1.0, 1.4)	**.01** (.01, .02)
Head circumference at birth, percentiles 1–10	**21** (51), *P* < .005	**1.4** (0.0, 1.7)	**.01** (.01, .02)
Placental, umbilical cord abnormalities			
Unevenly accelerated maturation	**24** (260), *P* < .05	**1.1** (1.0, 1.3)	**.02** (.01, .04)
Bipartite or tripartite placenta	**24** (16), *P* < .05	**1.5** (1.0, 2.0)	**.01** (.00, .02)
Velamentous insertion of cord	**39** (5), *P* < .05	**2.5** (1.1, 4.0)	**.01** (.00, .01)
Maternal pregnancy factor			
Cigarette smoking	**25** (397), *P* < .001	**1.4** (1.2, 1.6)	**.09** (.07, .11)
Population attributable risk			**.33** (.27, .39)

*Significant values are in boldface.
†Numbers of children who were hyperactive are in parentheses. P values compared with value in all cases category.

TABLE 11–12.

Risk Factors for Hyperactive Behavior With Accompanying Neurologic Abnormalities in Children at 7 Years of Age*

Risk Factors	No. of Hyperactive Children per 1,000 Children With Risk Factor†	Relative Risks (95% Confidence Intervals)	Attributable Risks (95% Confidence Intervals)
All cases	6 (314)		
Familial			
Sex: male	**12** (657), *P* < .001	**1.7** (1.5, 1.9)	**.24** (.22, .26)
Mother employed outside home	**9** (393), *P* < .001	**1.2** (1.0, 1.4)	**.06** (.05, .07)
Antenatal maldevelopment or damage			
Fetal abnormalities			
Birth weight, percentiles 1–10	**10** (115), *P* < .001	**1.4** (1.1, 1.6)	**.03** (.02, .04)
Umbilical cord abnormalities			
Green-colored umbilical cord	**8** (82), *P* < .001	**1.5** (1.1, 2.0)	**.05** (.01, .09)
Unusually long umbilical cord	**8** (29), *P* < .05	**1.2** (1.0, 1.4)	**.02** (.00, .04)
Maternal pregnancy factors			
Cigarette smoking	**9** (560), *P* < .001	**1.3** (1.2, 1.5)	**.13** (.11, .15)
Population attributable risk			**.52** (.50, .55)

*Significant values are in boldface.
†Numbers of children who had hyperactivity are in parentheses. P values compared with value in all cases category.

logic abnormalities (see Table 11–12). Meconium in the amniotic fluid is associated with several types of long term neurologic abnormalities (see Tables 11–5, 11–41, 11–43).

Fearful and Apprehensive Behavior

The levels of fearfulness exhibited by children during the seventh-year psychological examination were rated on a five-step scale: 1 = the child had no apparent

TABLE 11–13.
Risk Factors for Child Being Inhibited and Uneasy*

Risk Factors	No. of Inhibited, Uneasy Children per 1,000 Children With Risk Factor†	Relative Risks (95% Confidence Intervals)	Attributable Risks (95% Confidence Intervals)
All cases	138 (5,447)		
Familial			
Child: IQ value 60–79	**225** (1,335), *P*<.001	**2.0** (1.9, 2.2)	**.13** (.09, .11)
Siblings present who are <5 yr older than child being studied	**149** (3,605), *P*<.001	**1.6** (1.3, 1.5)	**.13** (.11, .15)
Father of child lives in home	**141** (4,331), *P*<.05	**1.2** (1.1, 1.3)	**.09** (.07, .12)
Low socioeconomic status	**141** (2,170), *P*<.01	**1.1** (1.0, 1.2)	**.06** (.04, .08)
Race: white	**147** (2,681), *P*<.001	**1.2** (1.1, 1.3)	**.04** (.03, .05)
Sex: female	**139** (2,784), *P*<.001	**1.1** (1.0, 1.2)	**.04** (.03, .05)
Antenatal maldevelopment or damage			
Placenta, umbilical cord abnormalities			
Diffuse subchorionic fibrin	**150** (1,432), *P*<.001	**1.2** (1.2, 1.3)	**.03** (.02, .04)
Unexplained neurologic abnormality at age 7 yr			
Poor coordination	**149** (513), *P*<.02	**1.2** (1.1, 1.3)	**.01** (.00, .02)
Population attributable risk			**.50** (.47, .53)

*Significant values are in boldface.
†Numbers of children who were inhibited and uneasy are in parentheses. P values compared with value in all cases category.

awareness of a strange situation, was completely unafraid, and displayed uninhibited behavior; 2 = the child had very little evidence of fear and was quickly at ease in the testing situation; 3 = the child had a normal amount of caution in the testing situation and was able to cope with it; 4 = the child was inhibited and uneasy throughout the testing and had some slowing of responses; 5 = the child was very fearful and apprehensive and displayed acute discomfort that significantly interfered with the test performance.[28]

Of the children in the study, 13.8% were inhibited and uneasy (category 4 behavior). Risk factors were identified for 50% of this behavior (Table 11–13). Only 4% was associated with risk factors for antenatal damage or maldevelopment. Familial factors dominated, the most important of which were being mildly mentally retarded, having one or more close-in-age older siblings, and having one's father in the home. These findings raise the possibility that interpersonal experiences in the home are a major factor in the genesis of inhibited and uneasy behavior.

One percent of the children were very fearful and apprehensive (category 5 behavior). Risk factors were identified for 62% of this behavior (Table 11–14). They were somewhat different from the risk factors for the less extreme, category 4 behavior. Whereas 4% of the risk factors for category 4 behavior were in the antenatal maldevelopment and damage category, 31% of the risk factors for very fearful (category 5) behavior were in this category. There were also some differences between the antecedents of category 4 and category 5 behavior in the familial category. Mild mental retardation was not a risk factor for category 5 behavior, but having older siblings and having one's father in the home remained major risk factors. This last set of findings reinforces the possibility that interactions between a child and other family members is a major cause of fearful behavior in children. The other main conclusion is that organic brain dysfunction may be a major antecedent of very fearful and apprehensive behavior but not of the milder inhibited and uneasy (category 4) behavior.

In the CPS a child who had fearful, apprehensive behavior increased the risk of the next child born into the family having the same behavior. However this behavior was considerably attenuated in the next-born child (Table 11–15). There

TABLE 11–14.

Risk Factors for Child Being Very Fearful and Apprehensive*

Risk Factors	No. of Fearful Children per 1,000 Children With Risk Factor†	Relative Risks (95% Confidence Intervals)	Attributable Risks (95% Confidence Intervals)
All cases	10 (365)		
Familial			
Siblings present who are <5 yr older than child being studied	12 (250), $P < .001$	**1.6** (1.1, 2.2)	**.25** (.21, .28)
Father of child lives in home	11 (293), $P < .05$	**1.2** (1.0, 1.5)	**.09** (.06, .13)
Antenatal maldevelopment or damage			
Placental, umbilical cord abnormalities			
Diffuse subchorionic fibrin	15 (124), $P < .001$	**1.7** (1.3, 2.0)	**.10** (.09, .12)
Unusually long umbilical cord	13 (44), $P < .02$	**1.3** (1.0, 2.0)	**.01** (.00, .02)
Bipartite or tripartite placenta	22 (11), $P < .01$	**1.9** (1.0, 3.4)	**.01** (.00, .01)
Unexplained neurologic abnormalities at age 7 yr			
Poor coordination	24 (65), $P < .001$	**2.0** (1.5, 2.6)	**.10** (.07, .12)
Other neurologic abnormalities	15 (73), $P < .001$	**3.0** (2.1, 4.2)	**.09** (.06, .11)
Population attributable risk			**.62** (.58, .66)

*Significant values are in boldface.
†Numbers of children who were very fearful and apprehensive are in parentheses. P values compared with value in all cases category.

are several likely explanations for this. First, the next-born children in the family had a much lower frequency of the antenatal maldevelopment and damage risk factors to which nearly a third of the very fearful behavior in the first-born was attributed. This is because very fearful behavior is so much more frequent in brain-damaged than in nondamaged children and many types of such damage and maldevelopment have no propensity to repeat in successive pregnancies. Second, the genetic composition of successive siblings is not the same and there is a genetic regression toward the mean in abnormal behavior. Finally, changes take place in family relationships as new children enter the family circle. Parents become more experienced in rearing children as new ones are added, and successive children progressively alter the environment in which all of the family members live.

A child displaying fearful, apprehensive behavior increased the risk of the next-born child in the family having very passive behavior, hostile behavior, and a long attention span (see Table 11–15). As mentioned earlier in this chapter, hostile behavior appears to be mainly environmental in origin. The children in the CPS who exhibited very fearful behavior did not have increased frequencies of low Apgar scores, meconium-stained amniotic fluid, or neonatal seizures in the absence of neonatal or subsequent neurologic abnormalities.

Emotional Reactivity

The emotional reactivity exhibited by children during their psychological examination at 7 years of age was rated on a five-step scale: 1 = the child was emotionally extremely flat with no changes in facial expression during testing or in the associated activities; 2 = the child had a somewhat flat affect and exhibited no change in emotional tone except for occasional small variations; 3 = the child was normally responsive and had an affect that was appropriate to the situation; 4 = the child had a somewhat unstable mood that varied more than average; the mood appeared to be motivated internally or to represent an exaggerated responsiveness to the testing situation; 5 = the child had extremely unstable emotional responses and overreacted to external situations or to unidentified, presumably internal, stimuli.[28]

TABLE 11–15.

Behavior Findings in Children at 7 Years of Age When Their Next-Older Sibling Displayed a Specified Behavior at the Same Age*

Behavior of Older Sibling†	Relative Risks (95% Confidence Intervals) for Younger Sibling‡
Fearful and apprehensive (555)	
Fearful and apprehensive	**1.2** (1.0, 1.4)
Very passive	**1.4** (1.1, 1.6)
Long attention span	**1.9** (1.1, 1.4)
Hostile	**1.5** (1.0, 2.0)
Emotionally flat (614)	
Emotionally flat	**1.6** (1.3, 1.9)
Very passive	**1.2** (1.0, 1.5)
Emotionally unstable (159)	
Emotionally unstable	1.2 (0.8, 1.7)
Very assertive	**2.1** (1.4, 3.2)
Rigid behavior	**1.6** (1.0, 2.6)
Withdrawal when frustrated (789)	
Withdrawal when frustrated	**1.6** (1.3, 1.9)
Very upset when frustrated (47)	
Very upset when frustrated	1.2 (0.7, 1.8)
Short attention span (419)	
Short attention span	**1.4** (1.1, 1.8)
Withdrawal when frustrated	**1.5** (1.2, 1.8)
Emotionally flat	**1.2** (1.0, 1.5)
Agreeable or ingratiating behavior	**1.3** (1.0, 1.9)

*Children with neurologic abnormalities were excluded from this analysis.
†Numbers of older siblings in a behavior category are in parentheses.
‡Significant values are in boldface.

Emotionally Flat Behavior

Of the children in the CPS, 15.5% had somewhat emotionally flat (category 2) behavior. Risk factors were identified for 54% of this behavior. Only 7 % of the risk was in the antenatal maldevelopment or damage category (Table 11–16). Familial factors dominated, the most important of which were being mildly mentally retarded, having one or more close-in-age older siblings, and being in a family with low socioeconomic status. One can speculate that these findings were influenced by inheritance and perhaps by suboptimal sociocultural stimulation.

Extremely flat (category 1) behavior was exhibited by 1.3% of the children in the study. Risk factors were identified for 75% of this behavior (Table 11–17). Seventeen percent was in the antenatal maldevelopment or damage category as compared with 7% of the risk in the less extreme, somewhat emotionally flat (category 2) behavior. This suggests that organic brain dysfunction played a larger role in the more extreme behavior. Fifty-eight percent of the more extreme (category 1) behavior was in the familial category (see Table 11–17). Many of the risk factors were the same as with the less severe category 2 behavior, but being black had a larger role with the more extreme behavior (see Tables 11–16, 11–17). One wonders if cultural barriers between the examiners and the children affected the flat behavior of the black children in the study.

Having one child with emotionally flat behavior (categories 1 and 2 combined) increased the risk for emotionally flat behavior in the next child born into the family (see Tables 11–15). As with other comparisons between consecutively born children, the abnormal behavior in the first-born was less frequent and less severe in the next-born. Children with flat emotional behavior did not have increased frequencies of low Apgar scores,

TABLE 11–16.

Risk Factors for Emotionally Flat Behavior*

Risk Factors	No. of Emotionally Flat Children per 1,000 Children With Risk Factor†	Relative Risks (95% Confidence Intervals)	Attributable Risks (95% Confidence Intervals)
All cases	155 (6,222)		
Familial			
Child: mild mental retardation	**320** (1,648), *P* < .001	**3.2** (3.0, 3.4)	**.18** (.16, .21)
Siblings present who are <5 yr older than child being studied	**174** (4,183), *P* < .001	**1.5** (1.4, 1.5)	**.12** (.10, .14)
Low socioeconomic status	**185** (2,875), *P* < .001	**1.4** (1.3, 1.5)	**.09** (.08, .11)
Race: black	**181** (3,618), *P* < .001	**1.4** (1.4, 1.5)	**.06** (.06, .07)
Sex: male	**161** (3,279), *P* < .001	**1.1** (1.1, 1.2)	**.03** (.02, .04)
Antenatal maldevelopment or damage			
Placental abnormality			
Diffuse subchorionic fibrin	**166** (1,575), *P* < .05	**1.1** (1.1, 1.2)	**.04** (.01, .02)
Unexplained neurologic abnormality at age 7 yr			
Poor motor coordination	**196** (672), *P* < .001	**1.4** (1.2, 1.5)	**.01** (.01, .02)
Severe mental retardation	**387** (54), *P* < .001	**4.3** (3.1, 6.0)	**.02** (.01, .03)
Neonatal, postneonatal periods			
Preterm birth	**181** (994), *P* < .001	**1.1** (1.0, 1.2)	**.01** (.00, .01)
Population attributable risk			**.54** (.51, .58)

*Significant values are in boldface.
†Numbers of children who were emotionally flat are in parentheses. P values compared with value in all cases category.

TABLE 11–17.

Risk Factors for Emotionally Extremely Flat Behavior*

Risk Factors	No. of Emotionally Extremely Flat Children per 1,000 Children With Risk Factor†	Relative Risks (95% Confidence Intervals)	Attributable Risks (95% Confidence Intervals)
All cases	13 (394)		
Familial			
Siblings present who are <5 yr older than child being studied	**16** (274), *P* < .001	**1.5** (1.1, 2.0)	**.23** (.19, .27)
Race: black	**17** (283), *P* < .001	**2.1** (1.7, 2.7)	**.20** (.18, .23)
Sex: male	**15** (241), *P* < .005	**1.3** (1.1, 1.6)	**.08** (.06, .11)
Congenital syndromes, disorders	**21** (110), *P* < .001	**1.7** (1.4, 2.1)	**.05** (.03, .08)
Parental mental retardation	**26** (21), *P* < .001	**1.5** (1.0, 2.4)	**.03** (.01, .05)
Antenatal maldevelopment or damage			
Fetal factor			
Twins	**29** (18), *P* < .001	**1.7** (1.0, 2.7)	**.02** (.00, .04)
Placental abnormality			
Unevenly accelerated maturation	**14** (303), *P* < .05	**1.3** (1.1, 1.6)	**.05** (.03, .07)
Unexplained neurologic abnormality at age 7 yr			
Cerebral palsy	**84** (11), *P* < .001	**2.2** (1.1, 4.2)	**.03** (.00, .07)
Other neurologic abnormalities	**22** (63), *P* < .001	**4.2** (3.1, 5.6)	**.07** (.05, .10)
Neonatal, postnatal periods			
CNS infections	**61** (7), *P* < .001	**2.7** (1.2, 5.9)	**.01** (.00, .02)
Population attributable risk			**.75** (.73, .78)

*Significant values are in boldface.
†Numbers of children who had extremely flat behavior are in parentheses. P values compared with value in all cases category.

meconium-stained amniotic fluid, or neo-natal seizures in the absence of neonatal or subsequent neurologic abnormalities.

Emotionally Unstable Behavior

Of the children in the CPS, 4.4% had emotionally somewhat unstable (category 4) behavior. Risk factors were identified for 44% of this behavior. Thirty-three percent of the risk was in the familial category (Table 11–18). The risk factors in this category were mild mental retarda-tion, being white, being male, and having one's father living apart from the family. The remaining 12% of identified risk was in the antenatal maldevelopment or dam-age category.

Emotionally extremely unstable (cate-gory 5) behavior was exhibited by 0.6% of the children in the study. Risk factors were identified for 52% of this behavior (Table 11–19). As with most other behavioral disorders, risks associated with markers for organic brain dysfunction played a much larger role in the more extreme than in the less severe behavior. More than two-thirds of the identified risk for ex-treme emotional unstability was in the antenatal maldevelopment or damage cat-egory. Only 19% of the risk was in the familial category. Being male and having adverse social conditions in the home

were responsible for all of the identified risk in the familial category.

Emotionally unstable behavior in one child did not increase the risk for this behavior in the next child born into a family (see Table 11–15). However, emo-tional instability in one child increased the risk of the next child being very assertive or having very rigid behavior (see Table 11–15). A likely explanation is that the unstable behavior of the first child unfa-vorably affected the psychological envi-ronment in which the next-born child was being reared. Children in the CPS with emotionally unstable behavior did not have increased frequencies of low Apgar scores, meconium-stained amniotic flu-id, or neonatal seizures in the absence of neonatal or subsequent neurologic abnormalities.

Reactions to Frustration

Tolerance to frustration during the 7-year psychological examination was rated on a five-step scale: 1 = the child withdrew completely and refused to at-tempt or to continue any task that ap-peared too difficult; 2 = the child occa-sionally withdrew from a task when a difficulty was encountered or when the task appeared too difficult for success;

TABLE 11–18.

Risk Factors for Child Being Emotionally Somewhat Unstable*

Risk Factors	No. of Emotionally Somewhat Unstable Children per 1,000 Children With Risk Factor†	Relative Risks (95% Confidence Intervals)	Attributable Risks (95% Confidence Intervals)
All cases	44 (1,710)		
Familial			
Child: mild mental retardation	**87** (448), *P* < .001	**2.5** (2.3, 2.8)	**.12** (.11, .13)
Race: white	**48** (947), *P* < .001	**1.4** (1.3, 1.5)	**.11** (.10, .13)
Sex: male	**48** (979), *P* < .001	**1.2** (1.1, 1.3)	**.06** (.05, .09)
Father not living with family	**49** (478), *P* < .001	**1.3** (1.2, 1.5)	**.04** (.04, .05)
Antenatal maldevelopment or damage			
Unexplained neurologic abnormality at age 7 yr			
Poor motor coordination	**91** (314), *P* < .001	**2.3** (2.1, 2.6)	**.09** (.08, .10)
Severe mental retardation	**467** (73), *P* < .001	**23.6** (17, 33)	**.03** (.02, .04)
Population attributable risk			**.44** (.41, .47)

*Significant values are in boldface.
†Numbers of children who were emotionally somewhat unstable are in parentheses. *P* values compared with value in all cases category.

3 = the child attempted to cope with difficult situations and did not become too upset if the task appeared to be too difficult; 4 = the child became very upset when difficulties were encountered and sometimes reacted with disorganized behavior, anger, or crying; 5 = the child exhibited extreme acting-out behavior including crying when a difficulty was encountered, displayed considerable anger, and behavior became so uncontrolled that continuation of the examination was difficult or impossible.[28]

Withdrawal

Children who occasionally withdrew when they encountered a difficulty (category 2 behavior) constituted 22.4% of the children in the study. Risk factors were identified for 47% of this behavior (Table 11–20). One-third of the identified risk was distributed among many different factors in the antenatal maldevelopment and damage category. The remaining two-thirds of identified risk was in the familial category and was associated with mild mental retardation, low socioeconomic status, and having older siblings.

One percent of the children in the CPS displayed extreme withdrawal behavior when a difficulty was encountered (category 1). Risk factors were identified for 57% of this behavior (Table 11–21). Just over half of the identified risk was in the antenatal maldevelopment or damage category and the rest was familial. Most of the antenatal risk was associated with neurologic abnormalities suggesting organic brain dysfunction, whereas almost all of the familial risk was in having older siblings. Thus, the two dominating causes of extreme withdrawal behavior are likely to be organic brain dysfunction and adverse interactions with older siblings.

A placental disorder, diffuse subchorionic fibrin beneath the chorionic plate of the placenta, was associated with children withdrawing when they were frustrated (see Chapter 7). This placental abnormality was also associated with very fearful and very passive behavior, suggesting that all three of these behaviors might sometimes have some common antenatal roots (see Tables 11–15, 11–14, 11–34, 11–35).

Having a child who withdrew when faced with difficulty (categories 1 and 2) increased the risk of this same behavior in the next child born into a family (see Table 11–15). However, as with other behavioral abnormalities, this behavior was less frequent and usually less severe in the next-born child. Since having older siblings was the most important risk factor for withdrawal behavior, unfavorable interactions with these older siblings is the likely reason why withdrawal behav-

TABLE 11–19.

Risk Factors for Child Being Emotionally Extremely Unstable*

Risk Factors	No. of Emotionally Extremely Unstable Children per 1,000 Children With Risk Factor†	Relative Risks (95% Confidence Intervals)	Attributable Risks (95% Confidence Intervals)
All cases	6 (184)		
Familial			
Sex: male	**8** (124), *P* < .001	**1.5** (1.1, 2.0)	**.13** (.11, .16)
Adverse social conditions in home	**10** (40), *P* < .001	**1.7** (1.2, 2.4)	**.06** (.05, .08)
Antenatal maldevelopment or damage			
Unexplained neurologic abnormalities at age 7 yr			
Poor coordination	**19** (46), *P* < .001	**2.8** (2.0, 4.0)	**.15** (.11, .19)
Cerebral palsy	**61** (7), *P* < .001	**1.5** (1.0, 2.9)	**.01** (.00, .01)
Other neurologic abnormalities	**50** (53), *P* < .001	**12.4** (8.9, 17.1)	**.19** (.16, .24)
Population attributable risk			**.52** (.49, .55)

*Significant values are in boldface.
†Numbers of children who were emotionally extremely unstable are in parentheses. P values compared with value in all cases category.

TABLE 11–20.

Risk Factors for Children Who Occasionally Withdrew When Frustrated*

Risk Factors	No. of Children Who Occasionally Withdrew per 1,000 Children With Risk Factor†	Relative Risks (95% Confidence Intervals)	Attributable Risks (95% Confidence Intervals)
All cases	224 (8,685)		
Familial			
Child: mild mental retardation	**398** (1,925), *P<.001*	**2.6** (2.5, 2.8)	**.12** (.11, .13)
Low socioeconomic status	**244** (3,757), *P<.001*	**1.2** (1.2, 1.3)	**.12** (.10, .14)
Siblings present who are <5 yr older than child being studied	**226** (5,444), *P<.001*	**1.2** (1.0, 1.3)	**.08** (.06, .10)
Antenatal maldevelopment or damage			
Placental, umbilical cord abnormality			
Diffuse subchorionic fibrin	**251** (2,386), *P<.001*	**1.3** (1.3, 1.4)	**.07** (.06, .08)
Fetal factors			
Major congenital malformations	**233** (818), *P<.001*	**1.1** (1.0, 1.2)	**.02** (.01, .03)
Birth weights, percentiles 1–10	**245** (823), *P<.001*	**1.2** (1.1, 1.4)	**.01** (.00, .01)
Twins	**286** (232), *P<.001*	1.4 (1.2, 1.6)	**.01** (.00, .01)
Unexplained neurologic abnormalities at age 7 yr			
Poor motor coordination	**284** (966), *P<.001*	**1.5** (1.3, 1.6)	**.03** (.03, .04)
Severe mental retardation	**598** (73), *P<.001*	**6.0** (4.2, 8.6)	**.01** (.00, .01)
Population attributable risk			**.47** (.44, .50)

*Significant values are in boldface.
†Numbers of children who occasionally withdrew when frustrated are in parentheses. P value compared with value in all cases category.

TABLE 11–21.

Risk Factors for Children Who Withdrew Completely When Frustrated*

Risk Factors	No. of Children Who Completely Withdrew per 1,000 Children With Risk Factor†	Relative Risks (95% Confidence Intervals)	Attributable Risks (95% Confidence Intervals)
All cases	10 (330)		
Familial			
Siblings present who are <5 yr older than child being studied	**12** (225), *P<.001*	**1.6** (1.1, 2.4)	**.25** (.21, .29)
Parental mental retardation	**17** (14), *P<.01*	**1.6** (1.0, 2.8)	**.01** (.00, .01)
Antenatal maldevelopment or damage			
Placental, umbilical cord abnormalities			
Diffuse subchorionic fibrin	**13** (96), *P<.005*	**1.4** (1.0, 1.9)	**.05** (.04, .06)
Unexplained neurologic abnormalities at age 7 yr			
Poor coordination	**31** (76), *P<.001*	**3.8** (2.8, 4.9)	**.12** (.09, .15)
Other neurologic abnormalities	**17** (61), *P<.001*	**8.4** (6.4, 11.0)	**.16** (.13, .19)
Population attributable risk			**.57** (.54, .60)

*Significant values are in boldface.
†Numbers of children who withdrew completely when frustrated are in parentheses. P values compared with value in all cases category.

ior repeated in the next-born sibling. Children with this behavioral pattern did not have increased frequencies of low Apgar scores, meconium-stained amniotic fluid, or neonatal seizures in the absence of neonatal or subsequent neurologic abnormalities.

Becoming Upset

Children in the CPS who reacted to difficulties by becoming very upset (combined categories 4 and 5) made up 1.8% of the children in the study. Risk factors were identified for 54% of this behavior. More than a third of the identified risk was

TABLE 11–22.

Risk Factors for Child Reacting to Frustration by Becoming Very Upset or Exhibiting Extreme Acting-out Behavior*

Risk Factors	No. of Upset Children per 1,000 Children With Risk Factor†	Relative Risks (95% Confidence Intervals)	Attributable Risks (95% Confidence Intervals)
All cases	18 (528)		
Familial			
Race: white	21 (308), $P < .001$	**1.5** (1.3, 1.7)	**.13** (.11, .15)
Sex: male	20 (328), $P < .005$	**1.3** (1.1, 1.5)	**.11** (.09, .13)
Mother blue collar worker	16 (278), $P < .02$	**1.1** (1.0, 1.3)	**.03** (.01, .05)
Adverse social conditions in home	26 (100), $P < .001$	**1.6** (1.3, 2.0)	**.03** (.02, .04)
Mental illness in parents	31 (17), $P < .02$	**1.6** (1.0, 2.6)	**.02** (.00, .05)
Antenatal maldevelopment or damage			
Unexplained neurologic abnormalities at age 7 yr			
Poor coordination	30 (75), $P < .001$	**1.2** (1.0, 1.5)	**.01** (.00, .01)
Other neurologic abnormalities	30 (57), $P < .001$	**10.6** (6.4, 17.5)	**.21** (.13, .29)
Population attributable risk			**.54** (.50, .58)

*Significant values are in boldface.
†Numbers of children who reacted to frustration by becoming very upset are in parentheses. P values compared with value in all cases category.

associated with markers for antenatal maldevelopment or damage and may have reflected organic brain dysfunction (Table 11–22). The remaining identified risk was in the familial category and likely reflects an admixture of genetic influences and personal interactions within the family and wider community. Being white and male predominated among these risk factors (see Table 11–22).

Becoming very upset when encountering a difficulty did not have a tendency to repeat in the next child born into a family (see Table 11–15). Children with this behavioral pattern also did not have increased frequencies of low Apgar scores, meconium-stained amniotic fluid, or neonatal seizures in the absence of neonatal or subsequent neurologic abnormalities.

Attention Span

The attention span exhibited by children during their seventh-year psychologic examination was graded on a five-step scale: 1 = the child attended to tasks very briefly, was highly distractible, attention was fleeting and sporadic, lack of concentration interfered significantly with test performance; 2 = the child spent a short time with tasks, was easily distracted, and frequently needed help to maintain attention; the brief attention span sometimes interfered with test performance; 3 = the child spent an adequate amount of time on tasks and was able to concentrate until success or failure was clear; 4 = the child had a long attention span, spent more than the average time on tasks, but was eventually able to turn to a new activity; 5 = the child was highly persevering; he or she was so fixated on one task that it required the examiner's intervention to change the activity.[28]

Short Attention Span

Genetic factors are reported to strongly predispose to both mild mental retardation and to a short attention span.[7,122,153,166,184] Short attention span is also one of the consequences of the fetal brain damage that sometimes occurs with a high maternal alcohol intake during pregnancy.[123,143]

Of the children in the CPS, 11.6% had a short attention span (category 2). Risk factors were identified for 71% of this behavior (see Table 11–23). More than half of the identified risk was in the

TABLE 11–23.

Risk Factors for Child Having a Short Attention Span*

Risk Factors	No. of Children Having Short Attention Span per 1,000 Children With Risk Factor†	Relative Risks (95% Confidence Intervals)	Attributable Risks (95% Confidence Intervals)
All cases	116 (4,652)		
Familial			
Child: mild mental retardation	**290** (1,516), *P* < .001	**4.2** (3.9, 4.5)	**.23** (.21, .24)
Low socioeconomic status	**140** (2,115), *P* < .001	**1.4** (1.3, 1.5)	**.04** (.03, .05)
Sex: male	**124** (2,518), *P* < .001	**1.3** (1.2, 1.3)	**.03** (.03, .04)
Adverse social conditions in home	**156** (790), *P* < .001	**1.1** (1.0, 1.2)	**.02** (.02, .03)
Mother working outside of home	**129** (2,799), *P* < .001	**1.1** (1.0, 1.1)	**.01** (.00, .01)
Antenatal maldevelopment or damage			
Placental abnormality			
Unevenly accelerated maturation	**122** (1,795), *P* < .001	**1.2** (1.1, 1.3)	**.02** (.01, .03)
Fetal abnormalities			
Fetal congenital malformations	**141** (491), *P* < .001	**1.3** (1.2, 1.5)	**.01** (.01, .02)
Head circumference at birth, percentiles 1–10	**167** (168), *P* < .001	**1.4** (1.2, 1.5)	**.01** (.01, .02)
Unexplained neurologic abnormalities at age 7 yr			
Other neurologic abnormalities	**214** (335), *P* < .001	**14.3** (11.5, 17.8)	**.17** (.13, .23)
Severe mental retardation	**873** (124), *P* < .001	**63.1** (38, 96)	**.16** (.11, .22)
Poor motor coordination	**205** (698), *P* < .001	**2.1** (1.9, 2.4)	**.02** (.01, .03)
Population attributable risk			*.71* (.69, .74)

*Significant values are in boldface.
†Numbers of children who had a short attention span are in parentheses. P value compared with value in all cases category.

antenatal brain maldevelopment or damage category and the rest was in the familial category. Taken together, severe and mild mental retardation accounted for 39% of the short attention span in the analyses.

Of the children in the CPS, 1.4% had a very short attention span (category 1). Risk factors were almost the same as for the less severe short attention span in category 2 (Tables 11–23 and 11–24). The major difference was that mental retardation, which was very important among the risk factors for short attention span, was not a risk factor for a very short attention span.

Short attention span in a child increased the risk for the same behavior in the next child born into a family (see Table 11–15). Short attention span also increased the risks of the next-born child having a flat affect, ingratiating behavior, and a withdrawal response to frustration (see Table 11–15). Children in the two short attention span categories did

not have increased frequencies of low Apgar scores, meconium in the amniotic fluid, or neonatal seizures in the absence of neonatal or subsequent neurologic abnormalities.

Most of the short attention spans identified in the 7-year-old CPS children may have continued into adult life since other studies have shown that short attention span persists at older ages.[55] Lou et al. reported that seven children who had short attention spans without neurologic abnormalities had a subnormal blood flow through the head of the caudate nucleus and posterior periventricular regions of their brains.[83]

Long Attention Span

Of the children in the CPS, 6.5% had a long attention span (category 4). Risk factors were identified for 34% of this behavior (Table 11–25). More than half of the identified risk was associated with being a male and most of the rest with mild mental retardation. It is noteworthy that

TABLE 11–24.

Risk Factors for Child Having a Very Short Attention Span*

Risk Factors	No. of Children Having Very Short Attention Span per 1,000 Children With Risk Factor†	Relative Risks (95% Confidence Intervals)	Attributable Risks (95% Confidence Intervals)
All cases	14 (448)		
Familial			
Sex: male	**18** (293), *P* < .001	**1.7** (1.4, 2.1)	**.18** (.16, .20)
Low socioeconomic status	**21** (251), *P* < .001	**2.0** (1.6, 2.4)	**.16** (.14, .18)
Race: black	**16** (262), *P* < .001	**1.2** (1.0, 1.5)	**.06** (.04, .08)
Adverse social conditions in home	**23** (88), *P* < .001	**1.6** (1.2, 2.0)	**.04** (.03, .04)
Antenatal maldevelopment or damage			
Fetal abnormality			
Fetal congenital malformations	**31** (84), *P* < .001	**2.1** (1.7, 2.7)	**.04** (.03, .04)
Unexplained neurologic abnormalities at age 7 yr			
Poor coordination	**59** (148), *P* < .001	**2.9** (2.4, 3.6)	**.13** (.12, .15)
Cerebral palsy	**282** (30), *P* < .001	**2.2** (1.4, 3.5)	**.02** (.00, .04)
Other neurologic abnormalities	**21** (192), *P* < .001	**14.3** (11.5, 17.8)	**.24** (.20, .27)
Population attributable risk			**.87** (.85, .90)

*Significant values are in boldface.
†Numbers of children who had a very short attention span are in parentheses. P value compared with value in all cases category.

TABLE 11–25.

Risk Factors for Child Having a Long Attention Span*

Risk Factors	No. of Children with a Long Attention Span per 1,000 Children With Risk Factor†	Relative Risks (95% Confidence Intervals)	Attributable Risks (95% Confidence Intervals)
All cases	65 (2,628)		
Familial			
Sex: male	**74** (1,517), *P* < .001	**1.4** (1.3, 1.5)	**.24** (.21, .26)
Child: mild mental retardation	**102** (514), *P* < .001	**1.9** (1.7, 2.1)	**.08** (.07, .10)
Child: IQ value > 120	**90** (175), *P* < .001	**1.6** (1.4, 1.8)	**.02** (.00, .04)
Parental mental illness	**77** (56), *P* < .05	**1.2** (1.0, 1.6)	**.01** (.00, .01)
Population attributable risk			**34** (.30, .39)

*Significant values are in boldface.
†Numbers of children who had a long attention span are in parentheses. P values compared with value in all cases category.

none of the risk was associated with markers for antenatal maldevelopment or damage.

Of the children in the CPS, 0.3% had a very long attention span (category 5). Risk factors were identified for 43% of this behavior (Table 11–26). In contrast to the less severe category 4 behavior, half of the identified risk for category 5 behavior was in the antenatal maldevelopment or damage category. The familial risk factors were similar for the two behavioral categories. Neither category 4 nor category 5 behavior in one child increased the likeli-

hood of this behavior repeating in the next child born into a family (Table 11–27). This is presumably because the behavior is not a reaction to interactions within the family and the organic brain dysfunction or damage responsible for so much of the category 5 behavior did not usually repeat in the fetuses of subsequent pregnancies.

Rigid/Impulsive Behavior

This was graded on a five-step scale: 1 = the child displayed extreme rigidity as evidenced by an inability to shift activity

TABLE 11–26.

Risk Factors for Child Having a Very Long Attention Span*

Risk Factors	No. of Children With Very Long Attention Span per 1,000 Children With Risk Factor†	Relative Risks (95% Confidence Intervals)	Attributable Risks (95% Confidence Intervals)
All cases	3 (186)		
Familial			
Sex: male	**4** (116), *P* < .02	**1.5** (1.0, 2.3)	**.16** (.15, .18)
Parental mental retardation	**8** (14), *P* < .005	**2.8** (1.3, 5.0)	**.04** (.02, .06)
Parental mental illness	**7** (8), *P* < .05	**2.3** (1.0, 4.4)	**.03** (.00, .07)
Antenatal maldevelopment or damage			
Maternal pregnancy factor			
Maternal diabetes mellitus	**10** (10), *P* < .005	**3.6** (1.5, 8.8)	**.03** (.00, .06)
Unexplained neurologic abnormalities at age 7 yr			
Poor coordination	**8** (48), *P* < .001	**2.7** (1.6, 4.4)	**.11** (.07, .14)
Other neurologic abnormalities	**5** (32), *P* < .005	**3.9** (2.1, 7.1)	**.08** (.04, .11)
Population attributable risk			**.43** (.38, .48)

*Significant values are in boldface.
†Numbers of children who had a very long attention span are in parentheses. P values compared with value in all cases category.

TABLE 11–27.

Behavior Findings in Children at 7 Years of Age When Their Next-Older Sibling Displayed a Specified Behavior at the Same Age*

Behavior of Older Sibling†	Relative Risks (95% Confidence Intervals) for Younger Sibling‡
Long attention span (221)	
Long attention span	1.3 (0.9, 1.8)
Rigid behavior (290)	
Very rigid behavior	1.1 (0.8, 1.4)
Withdrew when frustrated	**1.6** (1.3, 2.1)
Impulsive behavior (148)	
Very impulsive behavior	1.0 (0.6, 1.7)
Short attention span	**1.6** (1.0, 2.3)
Assertive and willful (82)	
Assertive and willful	**1.8** (1.0, 3.0)
Short attention span	**2.6** (1.7, 4.2)
Passive behavior (766)	
Passive behavior	**1.5** (1.3, 1.9)
Emotionally flat	**1.2** (1.0, 1.4)
Impulsive behavior	**1.3** (1.0, 1.7)
Hostile (78)	
Hostile	**2.2** (1.0, 5.0)
Agreeable and ingratiating	
Agreeable and ingratiating	1.1 (0.6, 2.0)

*Children with neurologic abnormalities were excluded from this analysis.
†Numbers of older siblings in a behavior category are in parentheses.
‡Significant values for younger siblings are in boldface.

or to alter his or her approach to a task; children in this category did not vary or adapt their responses and stayed with a single aspect of a task; 2 = the child tended to be inflexible in most situations but occasionally shifted approaches and made an appropriate response to a task; 3 = the child's behavior patterns were flexible and the child engaged in activities appropriate to different situations; 4 = the child's behavior was frequently impulsive, fluid, and sometimes uncontrolled;

5 = the child's behavior was extremely impulsive and often was explosive and uncontrolled.[28]

Rigid Behavior

Of the children in the CPS, 8.3% exhibited rigid (category 2) behavior (Table 11–28). Risk factors were identified for 58% of this behavior. Twenty-four percent of this risk was in the antenatal brain maldevelopment or damage category (see Table 11–28). Thirty-five percent was in the familial category. Half of this familial risk was attributable to mild mental retardation with most of the rest due to having older siblings and the family having a low socioeconomic status.

Of the children in the CPS, 0.3% exhibited extremely rigid behavior (category 1). Risk factors were identified for 49% of this behavior (Table 11–29). Almost all of the risk was attributable to markers of organic brain dysfunction.

Rigid or extremely rigid behavior in one child did not increase the risk for this behavior in the next child born into a family. However, the next child did have an increased risk for withdrawal behavior when faced with difficulties (see Table 11–27). Children with rigid or extremely rigid behavior did not have increased frequencies of low Apgar scores, meconium-stained amniotic fluid, or neonatal seizures in the absence of neonatal or subsequent neurologic abnormalities.

Impulsive Behavior

Impulsive behavior (category 4) was exhibited by 4.6% of the children in the CPS. Risk factors were identified for 49% of this behavior. Half of the identified risk was in the antenatal maldevelopment or damage category, and included unevenly accelerated placental maturation and markers for organic brain dysfunction (Table 11–30). The other half of the risk was in the familial category. The two major risk factors in this category were mild mental retardation and being male (see Table 11–30).

TABLE 11–28.

Risk Factors for Child Exhibiting Inflexible Behavior*

Risk Factors	No. of Children With Inflexible Behavior per 1,000 Children With Risk Factor†	Relative Risks (95% Confidence Intervals)	Attributable Risks (95% Confidence Intervals)
All cases	83 (3,340)		
Familial			
Child: mild mental retardation	**218** (1,088), *P* < .001	**4.1** (3.8, 4.4)	**.18** (.17, .19)
Siblings present who are <5 yr older than child being studied	**91** (2,204), *P* < .001	**1.3** (1.2, 1.4)	**.07** (.06, .08)
Low socioeconomic status	**104** (1,613), *P* < .001	**1.4** (1.3, 1.5)	**.07** (.06, .08)
Race: black	**91** (1,837), *P* < .001	**1.1** (1.0, 1.2)	**.02** (.01, .03)
Parental mental retardation	**95** (2,085), *P* < .001	**1.8** (1.5, 2.1)	**.01** (.00, .01)
Antenatal maldevelopment or damage			
Placental abnormalities			
Unevenly accelerated maturation	**87** (1,160), *P* < .001	**1.2** (1.1, 1.3)	**.08** (.03, .06)
Bipartite placenta	**114** (68), *P* < .001	**1.4** (1.1, 1.7)	**.01** (.00, .01)
Fetal factors			
Twins	**118** (96), *P* < .001	**1.5** (1.2, 1.8)	**.02** (.00, .03)
Congenital malformations	**93** (325), *P* < .001	**1.1** (1.0, 1.3)	**.01** (.00, .01)
Unexplained neurologic abnormalities at age 7 yr			
Poor motor coordination	**125** (429), *P* < .001	**1.7** (1.5, 1.9)	**.10** (.06, .08)
Severe mental retardation	**42** (57), *P* < .001	**10.9** (7.7, 15.3)	**.01** (.00, .01)
Neonatal			
CNS infections	**168** (2,204), *P* < .001	**2.2** (1.5, 3.3)	**.01** (.00, .01)
Population attributable risk			***.58*** (.53, .64)

*Significant values are in boldface.
†Numbers of children who had inflexible behavior are in parentheses. P value compared with value in all cases category.

Extremely impulsive behavior was exhibited by 0.3% of the children. Risk factors were identified for 77% of this behavior. More than half of the identified risk was in the antenatal brain maldevelopment or damage category and was due almost entirely to markers for organic brain dysfunction (Table 11–31). Being male was a major risk factor in the familial category.

Impulsive or extremely impulsive behavior in a child did not increase the risk for this behavior in the next child born into a family (see Table 11–27). However, the

TABLE 11–29.

Risk Factors for Child Exhibiting Extremely Rigid Behavior*

Risk Factors	No. of Children With Extremely Rigid Behavior per 1,000 Children With Risk Factor†	Relative Risks (95% Confidence Intervals)	Attributable Risks (95% Confidence Intervals)
All cases	3 (118)		
Familial			
Parental mental retardation	11 (10), *P* < .001	**2.9** (1.5, 5.5)	**.03** (.01, .05)
Antenatal maldevelopment or damage			
Fetal abnormality			
Congenital malformations	7 (21), *P* < .001	**1.9** (1.1, 1.3)	**.04** (.02, .06)
Unexplained neurologic abnormalities at age 7 yr			
Poor motor coordination	11 (34), *P* < .001	**3.9** (2.6, 5.8)	**.10** (.07, .13)
Other neurologic abnormalities	5 (55), *P* < .001	**16.6** (11.1, 24.8)	**.32** (.25, .39)
Population attributable risk			*.49* (*.43, .56*)

*Significant values are in boldface.
†Numbers of children who had extremely rigid behavior are in parentheses. P value compared with value in all cases category.

TABLE 11–30.

Risk Factors for Child Having Impulsive Behavior*

Risk Factors	No. of Children Having Impulsive Behavior per 1,000 Children With Risk Factor†	Relative Risks (95% Confidence Intervals)	Attributable Risks (95% Confidence Intervals)
All cases	46 (1,826)		
Familial			
Child: mild mental retardation	86 (417), *P* < .001	**2.2** (2.0, 2.5)	**.11** (.10, .12)
Sex: male	53 (1,073), *P* < .001	**1.5** (1.3, 1.6)	**.09** (.08, .10)
Father not living with family	54 (525), *P* < .001	**1.3** (1.2, 1.5)	**.03** (.02, .05)
Adverse social conditions in home	59 (300), *P* < .001	**1.3** (1.1, 1.5)	**.02** (.02, .03)
Antenatal maldevelopment or damage			
Placental abnormality			
Unevenly acclerated maturation	51 (1,348), *P* < .001	**1.4** (1.3, 1.6)	**.10** (.01, .02)
Fetal abnormality			
Head circumference at birth, percentiles 1–10	69 (158), *P* < .001	**1.5** (1.3, 1.8)	**.02** (.09, .11)
Maternal pregnancy factors			
Cigarette smoking	54 (424), *P* < .001	**1.2** (1.1, 1.4)	**.02** (.01, .03)
Seizure disorder	58 (73), *P* < .02	**1.2** (1.0, 1.5)	**.01** (.00, .01)
Unexplained neurologic abnormalities at age 7 yr			
Poor motor coordination	97 (333), *P* < .001	**2.8** (2.5, 3.1)	**.08** (.07, .09)
Severe mental retardation	528 (67), *P* < .001	**25.2** (18.0, 36.2)	**.03** (.02, .04)
Population attributable risk			*.49* (*.73, .80*)

*Significant values are in boldface.
†Numbers of children who exhibited impulsive behavior are in parentheses. P values compared with value in all cases category.

TABLE 11–31.

Risk Factors for Child Having Extremely Impulsive Behavior*

Risk Factors	No. of Children Having Extremely Impulsive Behavior per 1,000 Children With Risk Factor†	Relative Risks (95% Confidence Intervals)	Attributable Risks (95% Confidence Intervals)
All cases	3 (93)		
Familial			
Sex: male	4 (69), P < .001	**2.0** (1.4, 3.0)	**.21** (.18, .23)
Race: black	4 (59), P < .05	**1.7** (1.2, 2.4)	**.13** (.12, .15)
Antenatal maldevelopment or damage			
Fetal factor			
Twins	8 (5), P < .02	**2.4** (1.0, 4.8)	**.01** (.00, .01)
Unexplained neurologic abnormalities at age 7 yr			
Poor coordination	13 (37), P < .001	**6.0** (4.1, 9.0)	**.19** (.14, .25)
Other neurologic abnormalities	30 (38), P < .001	**18.1** (12.1, 27.0)	**.23** (.17, .29)
Population attributable risk			**.77** (.73, .80)

*Significant values are in boldface.
†Numbers of children who exhibited extremely impulsive behavior are in parentheses. P values compared with value in all cases category.

next child born did have an increased risk of having a short attention span. The children with impulsive and extremely impulsive behavior did not have increased frequencies of low Apgar scores, meconium in the amniotic fluid, or neonatal seizures in the absence of neonatal or subsequent neurologic abnormalities.

Assertiveness

Assertiveness was graded on a five-step scale: 1 = the child was extremely assertive and willful, dominating, aggressive, and lacking in reserve; he or she attempted to manipulate the testing situation and resisted externally imposed limitations; 2 = the child was forceful, unnecessarily rough, and careless in handling materials, was little inhibited by the presence of the examiner from doing what he or she wanted to do, and often ignored imposed limits; 3 = the child was self-assertive but accepted the testing situation and was capable of control and reserve when it was demanded; he or she looked for feedback and became less assertive and more pliant when such was indicated; 4 = the child accepted things passively and permitted himself or herself to be somewhat controlled by the examiner and the situation; this child rarely showed an inclination to do something different from what the examiner suggested; 5 = the child was extremely passive, malleable, overcompliant, and acquiesced to everything that was requested with no trace of resistance.[28]

Forceful and Rough Behavior

This category (category 2) included 2.1% of the children in the CPS. Risk factors were identified for 49% of this behavior (Table 11–32). Half of the identified risk was in the antenatal maldevelopment or damage category and included markers for organic brain dysfunction (see Table 11–32). There were two major familial risk factors: mild mental retardation in the child and being a male.

One-half of 1% of the children in the CPS were extremely assertive and willful (category 1). Risk factors were identified for 64% of this behavior (Table 11–33). Over two-thirds of the identified risk was in the antenatal maldevelopment or damage category. Most of the risk factors were markers for organic brain dysfunction. The most important familial risk factor was being a male.

Forceful and extremely assertive behavior in one child increased the risk for the same behavior in the next child born into a family (see Table 11–27). This next-born

TABLE 11–32.

Risk Factors for Child Being Forceful and Rough*

Risk Factors	No. of Forceful, Rough Children per 1,000 Children With Risk Factor†	Relative Risks (95% Confidence Intervals)	Attributable Risks (95% Confidence Intervals)
All cases	21 (829)		
Familial			
Child: mild mental retardation	**43** (230), P < .02	**2.5** (2.2, 2.9)	**.12** (.11, .14)
Sex: male	**26** (518), P < .001	**1.6** (1.4, 1.8)	**.10** (.09, .11)
Father of child not in home	**25** (242), P < .001	**1.2** (1.0, 1.4)	**.03** (.01, .04)
Antenatal maldevelopment or damage			
Placental abnormalities			
Unevenly accelerated maturation	**28** (299), P < .02	**1.3** (1.2, 1.6)	**09** (.08, .10)
Fetal abnormality			
Birth weight, percentiles 1–10	**25** (87), P < .05	**1.2** (1.0, 1.4)	**.01** (.00, .01)
Maternal pregnancy factors			
Cigarette smoking	**25** (188), P < .05	**1.2** (1.0, 1.4)	**.01** (.01, .02)
Convulsive disorder	**32** (40), P < .001	**1.5** (1.1, 2.1)	**.01** (.01, .02)
Unexplained neurologic abnormalities at age 7 yr			
Severe mental retardation	**388** (52), P < .001	**38.9** (22, 44)	**.05** (.03, .06)
Poor motor coordination	**43** (148), P < .001	**2.3** (1.9, 2.7)	**.06** (.04, .07)
Other neurologic abnormalities	**82** (115), P < .001	**1.2** (1.0, 1.5)	**.02** (.01, .04)
Population attributable risk			**.49** (.45, .53)

Significant values are in boldface.
†Numbers of children who were forceful and rough are in parentheses. P values compared with value in all cases category.

TABLE 11–33.

Risk Factors for Child Being Extremely Assertive and Willful*

Risk Factors	No. of Extremely Assertive and Willful Children per 1,000 Children With Risk Factor†	Relative Risks (95% Confidence Intervals)	Attributable Risks (95% Confidence Intervals)
All cases	5 (141)		
Familial			
Sex: male	**6** (85), P < .02	**1.4** (1.0, 12.0)	**.11** (.09, .13)
Father of child not in home	**7** (48), P < .005	**1.7** (1.2, 2.4)	**.09** (.07, .11)
Antenatal maldevelopment or damage			
Fetal abnormality			
Birth weight, percentiles 1–10	**9** (23), P < .001	**1.9** (1.1, 3.1)	**.05** (.03, .07)
Unexplained neurologic abnormality at age 7 yr			
Poor coordination	**15** (37), P < .001	**3.4** (2.3, 4.9)	**.13** (.09, .17)
Other neurologic abnormalities	**8** (44), P < .001	**11.1** (7.5, 16.1)	**.27** (.20, .34)
Population attributable risk			**.64** (.60, .68)

Significant values are in boldface.
†Numbers of children who had extremely assertive and willful behavior are in parentheses. P values compared with value in all cases category.

child also had an increased risk of having a short attention span. Twin studies have shown that assertiveness is strongly affected by the home environment and little influenced by genetic factors.[141] Forceful and extremely assertive behavior was not associated with increased frequencies of low Apgar scores, meconium in the amni-otic fluid, or neonatal seizures in the absence of neonatal or subsequent neurologic abnormalities.

Passive Behavior

Of the children in the CPS, 21.7% were passive in their behavior (category 4).[28] Risk factors were identified for 56% of this behavior (Table 11–34). Only 5% of this risk was in the antenatal maldevelopment or damage category. Being black and living in a family with low socioeconomic status were prominent risk factors in the familial category. One wonders if a cultural gap between the examiners and the children affected this behavior in children from poor and disadvantaged families. Having older siblings and a father living in the home were also risk factors. This raises the possibility that unfavorable interac-

tions within the family circle had a role in the behavior. Mild mental retardation in the child was also an antecedent of passive behavior.

One-half of 1% of the children in the CPS exhibited very passive behavior (category 5). Risk factors were identified for 39% of this behavior (Table 11–35). Over two-thirds of the identified risk was in the antenatal maldevelopment or damage category and included markers for organic brain dysfunction. Low socioeconomic

TABLE 11–34.

Risk Factors for Child Having Passive Behavior*

Risk Factors	No. of Passive Children per 1,000 Children With Risk Factor†	Relative Risks (95% Confidence Intervals)	Attributable Risks (95% Confidence Intervals)
All cases	217 (8,774)		
Familial			
Race: black	**246** (4,995), $P<.001$	**1.4** (1.3, 1.5)	**.13** (.12, .15)
Child: mild mental retardation	**353** (1,753), $P<.001$	**2.2** (2.1, 2.4)	**.11** (.10, .12)
Siblings present who are <5 yr older than child being studied	**226** (516), $P<.001$	**1.3** (1.2, 1.3)	**.10** (.08, .11)
Low socioeconomic status	**249** (3,846), $P<.001$	**1.2** (1.1, 1.2)	**.09** (.07, .10)
Father of child living with family	**228** (6,990), $P<.001$	**1.1** (1.1, 1.2)	**.06** (.03, .08)
Mother working outside of home	**233** (5,093), $P<.001$	**1.1** (1.0, 1.1)	**.02** (.01, .02)
Antenatal maldevelopment or damage			
Placental abnormality			
Diffuse subchorionic fibrin	**231** (2,164), $P<.001$	**1.1** (1.0, 1.1)	**.04** (.03, .05)
Unexplained neurologic abnormalities at age 7 yr			
Poor motor coordination	**246** (840), $P<.001$	**1.2** (1.1, 1.3)	**.01** (.01, .02)
Population attributable risk			**.56** (.35, .43)

*Significant values are in boldface.
†Numbers of children who had passive behavior are in parentheses. P value compared with value in all cases category.

TABLE 11–35.

Risk Factors for Child Having Very Passive Behavior*

Risk Factors	No. of Very Passive Children per 1,000 Children With Risk Factor†	Relative Risks (95% Confidence Intervals)	Attributable Risks (95% Confidence Intervals)
All cases	5 (156)		
Familial			
Low socioeconomic status	**6** (71), $P<.02$	**1.5** (1.1, 2.1)	**.11** (.10, .13)
Antenatal maldevelopment or damage			
Placental abnormality			
Diffuse subchorionic fibrin	**8** (58), $P<.001$	**1.9** (1.6, 2.2)	**.14** (.11, .16)
Unexplained neurologic abnormalities at age 7 yr			
Poor coordination	**10** (27), $P<.001$	**2.1** (1.4, 3.2)	**.05** (.04, .07)
Cerebral palsy	**41** (5), $P<.001$	**2.2** (1.0, 5.1)	**.01** (.00, .02)
Other neurologic abnormalities	**22** (26), $P<.001$	**4.3** (2.7, 6.9)	**.08** (.05, .11)
Population attributable risk			**.39** (.35, .43)

*Significant values are in boldface.
†Numbers of children who had very passive behavior are in parentheses. P values compared with value in all cases category.

status was the sole risk factor in the familial category.

Passive or very passive behavior in one child increased the risk for the same behavior in the next child born into a family (see Table 11–27). This next child also had increased risks of having a flat affect and impulsive behavior. The children who exhibited passive or very passive behavior had no increase in the frequencies of low Apgar scores, meconium in the amniotic fluid, or neonatal seizures in the absence of neonatal or subsequent neurologic abnormalities.

Hostile/Agreeable Behavior

The level of hostility was rated on a five-step scale: 1 = the child was very hostile and obstructive; he or she engaged in overt physical or verbal attacks on the examiner, test materials, or testing room objects, and some of these children had tantrums; 2 = the child exhibited an unusual amount of hostility, was uncooperative, and became angry when restrictions were imposed; some of these children introduced aggressive themes into their conversation; 3 = the child evidenced no

unusual amount of hostility; both affect and negative behavior were generally appropriate and controlled; 4 = the child was very agreeable and rarely displayed hostility, even when it might have been appropriate, and never balked or reacted in a displeased manner to imposed limitations; 5 = the child was ingratiating and the main determinant of behavior was a desire to please the examiner.[28]

Hostile Behavior

Of the children in the study, 2.2% were hostile (category 2). Risk factors were identified for 47% of this behavior (Table 11–36). Only one-fifth of the identified risk was in the antenatal maldevelopment or damage category. The remaining identified risk was in the familial category and included being male, being mildly mentally retarded, having a mother who worked outside of the home, having a father who lived apart from the family, and other adverse social conditions for the child (see Table 11–36).

One-tenth of 1% of the children in the CPS were very hostile (category 1). Risk factors were identified for 85% of this behavior and were different from the risk

TABLE 11–36.
Risk Factors for Child Being Hostile*

Risk Factors	No. of Hostile Children per 1,000 Children With Risk Factor†	Relative Risks (95% Confidence Intervals)	Attributable Risks (95% Confidence Intervals)
All cases	22 (878)		
Familial			
Sex: male	**26** (527), *P* < .001	**1.5** (1.3, 1.7)	**.14** (.12, .15)
Child: mild mental retardation	**45** (221), *P* < .001	**2.3** (2.0, 2.5)	**.12** (.10, .14)
Adverse social conditions in home	**29** (149), *P* < .001	**1.4** (1.2, 1.7)	**.04** (.03, .05)
Mother working outside of home	**24** (525), *P* < .05	**1.1** (1.0, 1.3)	**.04** (.03, .07)
Low socioeconomic status	**24** (363), *P* < .05	**1.1** (1.0, 1.1)	**.02** (.01, .04)
Father of child not in home	**25** (239), *P* < .05	**1.1** (1.0, 1.2)	**.01** (.00, .02)
Antenatal maldevelopment or damage			
Placental abnormality			
Bipartite placenta	**33** (20), *P* < .05	**1.6** (1.0, 2.5)	**.01** (.00, .01)
Maternal pregnancy factor			
Cigarette smoking	**27** (214), *P* < .001	**1.3** (1.2, 1.5)	**.04** (.03, .06)
Unexplained neurologic abnormalities at age 7 yr			
Poor motor coordination	**35** (119), *P* < .001	**1.7** (1.4, 2.1)	**.04** (.04, .05)
Severe mental retardation	**98** (13), *P* < .001	**4.3** (3.7, 5.0)	**.01** (.00, .02)
Population attributable risk			**.47** (.45, .49)

*Significant values are in boldface.
†Numbers of children who exhibited hostile behavior are in parentheses. P values compared with value in all cases category.

factors for the less severe category 2 behavior (Tables 11–36 and 11–37). About 30% of the identified risk for the very hostile behavior was in the antenatal maldevelopment or damage category and was associated with markers for organic brain dysfunction. The remaining identified risk was in the familial category and was associated with the mother working outside of the home and the father living apart from the family (Table 11–37). The fact that so much of the very hostile behavior was associated with parents working or living outside of the home is striking because absent parents had either a much smaller role or no role in the other types of abnormal behavior in the CPS. Hostile behavior in a child increased the risk for the same behavior in the next child born into a family (see Table 11–27). Twin studies have shown that hostile behavior is influenced by the home environment and little affected by genetic factors.[141] Results of the present analyses reinforce these findings in twins. Children in the CPS who were hostile had no increase in the frequencies of low Apgar scores, meconium-stained amniotic fluid, or neonatal seizures in the absence of neonatal or subsequent neurologic abnormalities.

Agreeable and Ingratiating Behavior

Children in the CPS classified as having this behavior (categories 4 and 5) constituted 5.7% of the children in the study.

Risk factors were identified for 45% of this behavior (Table 11–38). There was an interesting mix of familial and antenatal factors. The single most important familial factor was the presence of a child's father in the home with the family. The significance of this finding is reinforced by the finding that an absent father greatly increased the risk of a child being hostile (see Tables 11–36, 11–37). An unusually long umbilical cord was the next most important predictor of a child being agreeable and ingratiating. Unusually long umbilical cords are often markers for vigorous fetal motor activity, low neonatal mortality, and superior cognitive skills at 7 years of age (see Chapter 6).[105,108] The remaining important factor for ingratiating behavior was a child being female. Agreeable, ingratiating behavior in one child did not increase the likelihood of the same behavior in the next child born into a family (see Table 11–27). This is in contrast to hostile behavior, which tended to repeat in the next-born child. Twin studies have shown that agreeable behavior is greatly affected by the home environment and much less by genetic factors.[141]

Conclusions About Behavioral Disorders

The data base of the CPS permitted us to take into consideration a larger number of

TABLE 11–37.

Risk Factors for Child Being Very Hostile*

Risk Factors	No. of Very Hostile Children per 1,000 Children With Risk Factor†	Relative Risks (95% Confidence Intervals)	Attributable Risks (95% Confidence Intervals)
All cases	1.4 (56)		
Familial			
Mother employed outside home	**1.6** (50), *P* < .05	**2.3** (1.0, 5.0)	**.49** (.44, .54)
Father of child not in home	**1.2** (36), *P* < .05	**1.8** (1.0, 3.0)	**.13** (.09, .16)
Antenatal maldevelopment or damage			
Unexplained neurologic abnormalities at age 7 yr			
Poor motor coordination	**3.3** (11), *P* < .005	**2.6** (1.3, 5.1)	**.11** (.05, .16)
Other neurologic abnormalities	**2.2** (11), *P* < .001	**6.1** (3.0, 12.3)	**.13** (.05, .21)
Population attributable risk			**.85** (.82, .88)

*Significant values are in boldface.
†Numbers of children who exhibited very hostile behavior are in parentheses. P values compared with value in all cases category.

biologic factors, particularly antenatal disorders, than has been possible in most previous studies. Newly developed statistical methods have enabled us to present outcomes in a quantitative, easy-to-understand format. The analyses take many confounding risk factors into consideration and are not based on self-assessments. The credibility of the CPS findings is further supported by the good concordance of behavioral scoring by different teams of CPS psychologists on the same children.[122] A limiting feature of the CPS data needs also to be mentioned. The data that we analyzed were gathered in a single session rather than longitudinally. The very large number of children analyzed probably counterbalanced the limitations of a nonlongitudinal study because in general the CPS findings support the results of earlier twin studies.

Perhaps the most important feature of the current analyses is the quantitative information they provide on the roles of antenatal brain maldevelopment and damage on many types and degrees of abnormal childhood behavior. Indirect evidence of heritability was found for most but not all types of abnormal behavior. Evidence from twin studies indicates that heritability has less influence on children's hostility, assertiveness, and agreeableness than on most other personality characteristics.[141] Findings of the present study reinforce these observations on twins. Being a male was often a risk factor for abnormal behavior in the current analyses. Twin studies have shown a lower influence of heritability and a stronger effect of environmental factors on the behavior of boys than of girls.[153,154,166] Some of this difference between the sexes may be related to the fact that boys and girls often use different strategies for coping with adversity.[163]

The identification of individual risk factors for abnormal behavior is just the first step in the search for the roots of behavioral abnormalities. Rutter et al. have pointed to the multitude of possible gene-environmental interactions that may occur between such factors.[153] Genes operate through aspects of temperament, vulnerability to stress, a polygenic predisposition to particular disorders, and a shaping of the environment to exert their effects on human behavior.[153]

MOTOR DISORDERS

Poor Motor Coordination

This category includes all children who were found to have gross or fine abnormalities in motor coordination by a neurologic examination at 7 years of age.[28] Of the children in the study, 5.9% had findings that placed them in this category (Table 11–39). The only children excluded from the analyses in this table

TABLE 11–38.

Antecedents for Child Being Very Agreeable or Ingratiating*

Risk Factors	No. of Very Agreeable Children per 1,000 Children With Risk Factor†	Relative Risks (95% Confidence Intervals)	Attributable Risks (95% Confidence Intervals)
All cases	57 (1,824)		
Familial			
Father of child lives in home	**59** (1,774), *P* < .001	**1.2** (1.1, 1.4)	**.23** (.18, .28)
Sex: female	**60** (71), *P* < .02	**1.2** (1.1, 1.3)	**.04** (.03, .05)
Adverse social conditions in home	**63** (312), *P* < .02	**1.2** (1.1, 1.3)	**.01** (.00, .01)
Antenatal development			
Placental, umbilical cord findings			
Diffuse subchorionic fibrin	**60** (561), *P* < .001	**1.1** (1.0, 1.4)	**.01** (.00, .01)
Unusually long umbilical cord	**64** (192), *P* < .02	**1.4** (1.0, 2.1)	**.16** (.10, .23)
Population attributable risk			**.45** (.17, .73)

*Significant values are in boldface.
†Numbers of children who were very agreeable are in parentheses. P values compared with value in all cases category.

TABLE 11–39.

Risk Factors for Child Having Poor Motor Coordination*

Risk Factors	No. of Poorly Coordinated Children per 1,000 Children With Risk Factor†	Relative Risks (95% Confidence Intervals)	Attributable Risks (95% Confidence Intervals)
All cases	59 (3,516)		
Familial			
Sex: male	**113** (2,328), *P* < .001	**2.0** (1.9, 2.2)	**.22** (.21, .23)
Race: white	**106** (1,989), *P* < .001	**1.6** (1.5, 1.7)	**.13** (.12, .15)
≥ 2 older siblings	**92** (1,364), *P* < .001	**1.1** (1.0, 1.2)	**.08** (.03, .14)
Mother employed outside home	**88** (2,831), *P* < .005	**1.1** (1.0, 1.3)	**.07** (.03, .11)
Familial disorders	**106** (728), *P* < .001	**1.3** (1.2, 1.5)	**.03** (.02, .04)
Parental mental retardation	**110** (123), *P* < .005	**1.5** (1.2, 1.8)	**.01** (.00, .01)
Antenatal maldevelopment or damage			
Fetal abnormalities			
Birth weight, percentiles 1–10	**120** (407), *P* < .001	**1.4** (1.3, 1.6)	**.02** (.01, .03)
Head circumference at birth, percentiles 1–10	**117** (272), *P* < .001	**1.3** (1.1, 1.4)	**.01** (.00, .01)
Placental, umbilical cord abnormalities			
Diffuse subchorionic fibrin	**111** (1,067), *P* < .001	**1.4** (1.3, 1.5)	**.07** (.06, .09)
Unusually short umbilical cord	**113** (74), *P* < .01	**1.3** (1.0, 1.6)	**.01** (.00, .01)
Maternal pregnancy factors			
Cigarette smoking	**106** (835), *P* < .001	**1.2** (1.1, 1.3)	**.03** (.02, .04)
Gestational acetonuria	**110** (328), *P* < .001	**1.3** (1.2, 1.5)	**.01** (.01, .02)
Unexplained neurologic abnormalities at age 7 yr			
Other neurologic abnormalities	**144** (576), *P* < .001	**6.0** (5.5, 6.7)	**.11** (.10, .12)
Population attributable risk			**.78** (.74, .83)

*Significant values are in boldface.
†Numbers of children who had poor motor coordination are in parentheses. P values compared with value in all cases category.

are those who had cerebral palsy. Risk factors were identified for 78% of the children whose motor coordination was abnormal. One in seven of the affected children also had other neurologic abnormalities (see Table 11–39).

One-third of the identified risk for poor motor coordination was in the antenatal brain maldevelopment or damage category (see Table 11–39). The major risk factors in this category were other neurologic abnormalities which are often a marker for organic brain dysfunction. The remainder of the risk for poor motor coordination was in the familial risk category. The major risk factors were being male, white, having older siblings, and having a mother who worked outside of the home.

Children who had poor motor coordination had higher frequencies of low Apgar scores, neonatal seizures, and persisting neonatal neurologic abnormalities than children who had normal motor coordination. Some of the poor coordination observed in the CPS probably persisted. Gillberg et al. found that a third of children with such abnormalities at 7 years of age still had poor coordination at 13 years of age.[56]

Unclassified Awkwardness

This category includes all children who were judged to move in an awkward manner without having any specific motor or other neurologic abnormalities identified by a neurologic examination at 7 years of age.[28] Findings placed 6.4% of the children in the study in this category (Table 11–40). Risk factors were identified for 68% of this awkwardness. These risk factors were similar to the risk factors associated with poor motor coordination (see Table 11–39). One-fourth of the identified risk for unclassified awkwardness

TABLE 11–40.

Risk Factors for Children Having Unclassified Awkwardness at 7 Years of Age*

Risk Factors	No. of Awkward Children per 1,000 Children With Risk Factor†	Relative Risks (95% Confidence Intervals)	Attributable Risks (95% Confidence Intervals)
All cases	64 (2,603)		
Familial			
Sex: male	**87** (1,774), *P*<.001	**2.3** (2.1, 2.5)	**.34** (.32, .36)
Race: white	**74** (1,501), *P*<.001	**1.4** (1.3, 1.6)	**.17** (.15, .18)
Parental mental retardation	**130** (43), *P*<.001	**2.3** (1.4, 3.8)	**.01** (.00, .01)
Antenatal maldevelopment or damage			
Fetal abnormalities			
Birth weight, percentiles 1–10	**94** (317), *P*<.001	**1.5** (1.2, 1.8)	**.04** (.02, .05)
Congenital malformations			
CNS	**133** (102), *P*<.001	**2.6** (2.0, 3.2)	**.03** (.02, .03)
Non-CNS	**89** (257), *P*<.001	**1.3** (1.2, 1.5)	**.02** (.02, .03)
Maternal pregnancy factor			
Maternal seizure disorder	**94** (99), *P*<.001	**1.5** (1.2, 2.0)	**.01** (.01, .02)
Placental abnormalities			
Circumvallate placenta	**88** (86), *P*<.001	**1.3** (1.1, 1.6)	**.03** (.01, .05)
Subchorionic fibrin absent	**79** (372), *P*<.001	**1.2** (1.0, 1.4)	**.01** (.00, .02)
Retarded maturation	**94** (199), *P*<.001	**1.3** (1.0, 1.6)	**.02** (.01, .03)
Neonatal period			
Serum bilirubin >18 mg/dL	**109** (86), *P*<.001	**1.9** (1.5, 2.4)	**.02** (.01, .02)
Population attributable risk			**.68** (.65, .71)

*Cerebral palsy cases were excluded from these analyses. Significant values are in boldface.
†Numbers of children who were awkward are in parentheses. P value compared with value in all cases category.

was associated with markers for antenatal brain maldevelopment or damage and almost all of the remaining risk was in being male and white (see Table 11–39). Being male accounted for half of all of the identified risk.

Cerebral Palsy

Theories about the genesis of CP have a long history. For nearly a century the opinions of William J. Little dominated thinking about the origins of CP. In 1861 he made a presentation to the Obstetrical Society of London in which he implicated asphyxia during labor and delivery as the cause of CP.[81] Later in the century Sigmund Freud[52] and several German neuropathologists came closer to the truth when they concluded that CP probably originated early in gestation. Like Little, Freud noted that many children with CP had been in poor condition at birth, but he attributed their poor state to deprivation and enfeeblement that originated long before labor and delivery.[52]

For our studies we defined *cerebral palsy* as a chronic, nonprogressive disorder characterized by an abnormal control of movements or posture that appeared early in childhood and was often accompanied by spasticity or paralysis. We based the diagnosis on findings from the neurologic examination conducted on CPS children at 7 years of age. We picked the diagnosis made at 7 years because 71% of the CP diagnosed as mild and 39% diagnosed as moderate at 1 year of age in the CPS disappeared before 7 years.[116] Gross malformations are found in the brains of about a third of autopsied CP children and microscopic abnormalities are found in most of the rest. Lesions in full-term born CP victims commonly consist of narrowed gyri and sulci that have widened as the result of cortical neuron disappearance and laminar degeneration. Subcortical rather than cortical damage is characteristically present in CP that originates before 30 weeks of gestation. In such cases white matter is replaced by gliosis, often accompanied by cysts.

Cerebral Palsy in Full-Term Born Children

As just noted, the cerebral lesions usually responsible for CP in full-term born children are in the cortex. Severe damage can probably take place in the cortex early in gestation without producing CP. Resections of the cerebral cortex in monkeys at a gestational age corresponding to 25 to 29 weeks in humans causes very little functional change in subsequent motor performance, whereas a later resection of the same cortical areas produces permanent disabilities.[121]

The cerebral cortex and brainstem are highly sensitive to hypoxic damage late in gestation and during labor and delivery because they have high metabolic rates and high blood flows associated with rapid neurocellular differentiation and myelination. At that time cranial nerve nuclei in the brainstem have considerable glycogen which can protect them against hypoxia, whereas the cortex has almost no glycogen and is almost totally dependent on liver glycogen for fuel if hypoxia develops and is sustained. The cortical necrosis that develops in children exposed to severe late gestational or intrapartum hypoxia often resembles the lesions produced by prolonged partial asphyxia many years ago in monkeys by Myers and Brann.[12,100] This cortical necrosis is caused by edema compressing small blood vessels. The neural damage can involve most of the cortex, or it can be limited to the parasagittal cortex or to other localized sites. Intraventricular hemorrhage is rare in full-term born infants, and when it does occur, it usually originates in the thalamus rather than in the germinal matrix and subcortical gray matter as is the case in preterm, very low-birth-weight infants.[150] The thalamic hemorrhages in full-term infants are usually the consequence of venous infarction associated with sepsis, cyanotic congenital heart disease, or coagulopathy.

We analyzed the CPS data to try to identify and quantitate the antecedents of the most frequent types of CP in full-term born children. The analyses were based on specific disorders and factors that might damage a child's brain. The most widely discussed of these disorders is birth asphyxia, some claiming that it is a frequent, others that it is an uncommon cause of CP. In recent years the view has gained credence that it is an uncommon cause of CP because very few CP victims have had a specific disorder identified that can produce asphyxia or severe hypoxia during labor, delivery, or the early neonatal period.* The first goal of our studies was to determine how much of a role intrapartum hypoxia or asphyxia has in the genesis of the various types of CP in the CPS data base. A second goal was to quantitate the roles, if any, of chronic antenatal hypoxia disorders, congenital disorders, infections, trauma, hypoglycemia, oxytocin, and other risk factors in the development of CP (see Table 11–1).

Most studies that have attempted to evaluate the role of birth asphyxia as a cause of CP have used low Apgar scores and fetal distress to identify the asphyxia.† Low Apgar scores and fetal distress are often nonhypoxic in origin.[2,89,114,169] Their use as surrogates for birth asphyxia has resulted in misattributing to asphyxia many cases of brain damage that had a nonasphyxial origin.[114] Another goal of our studies was to determine if some of the major causes of CP produce clinical findings that are distinctive enough to make their use a valid method for identifying the cause of CP in individual CP victims. We particularly wanted to see if the neonatal clinical manifestations of asphyxia-initiated CP overlap the neonatal clinical manifestations of CP caused by other disorders. For example, neonatal apneic spells, newborn neurologic abnormalities, and early neonatal seizures are well-known consequences of birth asphyxia.[127,156] Is their presence proof that CP had an asphyxial origin, or are they sometimes manifestations of CP caused by other disorders?

---

* References 2, 12, 23, 40, 42, 80, 126, and 152.
† References 8, 46, 47, 50, 66, 119, 131, 147, 156, and 164.

Quadriplegic Cerebral Palsy. — There were 34 full-term born children in the CPS who had severe CP that affected all four extremities. Based on attributable risk estimates, explanations of varying specificity were found for 86% of this quadriplegic CP (Table 11–41).[114] Almost all of the identified risk was attributable to disorders or markers for antenatal brain maldevelopment. These disorders and markers included congenital malformations, congenital syndromes, short umbilical cords, and the absence of fibrin beneath the chorionic (fetal) plate of the placenta (see Table 11–41).[114] The only non-developmental risk factors for quadriplegic CP were meconium in the amniotic fluid (15%), birth asphyxial disorders (4%), postnatal central nervous system infections (3%), and severe neonatal respiratory distress (7%). Altshuler and Hyde have found evidence that meconium causes vasoconstriction in the placenta and umbilical cord which is a plausible explanation for the severe brain damage that sometimes follows its presence in the amniotic fluid (see Tables 11–5, 11–41).[3] As noted in Chapter 8, meconium in the amniotic fluid is also a marker for disorders that both stress and damage the fetus, particularly acute chorioamnionitis and congenital developmental disorders but also including birth asphyxial disorders. It is worth noting that 14% of the quadriplegic CP in the CPS was attributable to birth asphyxial disorders before meconium in the amniotic fluid was added to the risk analysis. After meconium had been added to the analysis, only 4% of the quadriplegic CP was attributable to birth asphyxia.[114]

Two other risk factors for quadriplegic CP, short umbilical cords and absent subchorionic fibrin, appear to often be the consequence of low fetal motor activity and thus are presumed markers for brain dysfunction that orginated before birth.[106,108,114] The CNS malformations that were most often associated with quadriplegic CP were hydrocephalus, meningomyelocele, and encephalocele. Cardiac malformations were the most frequent

TABLE 11–41.

Risk Factors for Quadriplegic Cerebral Palsy at 7 Years of Age in Children Who Were Born at Full Term*

Risk Factors	No. of Cases of Quadriplegic Cerebral Palsy per 1,000 Children With Risk Factor†	Relative Risks (95% Confidence Intervals)	Attributable Risks (95% Confidence Intervals)
All cases	0.5 (34)		
Familial			
Motor disorders, siblings	**4** (2), *P* < .01	**4.6** (1.1, 19.5)	.05 (.02, .11)
Antenatal maldevelopment or damage			
Fetal abnormalities			
Major malformations			
Central nervous system	**8** (7), *P* < .001	**6.6** (2.9, 17.0)	.13 (.03, .24)
Non–CNS	**4** (12), *P* < .01	**4.2** (2.0, 8.8)	.20 (.08, .33)
Minor malformations	**2** (12), *P* < .001	**1.7** (1.2, 2.3)	.08 (.05, .10)
Congenital syndromes	**9** (2), *P* < .001	**4.2** (1.1, 16.4)	.04 (.00, .08)
Meconium in amniotic fluid	**2** (13), *P* < .02	**1.6** (1.0, 2.9)	.14 (.09, .19)
Placental, umbilical cord abnormalities			
Absent subchorionic fibrin	**1** (6), *P* < .02	**1.5** (1.0, 3.1)	.05 (.01, .09)
Unusually short umbilical cord	**2** (2), *P* < .05	**1.8** (1.1, 2.6)	.04 (.02, .06)
Labor, delivery, neonatal, postneonatal periods			
Birth asphyxial disorders	**128** (6), *P* < .001	**2.3** (1.2, 6.4)	.04 (.00, .09)
CNS infections	**16** (3), *P* < .001	**5.4** (1.6, 9.8)	.03 (.00, .06)
Severe respiratory distress	**18** (5), *P* < .001	**27.1** (10.7, 68.7)	**.07** (.01, .14)
Population attributable risk			***.86*** (.77, .95)

Significant values are in boldface.
†Numbers of children who had quadriplegic palsy are in parentheses. P values compared with value in all cases category.

non-CNS malformations among the CP victims (five cases). Many developmental and acquired brain lesions have been identified in children with congenital cardiac malformations.[48,58,59]

The role of oxytocin in the genesis of quadriplegic CP is of particular interest because many claims have been made in legal proceedings that its use causes CP. In the CPS neonatal seizures were 35% more frequent after oxytocin was used than when it was not used, but there was no corresponding increase in the frequency of CP.[114] Fetal and neonatal hypoglycemia, the use of gas anesthesia at delivery, and chronic fetal hypoxic disorders were not associated with increased frequencies of quadriplegic CP.[114]

Hemiplegic Cerebral Palsy.—One side of the body is predominantly affected in hemiplegic CP. The arm is usually more severely affected than the leg. Fewer risk factors were identified for hemiplegic than for quadriplegic CP in full-term born CPS infants. The risk factors that were identified provided some information about the antecedents of 59% of this hemiplegic CP (Table 11–42). Three-fourths of the identified risk was attributable to disorders or markers for antenatal brain maldevelopment or damage. These included congen-

ital malformations, congenital syndromes, and microcephaly at birth (see Table 11–42). Six percent of the risk was associated with motor disorders in siblings, which may indicate a hereditary contribution to the disorder. The only nondevelopmental risk factor identified was postnatal CNS infections (10%). It is noteworthy that birth asphyxial disorders, non-CNS malformations, minor congenital malformations, meconium in the amniotic fluid, and placental disorders were not antecedents of hemiplegic cerebral palsy.

Paraplegic Cerebral Palsy.—Paraplegic CP usually involves both legs and spares the arms. It more often arises from spinal cord than from brain disorders. It was somewhat less frequent in full-term born children in the CPS than either quadriplegic or hemiplegic CP (Table 11–43). Risk factors were identified for 60% of the paraplegic CP in the CPS. The risk factors were similar to those associated with hemiplegic CP with the major addition of meconium in the amniotic fluid and severe neonatal respiratory distress. Altshuler and Hyde have found evidence that meconium causes vasoconstriction in the placenta and umbilical cord which is a plausible explanation for the severe brain damage that sometimes

TABLE 11–42.

Risk Factors for Hemiplegic Cerebral Palsy at 7 Years of Age in Children Who Were Born at Full Term*

Risk Factors	No. of Cases of Hemiplegic Cerebral Palsy per 1,000 Children With Risk Factor†	Relative Risks (95% Confidence Intervals)	Attributable Risks (95% Confidence Intervals)
All cases	1 (39)		
Familial			
Motor disorders, siblings	**4** (3), *P* < .05	**7.2** (1.7, 22.4)	**.06** (.00, .15)
Antenatal maldevelopment or damage			
Fetal abnormalities			
Congenital malformations of CNS	**5** (6), *P* < .001	**10.8** (4.0, 29.7)	**.22** (.06, .36)
Head circumference at birth, percentiles 1–10	**2** (7), *P* < .02	**3.8** (1.4, 10.4)	**.14** (.03, .25)
Congenital syndromes	**6** (2), *P* < .05	**6.8** (1.5, 31.8)	**.07** (.00, .16)
Neonatal, postneonatal periods			
CNS infections	**12** (3), *P* < .001	**20.9** (5.9, 74.4)	**.10** (.10, .21)
Population attributable risk			**.59** (.55, .64)

*Significant values are in boldface.
†Numbers of children who had hemiplegic cerebral palsy are in parentheses. P values compared with value in all cases category.

follows its presence in the amniotic fluid (see Tables 11–5, 11–41, and 11–43).[3] As noted in Chapter 8, meconium in the amniotic fluid is also a marker for disorders that both stress and damage the fetus, particularly acute chorioamnionitis and congenital developmental disorders. Seventeen percent of the risk was associated with motor disorders in siblings, which may represent a hereditary risk. The only nondevelopmental risk factor identified was postnatal CNS infections (4%). Birth asphyxial and placental disorders were not antecedents of paraplegic CP.

Cerebral Palsy That Disappears With Age

Nelson and Ellenberg found that many children in the CPS who had cerebral palsy at 1 year of age lost the disorder by 7 years.[116] We undertook analyses to identify the types and etiologies of the CP that disappeared before 7 years in the CPS. Just one of the 24 children who had spastic CP at 1 year of age lost the disorder by 7 years. The course of nonspastic CP was more variable. Those cases in which CP disappeared before age 7 years included 9 of the 16 cases of quadriplegic CP attributable to birth asphyxial disorders, 7 of the 37 quadriplegic CP cases attributable to congenital disorders, 25 of the 28 cases in children who had paraplegic CP and 20 of the 31 cases in children who had hemiplegic CP.

Spastic CP was much more often associated with impaired mental development than was nonspastic CP. At 1 year of age, 7 of the 24 children who had spastic CP were judged mentally normal but only 3 of the 24 had IQ values of 80 or more at 7 years. At 1 year of age, 94 of the 112 children with nonspastic CP were judged to have a normal mental development. Eighty of the 112 had IQ values of 80 or more at 7 years of age. The specific identified cause of the spastic or nonspastic CP did not significantly affect cognitive outcomes.

Cerebral Palsy in Preterm Born Children

Preterm born infants have a higher frequency of CP than full-term born infants. This is because children born preterm have many of the causes of CP found in full-term infants plus a substantial frequency of hypoxia-initiated subcortical white matter damage that is very rare in full-term born children. CP in the preterm born appears to be increasing in frequency because advances in obstetric and medical management have greatly improved the survival rate of very low-birth-

TABLE 11–43.
Risk Factors for Paraplegic Cerebral Palsy at 7 Years of Age in Children Who Were Born at Full Term*

Risk Factors	No. of Cases of Paraplegic Cerebral Palsy per 1,000 Children With Risk Factor†	Relative Risks (95% Confidence Intervals)	Attributable Risks (95% Confidence Intervals)
All cases	0.5 (30)		
Familial			
Motor disorders, siblings	4 (3), $P < .05$	**7.8** (1.0, 63.4)	**.17** (.03, .31)
Antenatal maldevelopment or damage			
Congenital malformations of CNS	3 (3), $P < .02$	**11.9** (2.6, 52.1)	**.15** (.00, .32)
Minor malformations	2 (5), $P < .05$	**4.5** (1.0, 20.6)	**.04** (.01, .10)
Meconium in amniotic fluid	1 (12), $P < .01$	**2.2** (1.1, 5.2)	**.14** (.04, .23)
Neonatal, postneonatal periods			
CNS infections	4 (3), $P < .05$	**12.7** (2.8, 58.0)	**.04** (.01, .15)
Severe respiratory distress	9 (3), $P < .05$	**22.2** (5.8, 89.0)	**.06** (.00, .13)
Population attributable risk			**.60** (.41, .80)

*Significant values are in boldface.
†Numbers of children who had paraplegic cerebral palsy are in parentheses. P values compared with value in all cases category.

weight preterm born children without counterbalancing reductions in the frequency of the antenatal disorders that are responsible for their CP.[69]

Cerebral palsy in preterm, low-birth-weight infants is usually the consequence of subcortical white matter necrosis. Cortical necrosis is so rare in very low-birth-weight preterm born infants that CP without mental retardation is usually assumed to be the result of injury before 35 weeks of gestation.[121] From studies in experimental animals it appears that preterm white matter necrosis is caused by the same intermittent or partial asphyxia that produces cortical necrosis in late gestational fetuses.[26]

Severe, diffuse placental villous edema appears to be the most frequent initiator of cerebral white matter necrosis before 30 weeks of gestation. It is the most frequent reason why very low-birth-weight infants are depressed at birth.[110] It probably makes fetuses hypoxic by compressing capillaries inside the villi and by imposing a new fluid barrier between maternal blood in the intervillous space and fetal blood in the intravillous capillaries.[110] When both severe and diffuse, villous edema is almost always associated with the need to resuscitate vigorously at birth, low Apgar scores at 5 and 10 minutes, and the need for prolonged mechanical ventilation after resuscitation.[110] The extent and severity of the villous edema correlates inversely with umbilical arterial blood oxygen and pH values.[110] The resulting hypoxia often damages type II pneumocytes in the fetal lungs. The resulting deficiency of surfactant predisposes to the development of hyaline membrane disease and the neonatal respiratory distress syndrome soon after birth.[110] The neonatal respiratory distress syndrome often continues and potentiates the hypoxia and acidosis initiated by the villous edema and predisposes to the development of periventricular leukomalacia (PVL).[87] The frequency of CP is particularly high when the neonatal respiratory distress syndrome evolves into chronic lung disease.[162]

Periventricular leukomalacia (PVL) occurs when the hypoxia and acidosis in conjunction with immaturity lead to a breakdown in the autoregulation of blood flow through the cerebral circulation. Vasoparalysis appears to be a major cause of this failure of autoregulation.[77] Fluctuations in blood pressure and blood flow sometimes then lead to bleeding from capillaries in the subependymal germinal matrix which often extends into a lateral ventricle and compresses blood vessels, leading to periventricular white matter infarction, which is termed *leukomalacia*.[79,177] This leukomalacia is responsible for most of the diplegic and quadriplegic CP that develops in preterm born, very low-birth-weight infants.

The germinal matrix capillary bed where the hemorrhages start is immature before 30 weeks of gestation. It subsequently matures and nearly disappears, so that germinal matrix hemorrhages are rare from late gestation onward. There are additional reasons why germinal matrix hemorrhages are rare late in gestation. Placental villi mature and resist becoming edematous as term approaches and autoregulation of the cerebral circulation is less easily disturbed than in preterm born infants.[110,176]

The sequential changes that follow PVL have been carefully observed. Leukomalacia is the only finding that is present in the first 7 days after the necrosis starts.[34] Cysts appear between 10 days and 9 weeks after the start of necrosis, and thereafter cysts, old glial scars, and a delay in myelination will usually be present.[34,148,174]

OTHER DISORDERS

Nonfebrile Seizures

It has been estimated that about one-third of nonfebrile childhood seizure disorders have their origin in brain lesions, malformations, or metabolic disorders.[20,25] Just how these various lesions and disorders initiate these seizures has not been determined, but more than one mechanism must be involved.[1] Among the well-established antenatal causes of nonfebrile seizure disorders are cerebral lesions caused by toxoplasmosis, cytomegalovirus infection, rubella, metabolic disorders, and hemorrhages. The most frequent intrapartum and neonatal causes of such seizure disorders are infections, hemorrhages, hypoxic-ischemic necrosis, cerebral infarcts, hypoglycemia, and hypocalcemia. The most frequent postneonatal causes of seizure disorders are infections, episodes of anoxia, trauma, and the consequences of prolonged seizures.[1] This last cause has been difficult to quantitate, but it is clear that severe, prolonged seizures sometimes potentiate brain damage and dysfunction.[1,149] Some investigators have claimed that even brief seizures can cause a deterioration of cognitive function.[11,43] Most neonatal seizures are not followed by a chronic seizure disorder, but there are exceptions. The usually cited exceptions are the seizures caused by cerebral malformations, meningitis, and hypoxic cerebral insults.[181]

Previous investigations have found that very few cases of nonfebrile seizure disorders in children can be explained by pregnancy events and disorders. Specifically, Nelson and Ellenberg identified gestational, intrapartum, and neonatal antecedents for less than 3% of nonfebrile seizures in children that did not have motor disorders.[117] We analyzed 26 risk factors and categories of risk factors in our search for the antecedents of nonfebrile seizure disorders in children. In the CPS, 1.2% of the children had a nonfebrile chronic seizure disorder at 7 years of age (Table 11–44). Risk factors were identified for 40% of these seizure disorders. Ten percent of the risk was in the antenatal brain maldevelopment or damage category (see Table 11–44). This risk was spread among a wide variety of factors. Being black and male were the most important risk factors in the familial risk category (see Table 11–44). Birth asphyxial disorders accounted for 3% of the risk.

Children who had nonfebrile seizures had higher frequencies of low 10-minute

TABLE 11–44.

Risk Factors for a Nonfebrile Seizure Disorder at 7 Years of Age*

Risk Factors	No. of Children With Nonfebrile Seizures per 1,000 Children With Risk Factor†	Relative Risks (95% Confidence Intervals)	Attributable Risks (95% Confidence Intervals)
All cases	12 (687)		
Familial			
Race: black	**15** (380), *P* <.001	**1.4** (1.2, 1.7)	**.16** (.15, .18)
Sex: male	**15** (373), *P* <.001	**1.2** (1.0, 1.4)	**.08** (.06, .10)
Other familial disorders	**23** (30), *P* <.001	**2.3** (1.6, 3.3)	**.02** (.01, .03)
Parental mental retardation	**26** (12), *P* <.001	**2.3** (1.3, 4.1)	**.01** (.00, .01)
Antenatal maldevelopment or damage			
Fetal abnormalities			
Hydramnios	**28** (25), *p* <.005	**1.7** (1.2, 2.6)	**.01** (.01, .02)
Maternal pregnancy factor			
Maternal seizure disorder	**19** (39), *P* <.001	**1.6** (1.1, 2.3)	**.02** (.01, .03)
Placental, umbilical cord abnormalities			
Opaque membrane, fetal surface	**19** (70), *P* <.001	**1.4** (1.1, 1.6)	**.03** (.01, .05)
Succenturiate lobe	**31** (22), *p* <.001	**2.7** (1.3, 4.1)	**.02** (.00, .05)
Meconium in amniotic fluid	**22** (25), *P* <.001	**1.6** (1.1, 2.3)	**.02** (.00, .04)
Labor, delivery, neonatal periods			
Birth asphyxial disorders	**41** (19), *P* <.001	**31.7** (18.4, 54.4)	**.03** (.01, .04)
Population attributable risk			**.40** (.38, .42)

*Significant values are in boldface.
†Numbers of children with nonfebrile seizures are in parentheses. P values compared with value in all cases category.

Apgar scores, neonatal seizures, and persisting neonatal neurologic abnormalities than children who did not have nonfebrile seizures.

Cocaine-Exposed Infants

A long list of abnormalities have been reported in the pregnancies and newborns of cocaine users. These include maternal episodes of severe hypertension and vasoconstriction that produce low uteroplacental blood flow and placental abruptions.[187] The characteristic gross and microscopic findings of this low uteroplacental blood flow are sometimes present in the placentas of cocaine users (see Chapter 7). The newborns of cocaine users are reportedly often growth-retarded, which raises the possibility of antenatal damage, maldevelopment, or poor maternal nutrition.[109] There are multiple reports associating congenital defects with fetal cocaine exposure, but a causal relationship is uncertain because cocaine is not a potent cytotoxin and most animal experiments have failed to document strong teratogenicity.[92,151] There are several reported cases of cerebral infarction in the newborns of mothers who used cocaine during pregnancy.[21,92]

A variety of behavioral abnormalities have been described in the children of cocaine users. These include lethargy, an abnormal cry, irritability, an erratic responsiveness to stimuli, a lack of alertness, poor sleep state regulation, and hypertonic reflex abnormalities.[22,72,129] There are claims that some of the children are easily upset in school and perform poorly unless they are carefully supervised and protected from unexpected stimuli and changes in routine. These reports are difficult to interpret because gravidas who use cocaine often smoke tobacco, drink alcohol, use other illicit drugs in addition to cocaine, and sometimes eat poorly during pregnancy. There is one report that children whose mothers used cocaine during pregnancy behave normally during the first year of life.[5] During the next few years efforts need to be made to determine which, if any, of the abnormalities reported in children of cocaine users are the consequences of in utero and postnatal exposure to the drug. Causation must not be inferred without taking confounding variables into consideration.[188]

THE ROLES OF HYPOXIA AND ASPHYXIA IN CENTRAL NERVOUS SYSTEM DISORDERS

Asphyxia

Asphyxia is a biochemical diagnosis in which the fetus or neonate lacks oxygen, retains carbon dioxide (respiratory acidosis), and is unable to adequately eliminate hydrogen ions (metabolic acidosis). A lack of blood flow to a tissue or organ (ischemia) is a related factor. The fetus initially responds to hypoxia or asphyxia much like deep-diving seals, with bradycardia, a reduction of blood flow to the lungs, skin, skeletal muscle, and most abdominal organs, while maintaining blood flow to the brain, heart, and adrenals. When the hypoxia becomes more severe, fetuses appear to maintain the perfusion of their brain stem centers that control heart rate, blood pressure, and respiratory drive at the expense of blood flow to the cerebral hemispheres. If the hypoxia becomes very severe, this autoregulation in the brain deteriorates so that blood flow responds only to blood pressure and not to the local mechanisms that normally regulate blood flow based on local tissue needs for oxygen.[85,86,144] At a still more advanced stage of hypoxia the heart fails and low blood pressure deprives all organs, including the brain, of oxygen and nutrients.

A number of mechanisms come into operation when the brain is damaged by acute hypoxia or asphyxia. Neuronal cellular membranes are depolarized, which diminishes the threshold for seizures and permits an excessive influx of calcium into the neuron.[78] The high levels of calcium trigger a series of events which can further damage or kill the cell.[78] Phospholipase A_2 is activated which leads to an accumulation of arachidonic acid within the cell.[161] If the hypoxia is relieved by reperfusion, the arachidonic acid metabolizes to vasoactive prostaglandins which constrict blood vessels and lead to platelet activation.[97] The liberation of superoxide radicals, which also takes place, often further injures the cell.[161,167] Oxygen deprivation and acidosis also lead to cellular energy failure and adenosine triphosphate (ATP) depletion. Glutamate and aspartate, released into the synaptic cleft, are not retaken up at neuronal junctions, which predisposes to seizures because the excitatory neurotransmitters then overbalance inhibitory neurotransmitters. The seizures in turn potentiate brain damage by increasing the metabolic rate of the brain in areas that participate in the seizures, which deprives other areas of the brain of oxygen and glucose. In the final stages neuronal membranes are disrupted and neuronal death takes place. Disruption of the blood-brain barrier leads to the formation of edema, which in turn sometimes compresses blood vessels and leads to infarction.[60,90,176]

Acute hypoxia or asphyxia can produce a variety of brain lesions, depending on its severity, duration, and the stage of gestation at which hypoxia or asphyxia takes place. Volpe has described these lesions in detail.[176,177] They fall into five categories: selective neuronal necrosis, parasagittal cerebral injury, status marmoratus, PVL, and focal or multifocal ischemic necrosis.

Selective Neuronal Necrosis

Selective neuronal necrosis is reported to be the most frequent lesion associated with hypoxic or asphyxial damage to the brain.[176] The disorder is characterized by individual neuron necrosis or small areas where many neurons are necrotic with little or no damage to other types of brain cells. The result is a reduced density of neurons in an area of the brain. The lesion differs from other brain lesions caused by hypoxia or asphyxia in that oligodendroglia, astrocytes, and microglia are often not affected, probably because they are

not as vulnerable to hypoxia as are neurons.[74] The areas where such selective neuronal necrosis is most frequent include the cerebral cortex, diencephalon, basal ganglia, midbrain, pons, medulla, and cerebellum.[176]

Associated clinical findings are diverse because of the widespread loci of the lesions, variations in the number of neurons destroyed, and because the disorder often coexists with other types of hypoxic and asphyxial brain damage. The neonatal findings can include seizures, hypotonia, alterations in the level of consciousness, and abnormalities in oculomotor movements, and in sucking, swallowing, and movements of the tongue. Because selective neuronal necrosis so often coexists with other types of injury, it is often uncertain to what extent the clinical findings in a child are related to selective neuronal necrosis and to what extent to other types of brain damage. Long-term consequences can include mental retardation, spastic motor deficits, seizure disorders, and impairments in sucking, swallowing, and facial movements.[176] The neuronal deficits found in the cranial nerve nuclei of some sudden infant death syndrome (SIDS) victims would appear to fall into the hypoxic selective neuronal necrosis category.[111]

Parasagittal Cerebral Injury

This is a disorder in which bilateral necrosis develops in the cerebral cortex and immediate subadjacent white matter. The lesion extends over the parasagittal and superomedial regions parallel to the midline of the brain.[176,178] It is the most frequent cause of severe ischemic brain damage in full-term born infants. The areas of necrosis are in the border zone between the termination of the anterior, middle, and posterior cerebral arteries so it seems clear that it is an ischemic disorder.[99,176] In the newborn period, affected children characteristically display weakness of their proximal limbs, arms being more affected than legs. In the long term, the most seriously damaged children have quadriplegic CP.[176] Many of the affected children also have cognitive deficits relating to language and visual-spatial functions.[176]

Status Marmoratus

According to Volpe, status marmoratus of the basal ganglia and thalamus is the least frequent lesion to follow neonatal hypoxic-ischemic brain damage.[176] Its characteristic features include neuronal loss, a reactive gliosis, and a hypermyelination that gives the basal ganglia and thalamus a marbled appearance. The excessive myelination is not of axons but of astrocytic processes.[10,176] It is mainly a disorder of full-term born infants.

The most frequent long-term consequence is choreoathetosis. This occurs when the caudate nuclei are damaged and the pyramidal tracts are intact.[93] Resting tremors and dystonia are less frequent features of the disorder. Bilateral involvement of the globus pallidus is responsible for the dystonia.[17] Choreoathetosis, tremors, and dystonia characteristically appear between 1 and 4 years of age. Associated hypoxic injury to the cerebral cortex is often responsible for the cognitive impairments that are sometimes present. About one-third of the surviving children with the disorder reportedly exhibit spastic quadriparesis.[93]

Periventricular Leukomalacia

This lesion is characterized by white matter necrosis adjacent to the external angles of the lateral ventricles. It typically develops in children born before 32 weeks of gestation who experienced severe hypoxia before birth. The most frequent cause of this hypoxia is severe, diffuse, placental, villous edema.[110,115] The white matter necrosis usually develops after birth following a series of events that include neonatal pulmonary insufficiency and a breakdown of the autoregulation of the cerebral circulation.[86,87,144] These events are described in Chapter 7. The white matter lesions of PVL develop in zones at the end of arterial distributions and are thus presumed to be ischemic in origin.[176,177] The lesions are most evident around the anterior and posterior ends of the lateral ventricles, in the acoustic radiations adjacent to the temporal horns, in the optic radiations adjacent to the occipatal horns, and in the centrum semiovale near the ventricles.[176] Hemorrhage often coexists with PVL. It can vary from petechiae to the massive escape of blood into the brain parenchyma and ventricles.[41,171]

Long-term lesions of PVL occur in a continuum from small foci of gliosis, to a reduction in myelin with consequent ventricular dilatation, to devastating multicystic encephalomalacia in which only a thin rim of cerebral cortex surrounds massively enlarged ventricles. Long-term consequences of the lesions include spastic diplegic and quadriplegic spastic CP in which the lower limbs are usually more affected by motor abnormalities than the upper limbs.[157] Severe cognitive and sensory impairments can also be present.

Focal or Multifocal Ischemic Necrosis

These are sizable but localized areas of necrosis that develop within the distribution of major cerebral blood vessels.[94,176] They evolve into cavities that are variously termed *porencephaly, hydranencephaly,* and *multicystic encephalomalacia.* Porencephaly refers to a single cavity, hydranencephaly to massive, bilateral cavities, and multicystic encephalomalacia to multiple cavities. These lesions are the result of necrosis that develops between the sixth month of gestation and the early months after birth.[94,99,176] Necrosis before the sixth month of gestation leads to gyral deformities without cavitation.[176] Because of their location and cavitary character, Volpe and others surmise that most of the lesions are due to vascular occlusion or maldevelopment.[176] Intrapartum or neonatal hypoxia may play a role in a few cases in which there are other types of cortical injury and in cases in which a specific hypoxic insult has been documented.[173,179] As previously mentioned, PVL sometimes evolves into multicystic encephalomalacia. Clinical findings associated with focal or multifocal ischemic necrosis depend on the size, number, and locations of the cystic lesions. If the lesion is large, single, and in the distribution of the middle cerebral artery, the neonate will usually be hemiparetic. Large bilateral lesions often produce quadriplegia. When they are present, impairments in cognitive function usually reflect the presence of bilateral lesions that affect the cortex.

Neonatal Clinical Manifestations of Acute Hypoxic and Asphyxial Disorders

Analysis of Blood Before or at Birth

Intrapartum hypoxia or asphyxia can only be confirmed by an analysis of fetal or neonatal blood. This is usually done by sampling fetal scalp or umbilical arterial blood. The determination can also be made by examining capillary blood from the neonate immediately after birth. The postnatal capillary origin of the sample should be recorded in the child's chart because the values for identifying hypoxia or asphyxia in capillary blood differ from those for umbilical arterial blood. The extremity from which the postnatal capillary blood is removed must be warmed for at least 10 minutes before the sample is taken to insure that the blood being examined has not been oxygen-depleted by stagnating in the capillaries from which it is removed.

By itself, a history of low oxygen level or acidosis in fetal or neonatal blood is not proof that birth asphyxia was the cause of motor or cognitive abnormalities that may be present. Almost no correlation has been found between such acidosis and the presence of neurologic abnormalities in the neonatal period.[35,36,134] There are several reasons for this finding. First, cord blood gases and pH values are profoundly affected by maternal acid-base status. Second, the duration of bearing down during labor has a positive correlation with fetal acidosis, but there is no evidence that a long period of bearing down produces irreversible brain damage.[168] Third, intrapartum hypoxia at term that is severe enough to damage the fetal brain damages other organs as well and the multiorgan damage usually causes stillbirth or neonatal death.[50,114,124,135,136,159,170]

Electronic Fetal Monitoring

The finding of a fetal heart rate abnormality by auscultation or electronic fetal monitoring should not automatically be assumed to be a manifestation of acute fetal hypoxia or asphyxia. In many instances the cause is acute chorioamnionitis or preexisting brain damage or maldevelopment.[155] In the case of earlier gestational brain damage or maldevelopment, heart rate abnormalities often occur as manifestations of brain dysfunction that has been present long before labor and delivery. To attribute monitored abnormalities in fetal heart rate to acute hypoxic or asphyxial brain injury, the following must also be present: (a) the biochemical findings characteristic of intrapartum hypoxia or asphyxia, (b) a depressed newborn, (c) neonatal renal dysfunction, and (d) long-term neurologic abnormalities that are compatible with intrapartum hypoxia or asphyxia. In addition, nonhypoxic disorders that might explain the fetal heart rate abnormalities should be absent.

Apgar Scores

Most of the older studies that have attempted to assess the role of antenatal hypoxia in the genesis of brain damage have used low Apgar scores as a major criterion for identifying antenatal intrapartum hypoxia and asphyxia.* In the CPS, low 5- and 10-minute Apgar scores were severalfold more often associated with congenital disorders than with birth asphyxial disorders in children who developed CP (Table 11–45).[114] This reinforces the point that abnormal Apgar scores can have many different causes, many of which are unrelated to intrapartum hypoxia or asphyxia. In one very large study only 20% of the neonates with 5-minute

---

* References 8, 46, 47, 50, 66, 118, 119, 131, 147, 156, and 164.

TABLE 11–45.

The Ratio of Clinical Findings in Children With Congenital Disorders vs. Children Exposed to Asphyxial Disorders*

Clinical findings	Ratio of Congenital Disorders to Birth Asphyxial Disorders When Clinical Finding Was Present
	Cerebral Palsy Present
Meconium in amniotic fluid	11:1 (34:3)
Apgar Scores at 1 and 10 Minutes	
0–3, 0–5	2:1 (9:6)
0–3, 6–10	3:1 (6:2)
Neonatal hypotonia	3:1 (13:5)
Neonatal seizures	1.2:1 (11:9)
Neonatal apneic episodes	3:1 (10:3)
Persistent neurologic abnormalities in neonatal period	4:1 (36:9)
Neurologic abnormalities redeveloping during 1st year of life	>100:1 (13:0)
Head circumference at birth, percentiles 1–10	>100:1 (13:0)
Head circumference increase <10 cm in 1st year of life	3:1 (13:5)

Numbers of affected children are in parentheses.

Apgar scores less than 7 had umbilical arterial blood pH values less than 7.10.[169]

Neonatal Seizures

An early neonatal seizure that follows biochemical evidence of intrapartum hypoxia or asphyxia is an indication of brain dysfunction, but rarely is this dysfunction permanent.[127] To be interpreted as hypoxic or asphyxial in origin, seizures should first appear between 6 and 48 hours after birth.[91] If they appear at less than 6 hours of age, they usually have a nonhypoxic origin, or else the hypoxia that damaged the brain antedated labor and delivery. Neonatal seizures are not always tonic-clonic. They can manifest as lip smacking, eye-rolling, bicycling (pedaling), or other unexplained movements. To be attributed with reasonable certainty to hypoxia or asphyxia, seizures should meet the same biochemical and clinical criteria for intrapartum hypoxia or asphyxia as were outlined to attribute fetal heart rate abnormalities to intrapartum hypoxia or asphyxia. The risk factors for neonatal seizures in the CPS are found in Table 11–46.

Neonatal Neurologic Abnormalities

Neonates with brain damage due to intrapartum hypoxia or asphyxia have a well-known sequence of behavioral and neurologic abnormalities. First, they have an altered level of consciousness. If the brain damage is mild, the neonate may be excessively irritable. If the damage is more severe the child will be lethargic or unresponsive, initially hypotonic or floppy, and only later hypertonic or stiff. If the child was hypertonic at birth, it is very unlikely that intrapartum hypoxia or asphyxia was the cause. Deep tendon reflexes can be accentuated or depressed by intrapartum hypoxic or asphyxial brain damage. The Moro reflex, the grasp reflex, and suck are usually depressed in the early neonatal period.

Other Organ Dysfunction in the Neonatal Period

The heart is sometimes damaged by intrapartum hypoxia or asphyxia.[19] With increases in protein breakdown and renal failure, the hypoxia-damaged neonate will have increased serum levels of potassium, urea nitrogen, and creatinine.

TABLE 11–46.

Risk Factors for Neonatal Seizures in Full Term Born Infants*

Risk Factors	No. of Children With Neonatal Seizures per 1,000 Children With Risk Factor†	Relative Risks (95% Confidence Intervals)	Attributable Risks (95% Confidence Intervals)
All cases	4 (183)		
Neonatal hypoxic disorders	**69** (72), *P* < .001	**13.4** (9.5, 19.1)	**.22** (.18, .26)
Congenital malformations	**8** (113), *P* < .001	**2.5** (1.8, 3.4)	**.18** (.16, .20)
Birth asphyxial disorders	**11** (70), *P* < .001	**2.1** (1.6, 2.9)	**.10** (.08, .11)
Bacterial infections	**38** (46), *P* < .001	**4.0** (2.8, 5.9)	**.09** (.07, .11)
Meconium in amniotic fluid	**12** (73), *P* < .001	**2.5** (1.6, 3.4)	**.12** (.09, .15)
Metabolic disorders	**25** (32), *P* < .005	**3.7** (2.4, 5.7)	**.07** (.04, .11)
Intracranial hemorrhage	**253** (24), *P* < .001	**18.5** (10.3, 33.4)	**.07** (.04, .11)
Population attributable risk			**.84** (.80, .88)

Significant values are in bold print.
†Number of children with neonatal seizures are in parentheses. P values compared with value in all cases category.

Hypoglycemia appears as glycogen stores are exhausted and hypocalcemia sometimes develops as the result of parathormone deficiency. It is very important to assess renal function in cases where there is suspicion that intrapartum hypoxia or asphyxia may have damaged the fetal brain. Since the kidneys are more vulnerable to hypoxic damage during labor and delivery than the brain, hypoxic brain damage is almost always accompanied by evidence of renal damage.[114,135,136,159,170] Such renal damage almost always produces hematuria and reduces urine output.[135] If there is reluctance to attach a bag to measure a newborn's urine output, weighing the diaper intermittently will give an estimate of urine output, and a dipstick applied to a wet diaper can be used to test for hemoglobin. In my experience hematuria is always present in cases in which intrapartum hypoxia or asphyxia damaged the kidneys. If there is any suspicion of renal damage, serum blood urea nitrogen (BUN) and creatinine values should be determined on the first day of life and followed until the issue is resolved.

Other Clinical Findings

Several other clinical findings that characteristically follow birth asphyxia were severalfold more frequently related to congenital disorders than to birth asphyxia in CP victims in the CPS. These included meconium in the amniotic fluid, neonatal apnea spells, neurologic abnormalities persisting through the neonatal period, and neurologic disorders that disappeared during the neonatal period and then reappeared later in the first or second years of life (see Table 11–45).[114] Slow head growth after birth and microcephaly at birth were also often manifestations of congenital or developmental disorders in children with CP (see Table 11–45).[114] This leads to the conclusion that these clinical findings, by themselves, cannot be trusted to identify antenatal asphyxia or to distinguish CP of asphyxial origin from CP due to other causes.

Consequences of Birth Asphyxial Disorders in the Collaborative Perinatal Study

In our analyses of the CPS data we required that one or more early neonatal seizures follow a specifically identified birth asphyxial disorder for a child to be placed in the birth asphyxial category. Using this definition, birth asphyxia appears to have caused only 1% of the CP in full-term born infants in the CPS. This might seem inconsistent with the frequent findings at autopsy of acute asphyxial lesions in the brains of children who were stillborn or who died in the newborn period. There is a simple explanation for the presence of these lesions. Birth asphyxia or hypoxia that is severe enough to damage the fetal brain usually kills before or soon after birth.[45,50,124] This is what apparently happened in the CPS. Almost half of the 1,349 CPS children who were stillborn or who died in the neonatal period died as the consequence of a birth asphyxial disorder. Only 24 of the children in the birth asphyxial category survived to 7 years of age.[114] Eleven of the 24 had CP or other neurologic abnormalities.[114]

From these findings it seems that the margin between the level at which intrapartum hypoxia or asphyxia begins to damage the fetal brain and the level at which it kills is very narrow in late gestation.[50,124] The ability of Myers and his associates to produce severe brain damage in monkeys by inducing perinatal asphyxia might seem inconsistent with this view, but in fact the findings of Myers and co-workers support it because many of the monkeys died and most of the survivors had no neurologic abnormalities.[100–103] A 1984 Oxford study produced still more evidence that CP is rarely the result of birth asphyxia.[127] A failure of medical personnel to react to evidence of intrapartum hypoxia and asphyxia was followed by an increased frequency of neonatal apnea and seizures, but not of CP.

As previously mentioned in this chapter, our criteria for diagnosing asphyxia in the CPS required the presence of a disorder capable of causing birth asphyxia followed by early neonatal seizures. Do these criteria exclude many cases of asphyxial brain damage? The question is important because cerebral palsy and other motor and cognitive disorders have often been attributed to umbilical cord compression or some other asphyxial disorder even though no such disorder was identified at delivery. Attributing brain dysfunction to such an occult disorder is usually a mistake because birth asphyxial disorders that were severe enough to damage the fetal brain were not missed in the CPS. Specifically, no psychomotor disorder for which birth asphyxial disor-

ders were a risk increased in frequency following a birth asphyxial disorder in the absence of neonatal seizures (see Table 11–47). All 49 CP victims in the CPS who had neonatal neurologic abnormalities had an explanation for the etiology of their neurologic impairments.[114] Nine had experienced birth asphyxial disorders, 36 had congenital disorders, and 4 had recognized CNS infections. Oxytocin, whose use was associated with an increased frequency of neonatal seizures in the CPS, was not followed by an increased frequency of CP.[114] The use of gas anesthesia during delivery, a chronic maternal seizure disorder, maternal diabetes mellitus, and neonatal or presumed fetal hypoglycemia were also not associated with an increased frequency of CP.[114]

Did the criteria that we adopted to identify potentially brain-damaging birth asphyxia include many undamaged children? The answer is no. Eighty-three percent of the children who experienced birth asphyxial disorders followed by neonatal seizures had neurologic abnormalities in the neonatal period (see Table 11–47). Half of these children lost their motor disorder by 7 years of age. Children who were exposed to birth asphyxial disorders but did not have neonatal seizures did not have an increased frequency of any central nervous system disorder at 7 years of age (see Table 11–47). Findings were similar for children who were exposed to meconium in the amniotic fluid. If neonatal seizures were absent there was no long term increase in the frequency of cognitive or motor disorders. If neonatal seizures had been present these children had an increased frequency of CNS abnormalities at 7 years of age, particularly non-febrile seizure disorders (see Table 11–47).

According to our analyses, birth asphyxial disorders had a role in only three CNS disorders in the CPS. These were quadriplegic CP, severe mental retardation with motor abnormalities other than CP, and a nonfebrile seizure disorder (see Tables 11–5, 11–41, 11–44).[114] The relative risk that birth asphyxia posed for these disorders was significant, but only a few

TABLE 11–47.

The Role of Neonatal Seizures in Identifying Children Whose Brains Were Damaged by Birth Asphyxial Disorders and by Meconium in the Amniotic Fluid.*

Central Nervous System Disorders	(A)†	(B)*	(C)*	(D)*	(E)*
	Frequency of Brain Disorder per 1,000 Full Term Births				
Neonatal neurologic abnormalities	**53** (1581), *P*<.01	**70** (276)	**834** (10)	**54** (395)	**558** (10)
At age 7 yr					
Quadriplegic cerebral palsy	**0.4** (13), *P*<.01	**0.3** (1)	**178** (3)	**0.4** (3)	**111** (2)
IQ <60 + motor disorders	**7** (192), *P*<.01	**7** (29)	**167** (2)	**8** (55)	**111** (2)
Non-febrile seizure disorders	**12** (346), *P*<.01	**11** (45)	**583** (3)	**11** (77)	**667** (12)

*Significant values are in boldface. (A) = no asphyxial disorder, no neonatal seizures, no meconium in amniotic fluid; (B) = birth asphyxial disorders present, no neonatal seizures, no meconium in amniotic fluid; (C) = birth asphyxial disorders present, neonatal seizures present, no meconium in amniotic fluid; (D) = meconium in amniotic fluid, no neonatal seizures, birth asphyxial disorders excluded; (E) = meconium in amniotic fluid, neonatal seizures present, birth asphyxia disorders excluded.
†The number of children are in parentheses. P values compared with values in (A) category. Children with congenital malformations and congenital syndromes were excluded from the analyses.

children who were exposed to hypoxia or asphyxia severe enough to damage their brains survived. As a result, the proportion of these disorders attributable to birth hypoxia or asphyxia was small.

Conclusions

All of the aforementioned information underscores the importance of making accurate measurements and observations on neonates to avoid misattributing nonasphyxial CP to asphyxia. First, CP should never be attributed to birth asphyxia without the identification of a specific asphyxial disorder. Next, carefully recorded observations of a neonate's kidney, heart, and lung function should be noted because birth asphyxia that is severe enough to damage the brain usually damages the kidneys and often the lungs and the heart.[19,114,135,136,159,170] If a child was not seriously depressed at birth or was easy to resuscitate, there is no basis for attributing subsequent psychomotor impairments to birth asphyxial disorders. Many nonasphyxial causes of severe brain dysfunction produce low Apgar scores at birth.

Consequences of Meconium in the Amniotic Fluid

In our analyses, meconium in the amniotic fluid was a major risk factor for three disorders: (1) quadriplegic cerebral palsy, (2) lesser motor impairments accompanied by severe mental retardation, and (3) chronic, nonfebrile seizure disorders (see Tables 11–5, 11–6, 11–41, and 11–44). Several types of evidence suggest that hypoxia was the mechanism through which meconium acted to produce these disorders. First, the above mentioned three disorders are the same as those that followed acute birth asphyxial disorders in the CPS, raising the possibility of a common hypoxic origin. How might meconium produce acute or subacute fetal hypoxia? Altshuler and Hyde have provided a clue in their observations that meconium both causes umbilical cord blood vessels to constrict and is associated with necrosis in the walls of these blood vessels.[3]

Findings in the CPS support those of Altshuler and Hyde. First, necrosis was three times more frequent in umbilical and placental surface blood vessels when meconium-filled macrophages were present than when they were absent. The respective rates of this necrosis were 9/1,000 (13 cases) and 3/1,000 (85) (*P*<.001). Second, thrombi were more frequent in umbilical cord and placental surface vessels when meconium was present than when it was absent. The respective rates were 41/1,000 (59 cases) and 25/1,000 (742 cases) (*P*<.001). There is still other evidence that meconium-initiated vasoconstriction can cause severe fetal hypoxia and acidosis. I have reviewed six cases of quadriplegic cerebral palsy in which a heavy deposition of meconium in the amniotic fluid was associated with umbilical arterial blood pH values lower than 7.0. In all six cases there was no other identified cause for fetal acidosis.

Clinical findings in the neonatal period suggest that meconium-initiated brain damage may be a subacute rather than an acute process. In Table 11–48, clinical findings from the CPS are shown that characteristically follow birth asphyxia severe enough to cause permanent damage to fetal brains. All of the children whose cases are enumerated in the table had one or more of the three disorders that are characteristic manifestations of such damage: (1) quadriplegic cerebral palsy, (2) lesser motor impairments accompanied by severe mental retardation, and (3) chronic, nonfebrile seizure disorders. In each vertical column, cases in which either of the other two risk factors for psychomotor impairments were present were excluded from the analysis. For example, the column that includes children with congenital malformations includes no children who were exposed to

birth asphyxial disorders or to meconium. As might be expected, children with brain damage following a birth asphyxial disorder were difficult to resuscitate at birth, had Apgar scores that were still low at 10 minutes, were hypotonic, and had multiple other neonatal neurologic and behavioral abnormalities. These neonatal abnormalities were present but less frequent in brain-impaired children who had been exposed to meconium or had major congenital malformations (see Table 11–48).

Only 3 of 31 non-CPS children with meconium-associated quadriplegic cerebral palsy whose cases I have reviewed have had more than very brief occurrences of neonatal renal or myocardial failure. This frequent absence of renal and cardiac failure may be an indication that the hypoxia to which these children had been exposed was subacute rather than acute. It is also possible that mechanisms other than hypoxia were responsible for some of their brain dysfunction.

Disorders That Cause Chronic Fetal Hypoxia

In the CPS, disorders that produced chronic low blood flow from the uterus to

TABLE 11–48.

Rates of Clinical Findings in Neonates When Disorders That Are the Characteristic Consequences of Birth Asphyxial Disorders Were Present at Age 7 Years*

Neurologic Examination	Birth Asphyxial Disorders	Meconium in Amniotic Fluid	Major Malformations in Neonate
	Frequency/1,000 Births When Specified Risk Factors Were Present		
Vigorous resuscitation at birth	929 (13), $P<.001$	173 (25), $P<.001$	83 (10), $P<.05$
Apgar scores at 1 and 10 min			
0–3, 0–5	643 (9), $P<.001$	125 (18)	143 (17), $P<.001$
0–3, 6–10	214 (3)	382 (55)	571 (69), $P<.001$
4–10, 6–10	143 (2)	493 (71)	286 (34), $P<.001$
Respiratory distress	429 (6)	56 (8)	42 (5)
Neonatal seizures	–	153 (22), $P<.001$	92 (11), $P<.02$
Jitters/tremulous	500 (7), $P<.001$	90 (13)	183 (22), $P<.001$
Myoclonus	214 (3), $P<.001$	35 (5)	50 (6), $P<.02$
Hypotonia	571 (8), $P<.001$	139 (20), $P<.001$	317 (38), $P<.001$
Lethargy	429 (6)	76 (11), $P<.001$	58 (7), $P<.005$
Hypertonia	500 (7), $P<.001$	63 (9)	75 (9), $P<.01$
Abnormal reflexes	643 (9), $P<.001$	125 (18), $P<.05$	267 (32), $P<.001$
Abnormal cry	571 (8), $P<.001$	90 (13), $P<.02$	100 (12), $P<.001$
Abnormal suck	286 (4), $P<.001$	76 (11), $P<.001$	75 (9), $P<.001$

*P values compared with all cases in the analysis. Number of cases with neonatal abnormality are in parentheses.

TABLE 11–49.

Types of Central Nervous System Dysfunction That Followed Chronic Low Uteroplacental Blood Flow (Collaborative Perinatal Study)

Brain Dysfunction	Relative Risks of Low Blood Flow for Brain Dysfunction*	Attributable Risks of Low Blood Flow to Brain Dysfunction*
Mild mental retardation		
No motor abnormalities	**1.2** (1.1, 1.3)	**.05** (.03, .07)
Severe mental retardation		
No motor abnormalities	**1.2** (1.1, 1.3)	**.03** (.00, .06)
With motor abnormalities	**1.3** (1.1, 1.7)	**.07** (.05, .09)
Learning disorder with normal IQ	**1.2** (1.0, 1.4)	**.05** (.04, .07)
Hyperactivity without neurologic abnormalities	**1.1** (1.0, 1.3)	**.02** (.01, .04)
Emotionally flat	**1.3** (1.1, 1.6)	**.05** (.03, .07)

Significant values are in boldface; 95% confidence intervals are in parentheses.

the placenta appear to have affected the long-term brain function of many more children than did birth asphyxial disorders. Birth asphyxial disorders had their largest impact on motor function, whereas chronic low uteroplacental blood flow mainly affected cognitive functions and behavior. The impact on cognitive function was broad, appearing in every category that measured these functions, and it was independent of many familial and postnatal environmental factors that also affect a child's scores on tests of cognition (Table 11–49). Placental findings characteristic of chronic low uteroplacental blood flow also correlated with increased frequencies of two behavioral disorders, hyperactivity and emotionally flat affect, independent of confounding factors that affect behavior (see Table 11–49).

By what mechanisms might chronic low uteroplacental blood flow damage the fetal brain or otherwise impair its development? The delivery of oxygen and nutrients to the fetus is almost entirely dependent on the volume of blood that flows from the uterus to the placenta. If an inadequate delivery of nutrients and oxygen to the fetus is responsible for the just-mentioned cognitive and behavioral abnormalities, the injury or maldevelopment may occur late in gestation because it is then that a mismatch most often develops between the needs of the fetus for nutrients and oxygen and the ability

of uteroplacental blood flow and the placenta to meet these needs (see Chapter 3). The settings in which this mismatch most often occurs are preeclampsia, chronic maternal hypertension, twins, and gestations that extend beyond 42 weeks.[37,54,61,65,98,104]

Relevance of the Collaborative Perinatal Study (CPS) Findings

Finally, it must be asked if obstetric and neonatal clinical advances since 1966 make the findings that relate to brain dysfunction in the CPS obsolete. The answer is no because medical and obstetric advances since 1966 have not produced a decrease in the frequency of CP or most other CNS disorders.[32,63,68,71,73,91,130,138,165] All of the CP that we analyzed was in full-term born children, and it is unlikely that current obstetric and pediatric management could have prevented this CP because most of the responsible disorders developed long before labor and delivery and were unrecognized at the time the maldevelopment or damage took place. Electronic fetal monitoring has come into widespread use since the CPS data were collected. Many have assumed that such monitoring is preventing some cases of CP by warning of asphyxia or hypoxia before irreversible brain damage takes place. There is no good evidence that this damage is being prevented.[89,91,160] The same is true for perinatal mortality. Eight randomized clinical trials have found no evidence that it is being reduced by electronic fetal monitoring.[51,160] The main reason for these failures is that almost all of the damage and maldevelopment is taking place before labor and delivery. Analyses of the teeth and bones of children with neurodevelopmental handicaps confirm this thesis. Fifty percent to 70% of such children have reportedly had hypoplastic enamel in their teeth.[27,175] The location and extent of the hypoplasia presumably reflects the time and duration of the damaging insult. In a large study of stillbirths and neonatal deaths, over two-thirds of the children had cartilage abnormalities that indicated significant injury long before death.[44]

REFERENCES

1. Aicardi J: Epilepsy in brain-injured children. *Dev Med Child Neurol* 1990; 32:191–202.

2. American Academy of Pediatrics, Committee on Fetus and Newborn: Use and abuse of the Apgar score. *Pediatrics* 1986; 78:1148–1149.

3. Altshuler G, Hyde S: Meconium-induced vasocontraction: A potential cause of cerebral and other fetal hypoperfusion and of poor pregnancy outcome. *J Child Neurol* 1989; 4:137–142.

4. Anastopoulos AD, Barkley RA: Biological factors in attention deficit hyperactivity disorder. *Behav Ther* 1988; 11:47–53.

5. Baar AL, Fleury P, Ultee CA: Behaviour in first year after drug dependent pregnancy. *Arch Dis Child* 1989; 64:241–245.

6. Benichou J, Gail MH: Variance calculations and confidence intervals for estimates of the attributable risk based on logistic models. *Biometrics* 1990; 46:991–1003.

7. Biederman J, Munir K, Knee D, Habelow W, Armentano M, Autor S, Hoge SK, Waternaux C: A family study of patients with attention deficit disorder and normal controls. *J Psychiatr Res* 1986; 20:263–274.

8. Blair E, Stanley FJ: Intrapartum asphyxia: A rare cause of cerebral palsy. *J Pediatr* 1988; 112:515–519.

9. Blidner IN, McClemont S, Anderson GD, Sinclair JC: Size-at-birth standards for an urban Canadian population. *Canad Med Assoc J* 1984; 130:133–140.

10. Borit A, Herndon RM: The fine structure of plaques fibromyeliniques in ulegyria and in status marmoratus. *Acta Neuropathol* 1970; 14:304–311.

11. Bourgeois BFD, Prensky AL, Palkes HS, Talent BK, Busch SG: Intelligence in epilepsy: A prospective study in children. *Ann Neurol* 1983; 14:438–444.

12. Brann AW Jr: Factors during neonatal life that influence brain disorders, in Freeman J (ed): *Prenatal and Perinatal Factors Associated with Brain Disorders*. Bethesda, Md, US Department of Health and Human Services, 1985, publication no. 85–1149, pp 302–316.

13. Brann AW Jr, Myers RE: Central nervous system findings in the newborn monkey following severe in utero partial asphyxia. *Neurology* 1975; 25:327–328.

14. Brazelton TB, Snyder DM, Yogman MW: A developmental approach to behavioral problems, in Hoekelman RA (ed): *Primary Pediatric Care*. St Louis, CV Mosby Co, 1987, p 700.

15. Broman S: The Collaborative Perinatal Project: An overview, in Mednick SA, Harway M, Finello KM (eds): *Handbook of longitudinal Research*, vol 2. New York, Praeger, 1984, pp 185–215.

16. Broman SH, Nichols PL, Kennedy WA: *Preschool IQ, Prenatal and Early Developmental Correlates*. Hillsdale, NJ, Lawrence Erlbaum, 1975.

17. Brun A, Kyllerman M: Clinical, pathogenetic and neuropathological correlates in dystonic cerebral palsy. *Eur J Pediatr* 1979; 131:93–104.

18. Bruzzi P, Green SB, Byar DP, Brinton LA, Schairer C: Estimating the population attributable risk for multiple risk factors using case-control data. *Am J Epidemiol* 1985; 122:904–914.

19. Cabal LA, Devaskar U, Siassi B, Hodgman J, Emmanouilides G: Cardiogenic shock associated with perinatal asphyxia in preterm infants. *J Pediatr* 1980; 96:705–710.

20. Cavazzuti GB: Epidemiology of different types of epilepsy in school age children of Modena, Italy. *Epilepsia* 1980; 21:57–62.

21. Chasnoff I, Bussey M, Savid R, Stack C: Perinatal cerebral infarction and maternal cocain use. *J Pediatr* 1986; 108:456–459.

22. Chasnoff I, Grioffith DR, MacGregor S, Dirkes K, Burns KA: Temporal patterns of cocaine use in pregnancy. Perinatal outcome. *JAMA* 1989; 261:1741–1744.

23. Chefetz MD: Etiology of cerebral palsy: Role of reproductive insufficiency and the multiplicity of factors. *Obstet Gynecol* 1965; 25:635–647.

24. Chess S: Evolution of behavior disorder in a group of mentally retarded children. *J Am Acad Child Psychiatry* 1977; 16:4–18.

25. Chevrie JJ, Aicardi J: Convulsive disorders in the first year of life: Etiologic factors. *Epilepsia* 1977; 18:489–498.

26. Clapp JF, Peress NS, Wesley M, Mann LI: Brain damage after intermittent partial cord occlusion in the chronically instrumented fetal lamb. *Am J Obstet Gynecol* 1988; 159:504–509.

27. Cohen HJ, Diner H: The significance of developmental dental enamel defects in neurological diagnoses. *Pediatrics* 1970; 46:737–747.

28. *The Collaborative Perinatal Study on Cerebral Palsy, Mental Retardation and Other Neurological and Sensory Disorders of Infancy and Childhood Manual.* Bethesda, Md, US Department of Health, Education and Welfare, 1966.

29. Conboy TJ, Pass RF, Stagno S, Alford CA, Myers GJ, Britt WJ, McCollister FP, Summers MN, McFarland CE, Boll TJ: Early clinical manifestations and intellectual outcome in children with symptomatic congenital cytomegalovirus infection. *J Pediatr* 1987; 111:343–348.

30. Costeff H, Cohen BE, Weller LE: Biological factors in mild mental retardation. *Dev Med Child Neurol* 1983; 25:580–587.

31. Cunningham L, Cadoret RJ, Loftus R, Edwards JE: Studies of adoptees from psychiatrically disturbed biological parents: Psychiatric conditions in childhood and adolescence, *Br J Psychiatry* 1975; 126:534–549.

32. Dale A, Stanley FJ: An epidemiological study of cerebral palsy in Western Australia, 1956–1975. II: Spastic cerebral palsy and perinatal factors. *Dev Med Child Neurol* 1980; 22:13–25.

33. Delaney-Black V, Camp BW, Lubchenco LO, Swanson C, Roberts L, Gaherty P, Swanson B: Neonatal hyperviscosity association with lower achievement and IQ scores at school age. *Pediatrics* 1989; 83:662–667.

34. DeVries LS, Wigglesworth JS, Regev R, Dubowitz LMS: Evolution of periventricular leukomalacia during the neonatal period and infancy: correlation of imaging and postmortem findings. *Early Hum Dev* 1988; 17:205–219.

35. Dijxhoorn MJ, Visser GHA, Fidler VJ, Touwen BCL, Huisjes HJ: Apgar score, meconium and acidaemia at birth in relation to neonatal neurological morbidity in term infants. *Br J Obstet Gynaecol* 1986; 93:217–222.

36. Dijxhoorn MJ, Visser GHA, Huisjes HJ, Fidler V, Touwen BCL: The relation between umbilical pH values and neonatal neurological morbidity in full-term appropriate for dates infants. *Early Hum Dev* 1985; 11:33–42.

37. Dixon HG, Browne JCM, Davey DA: Choriodecidual and myometrial blood flow. *Lancet* 1963; 2:369–373.

38. Drillien CM: Studies in mental handicap. II. Some obstetric factors of possible aetiological significance. *Arch Dis Child* 1968; 43:283–294.

39. Drillien CM, Jameson S, Wilkinson EM: Studies in mental handicap. I. Prevalence and distribution by clinical type and severity of defect. *Arch Dis Child* 1966; 41:528–538.

40. Durkin MV, Kaveggia E, Pendleton E, Neuhause G, Opitz JM: Analysis of etiological factors in cerebral palsy with severe mental retardation: Analysis of gestational, parturitional and neonatal data. *Eur J Pediatr* 1976; 123:67–81.

41. Dykes FD, Dunbar B, Lazarra A, Ahrmann PA: Posthemorrhagic hydrocephalus in high-risk preterm infants: Natural history, management, and long-term outcome. *J Pediatr* 1989; 114:611–618.

42. Eastman NJ, Kohl SG, Maisel JE, Kavaler F: The obstetrical background of 753 cases of cerebral palsy. *Obstet Gynecol Surv* 1962; 17:459–500.

43. Ellenberg JH, Nelson KB: Do seizures in children cause intellectual deterioration? *N Engl J Med* 1986; 314:1085–1088.

44. Emery JL, Kalpaktsoglou PK: The costochondrial junction during later stages of intrauterine life, and abnormal growth patterns found in association with perinatal death. *Arch Dis Child* 1967; 42:1–13.

45. Fenichel G: *Neonatal Neurology.* New York, Churchill Livingstone Inc, 1985.

46. Finer NN, Robertson CM, Peters KL: Factors affecting outcome in hypoxic-ischemic encephalopathy in term infants. *Am J Dis Child* 1983; 137:21–25.

47. Finer NN, Robertson CM, Richards RT, Pinnell LE, Peters KL: Hypoxic-ischemic encephalopathy in term infants: Perinatal factors and outcome. *J Pediatr* 1981; 98:112–117.

48. Fitz C: Computed tomography, state of the art, in Pape KE, Wigglesworth JS (eds): *Perinatal Brain Lesions.* Boston, Blackwell Scientific Publications, 1989, p 47.

49. Flyer DC, Buckley LP, Hellenbrand WE, Cohn HE, Kirklin JW, Nadas AS, Cartier JM, Breihart MH: Report of the New England Regional Infant Cardiac Program. *Pediatrics* 1980; 65:375–461.

50. Freeman JM, Nelson KB: Intrapartum asphyxia and cerebral palsy. *Pediatrics* 1988; 82:240–249.

51. Freeman R: Intrapartum fetal monitoring, a disappointing story. *N Engl J Med* 1990; 322:624–626.

52. Freud S: *Infantile Cerebral Paralysis.* Coral Gables, Fla, University of Miami Press, 1968, p 142.

53. Gailey E, Kantola-Sorsa E, Granstrom ML: Intelligence of children of epileptic mothers. *J Pediatr* 1988; 113:677–684.

54. Gallery EDM, Hunyor SN, Gyory AZ: Plasma volume contraction, a significant factor in both pregnancy-associated hypertension and chronic hypertension in pregnancy. *Q J Med* 1979; 48:593–602.

55. Gillberg IC, Gillberg C: Children with preschool minor neurodevelopmental disorders, IV. Behavior and school achievement at age 13. *Dev Med Child Neurol* 1989; 31:3–14.

56. Gillberg IC, Gillberg C, Groth J: Children with preschool minor neurodevelopmental disorders, V. Neurodevelopmental profiles at age 13. *Dev Med Child Neurol* 1989; 31:14–24.

57. Gittelman R, Mannuzza S, Shenker R, Bonagura N: Hyperactive boys almost grow up. I. Psychiatric status. *Arch Gen Psychiatry* 1985; 42:937–947.

58. Glauser TA, Rorke LB, Weinberg PM, Clancy RR: Congenital brain anomalies associated with the hypoplastic left heart syndrome. *Pediatrics* 1990; 85:984–990.

59. Glauser TA, Rorke LB, Weinberg PM, Clancy RR: Acquired neuropathologic lesions associated with hypoplastic left heart syndrome. *Pediatrics* 1990; 85:991–1000.

60. Goldstein GW: Pathogenesis of brain edema and hemorrhage: Role of the brain capillary. *Pediatrics* 1979; 64:357–360.

61. Goodlin RC, Dobry CA, Anderson JC, Woods RE, Quaife M: Clinical signs of normal plasma volume expansion during pregnancy. *Am J Obstet Gynecol* 1983; 145:1001–1009.

62. Goodman R, Stevenson J: A twin study of hyperactivity, I. An examination of hyperactivity scores and categories derived from Rutter teacher and parent questionnaires. *J Child Psychol Psychiatry* 1989; 30:671–689.

63. Grant A: The relationship between obstetrically preventable intrapartum asphyxia, abnormal neonatal neurologic signs and subsequent motor impairment in babies born at or after term, in Kubli F (ed): *Perinatal Events and Brain Damage in Surviving Children.* Berlin, Springer-Verlag 1988, pp 149–159.

64. Greenwood RD, Rosenthal A, Parisi L, Flyer DC, Nadas AS: Extracardiac abnormalities in infants with congenital heart disease. *Pediatrics* 1975; 55:485–492.

65. Grunberger W, Leodolter S, Parshalk O: Maternal hypotension: Fetal outcome in treated and untreated cases. *Gynecol Obstet Invest* 1979; 10:32–38.

66. Hagberg B, Hagberg G. Prenatal and perinatal risk factors in a survey of 681 Swedish cases, in: Stanley F, Alberman A (eds): *Epidemiology of the Cerebral Palsies. Clinics in Developmental Medicine* No. 87. London, Heinemann Medical Books Ltd, 1984, pp 116–133.

67. Hagberg B, Hagberg G, Lewerth A, Lindberg U: Mild mental retardation in Swedish school children. II. Etiologic and pathogenetic aspects. *Acta Pediatr Scand* 1981; 70:445–452.

68. Hagberg B, Hagberg G, Olow I: The changing panorama of cerebral palsy in Sweden. *Acta Paediatr Scand* 1984; 73:433–440.

69. Hagberg B, Hagberg G, Zetterstrom R: Decreasing perinatal mortality, increase in cerebral palsy morbidity? *Acta Paediatr Scand* 1989; 78:664–670.

70. Hastings RP (ed): *SUGI Supplemental Library User's Guide,* ed 5. Cary, NC, SAS Institute, 1986.

71. Hensleigh PA, Fainstat T, Spencer R: Perinatal events and cerebral palsy. *Am J Obstet Gynecol* 1986; 154:978–981.

72. Hume RF Jr, O'Donnell KJ, Stanger CL, Killam AP, Gingras JL: In utero cocaine exposure: Observations of fetal behavioral state may predict neonatal outcome. *Am J Obstet Gynecol* 1989; 161:685–690.

73. Jarvis SN, Holloway JS, Hey EN: Increase in cerebral palsy in normal birthweight babies. *Arch Dis Child* 1985; 60:1113–1121.

74. Kim SU: Brain hypoxia studied in mouse central nervous system cultures. I. Sequential cellular changes. *Lab Invest* 1975; 33:658–669.

75. Lamont MA, Dennis NR: Aetiology of mild mental retardation. *Arch Dis Child* 1988; 63:1032–1038.

76. Lehtovirta P, Forss M: The acute effect of smoking on intervillous blood flow of the placenta. *Br J Obstet Gynaecol* 1978; 85:729–731.

77. Levene MI, Fenton AC, Evans DH, Archer LNJ, Shortland DB, Gibson NA: Severe birth asphyxia and abnormal cerebral blood flow velocity. *Dev Med Child Neurol* 1989; 31:427–434.

78. Levene MI, Gibson NA, Fenton AC, Papathoma E, Barnett D: The use of a calcium-

channel blocker, nicardipine, for severe asphyxiated newborn infants. *Dev Med Child Neurol* 1990; 32:567–574.

79. Leviton C, VanMarter L, Kuban KCK: Respiratory distress syndrome and intracranial hemorrhage: Cause or association? Inference from surfactant clinical trials. *Pediatrics* 1989; 84:915–922.

80. Lilienfeld AM, Parkhurst E: A study of the association of factors of pregnancy and parturition with the development of cerebral palsy: A preliminary report. *Am J Hyg* 1951; 53:262–282.

81. Little WJ: On the influence of abnormal parturition, difficult labour, premature birth, and asphyxia neonatorum on the mental and physical condition of the child, especially in relation to deformities. *Lancet* 1861; 2:378–379.

82. Lou HC, Henriksen L, Bruhn P: Focal cerebral hypoperfusion in children with dysphasia and/or attention deficit disorder. *Arch Neurol* 1984; 41:825–829.

83. Lou HC, Henriksen L, Bruhn P: Focal cerebral dysfunction in developmental learning disabilities. *Lancet* 1990; 335:8–11.

84. Lou HC, Henriksen L, Bruhn P, Borner H, Nielson JB: Striatal dysfunction in attention deficit and hyperkinetic disorder. *Arch Neurol* 1989; 46:48–52.

85. Lou HC, Lassen NA, Friis-Hansen B: Impaired autoregulation of cerebral blood flow in the distressed newborn infants. *J Pediatr* 1979; 94:118–121.

86. Lou HC, Skov H, Henriksen L: Intellectual impairment with regional cerebral dysfunction after low neonatal cerebral blood flow. *Acta Paediatr Scand [Suppl]* 1989; 360:72–82.

87. Low JA, Froese AF, Galbraith RS, Sauerbrei EE, McKinven JP, Karchmar EJ: The association of fetal and newborn metabolic acidosis with severe periventricular leukomalacia in the preterm newborn. *Am J Obstet Gynecol* 1990; 162:977–982.

88. Lucas A, Morley R, Cole TJ, Gore SM, Lucas PJ, Crowle P, Pearse R, Boon AJ, Powell R: Early diet in preterm babies and developmental status at 18 months. *Lancet* 1990; 335: 1477–1481.

89. Lumley J: Does continuous intrapartum fetal monitoring predict long-term neurological disorders? *Paediatr Perinat Epidemiol* 1988; 2:299–307.

90. Lupton BA, Hill A, Roland EH, Whitefield MF, Flodmark O: Brain swelling in the asphyxiated term newborn: Pathogenesis and outcome. *Pediatrics* 1988; 82:139–146.

91. MacDonald D, Grant A, Sheridan-Pereira M, Boylan P, Chalmers I: The Dublin randomized controlled trial of intrapartum fetal heart rate monitoring. *Am J Obstet Gynecol* 1985; 152:524–539.

92. Macgregor S, Keith L, Chasnoff I, et al: Cocaine use during pregnancy; adverse perinatal outcome. *Am J Obstet Gynecol* 1987; 157:686–690.

93. Malamud N: Status marmoratus: A form of cerebral palsy following either birth injury or inflammation of the central nervous system. *J Pediatr* 1950; 37:610–619.

94. Mannino FL, Trauner DA: Strokes in neonates. *J Pediatr* 1983; 102:605–610.

95. McClearn GE, Plomin R, Nesselroade RJ, Pedersen N, Friberg I, DeFaire U: The Swedish adoptive twin study on aging: Individual differences in personality, in press.

96. Mesulam MM: Frontal cortex and behavior. *Ann Neurol* 1986; 19:320–325.

97. Moncada S, Vane JIR: Unstable metabolites of arachidonic acid and their role in haemostasis and thrombosis. *Br Med Bull* 1978; 34:129–135.

98. Morris N, Osborn SB, Wright HP: Effective circulation of the uterine wall in late pregnancy. *Lancet* 1955; 1:323–325.

99. Myers RE: Über die Lokalisation Frühkindlicher Hirnschäden in arteriellen Grenzgebieten. *Arch Psychiatr Nervenckr* 1953; 190:328–341.

100. Myers RE: Two patterns of perinatal brain damage and their conditions of occurrence. *Am J Obstet Gynecol* 1972; 112:246–276.

101. Myers RE: Experimental models of perinatal brain damage: Relevance to human pathology, in Gluck L (ed): *Intrauterine Asphyxia and the Developing Fetal Brain.* Chicago, Year Book Medical Publishers, Inc, 1977, pp 37–97.

102. Myers RE, Adamsons K: Obstetric considerations of perinatal brain injury. *Rev Perinat Med* 1981; 4:222–245.

103. Myers RE, Wagner KR, DeCourten GM: Lactic acid accumulation in tissue as cause of brain injury and death in cardiogenic shock from asphyxia, in Lauerser NH, Hockberg HM (eds): *Perinatal Biochemical Monitoring.* Baltimore, Williams & Wilkins Co, 1981, p 11.

104. Naeye RL: Causes of perinatal mortality excess in prolonged gestations. *Am J Epidemiol* 1978; 108:429–433.

105. Naeye RL: Umbilical cord length: Clinical significance. *J Pediatr* 1985; 107:278–282.

106. Naeye RL: When and how does antenatal brain damage occur?, in Iffy L (ed): *Second Perinatal Practice and Malpractice Symposium.* New York, Healthmark Communications, 1986, p 125.

107. Naeye RL: How and when does antenatal hypoxia damage fetal brains?, in Kubli F, Patel N, Schmidt W, Linderkamp O (eds): *Perinatal Events and Brain Damage in Surviving Children.* New York, Springer-Verlag, 1988, pp 70–80.

108. Naeye RL: The clinical significance of absent subchorionic fibrin in the placenta. *Am J Clin Pathol* 1990; 94:196–198.

109. Naeye RL: Maternal body weight and pregnancy outcome. *Am J Clin Nutr* 1990; 52:273–279.

110. Naeye RL, Maisels MJ, Lorenz RP, Botti JJ: The clinical significance of placental villous edema. *Pediatrics* 1983; 71:588–594.

111. Naeye RL, Olsson JM, Combs JW: New brain stem and bone marrow abnormalities in victims of the sudden infant death syndrome. *J Perinat* 1989; 9:180–183.

112. Naeye RL, Peters EC: Mental development of children whose mothers smoked during pregnancy. *Obstet Gynecol* 1984; 64:601–607.

113. Naeye RL, Peters EC: Antepartum events and cerebral handicap, in Kubli F, Patel N, Schmidt W, Linderkamp O (eds): *Perinatal Events and Brain Damage in Surviving Children.* New York, Springer-Verlag, 1988, pp 83–91.

114. Naeye RL, Peters EC, Bartholomew M, Landis JR: Origins of cerebral palsy. *Am J Dis Child* 1989; 143:1154–1161.

115. Naeye RL, Tafari N: *Risk Factors in Pregnancy and Diseases of the Fetus and Newborn.* Baltimore, Williams & Wilkins Co, 1983.

116. Nelson KB, Ellenberg JH: Children who "outgrew" cerebral palsy. *Pediatrics* 1982; 69:529–536.

117. Nelson KB, Ellenberg JH: Obstetric complications as risk factors for cerebral palsy or seizure disorders. *JAMA* 1984; 251:1843–1848.

118. Nelson KB, Ellenberg JH: Antecedents of cerebral palsy. I. Univariate analysis of risks. *Am J Dis Child* 1985; 139:1031–1038.

119. Nelson KB, Ellenberg JH: Antecedents of cerebral palsy, *N Engl J Med* 1986; 315:81–86.

120. New England Congenital Hypothyroidism Collaborative: Elementary school performance of children with congenital hypothyroidism. *J Pediatr* 1990; 116:27–32.

121. Newton ER: The relationship between intrapartum obstetric care and chronic neurodevelopmental handicaps in children. *Reprod Toxicol* 1990; 4:85–94.

122. Nichols PL: Familial mental retardation. *Behav Genet* 1984; 14:161–170.

123. Nichols PL, Chen T: *Minimal Brain Dysfunction: A Prospective Study.* Hillsdale, NJ, Lawrence Erlbaum. 1981.

124. Niswander KR: Asphyxia in the fetus and cerebral palsy, in Mishell DR, Kirschbaum TH, Morrow CP (eds): *Year Book of Obstetrics and Gynecology.* Chicago, Year Book Medical Publishers, Inc, 1983, pp 107–125.

125. Niswander KR, Gordon M: *The Women and Their Pregnancies.* Philadelphia, WB Saunders Co, 1972.

126. Niswander KR, Gordon M, Drage JS: The effect of intrauterine hypoxia on the child surviving to 4 years. *Am J Ob Gyn* 1975; 121:892–899.

127. Niswander K, Henson G, Elbourne D, Chalmers I, Redman C, MacFarlane A, Tizard P: Adverse outcome of pregnancy and the quality of obstetric care. *Lancet* 1984; 2:827–831.

128. Okada R, Johnson D, Lev M: Extracardial malformations associated with congenital heart disease. *Arch Pathol* 1968; 85:649–657.

129. Oro AS, Dixon SD: Perinatal cocaine and methamphetamine exposure: Maternal and neonatal correlates. *J Pediatr* 1987; 111:571–578.

130. Paneth N, Kiely J: The frequency of cerebral palsy: A review of population studies in industrial nations since 1950, in Stanley F, Alberman E (eds): *The Epidemiology of the Cerebral Palsies.* Philadelphia, JB Lippincott Co, 1984, pp 46–56.

131. Paneth N, Stark RI: Cerebral palsy and mental retardation in relation to indicators of perinatal asphyxia. *Am J Obstet Gynecol* 1983; 147:960–966.

132. Parks YA, Wharton BA: Iron deficiency and the brain. *Acta Paediatr Scand [Suppl]* 1989; 361:71–77.

133. Penrose LS: *The Biology of Mental Defects*, ed 3. London, Sedgwick & Jackson, 1983.

134. Perkins RP: Perspectives on perinatal brain damage. *Obstet Gynecol* 1987; 69:807–819.

135. Perlman JM, Tack ED: Renal injury in the asphyxiated newborn infant: Relationship to neurologic outcome. *J Pediatr* 1988; 113:875–879.

136. Perlman JM, Tack ED, Martin T, Shackleford G, Amon E: Acute systemic organ injury in term infants after asphyxia. *Am J Dis Child* 1989; 143:617–620.

137. Perrin EC, Gerrity PS: Development of children with a chronic illness. *Pediatr Clin North Am* 1984; 31:19–31.

138. Pharoah POD, Cooke T, Rosenbloom I, Cooke RWI: Trends in birth prevalence of cerebral palsy. *Arch Dis Child* 1987; 62:379–384.

139. Pless IB: Clinical assessment: Physical and psychological functioning. *Pediatr Clin North Am* 1984; 31:33–45.

140. Plomin R: Genetic risk and psychosocial disorders: Links between the normal and abnormal, in Rutter M, Casaer P (eds): *Biological Risk Factors for Psychosocial Disorders*. New York, Cambridge University Press, 1991, pp 101–138.

141. Plomin R, Chipuer HM, Loehlin JC: Behavior genetics and personality, in Pervin LA (ed): *Handbook of Personality, Theory and Research*. New York, Guilford Press, 1990, pp 225–243.

142. Plomin R, DeFries JC, McClearn GE: *Behavioral Genetics: A Primer*, ed 2. New York, WH Freeman Co, 1990.

143. Porter R, O'Connor J, Whelan J (eds): *Mechanisms of Alcohol Damage in Utero. Ciba Foundation Symposium 105*. London, Pitman, 1984.

144. Ramaekers VT, Casaer P: Defective regulation of cerebral oxygen transport after severe brain asphyxia. *Dev Med Child Neurol* 1990; 32:56–62.

145. Raynaud C, Billard C, Tzonrig N, et al: Study of CBF developmental dysphasic children at rest and during verbal stimulation. *Cereb Blood Flow Metab* 1989; 9(suppl 1):S323.

146. Rizzolatti G, Matelli M, Pavesi G: Deficits in attention and movement following the removal of postarcuate (area 6) and prearcuate (area 8) cortex in macaque monkeys. *Brain* 1983; 106:655–653.

147. Robertson C, Finer N: Term infants with hypoxic-ischemic encephalopathy: Outcome at 3.5 years. *Dev Med Child Neurol* 1985; 27:473–484.

148. Rodriguez J, Claus D, Verellen G, Lyon G: Periventricular leucomalacia: Ultrasonic and neuropathological correlations. *Dev Med Child Neurol* 1990; 32:347–355.

149. Roger J, Dravet C, Bureau M: Unilateral seizures, hemiconvulsions-hemiplegia syndrome (HH) and hemiconvulsions-hemiplegia-epilepsy syndrome (HHE), in Broughton R (ed): *Henri Gastaut and the Marseille school's contribution to the neurosciences, electroencephalography and clinical neurosciences. Electroencephalogr Clin Neurophysiol* 1982: (suppl 35):211–221.

150. Roland EH, Flodmark O, Hill A: Thalamic hemorrhage with intraventricular hemorrhage in the full term newborn. *Pediatrics* 1990; 85:737–742.

151. Roland EH, Volpe JJ: Effect of maternal cocaine use on the fetus and newborn: Review of the literature. *Pediatr Neurosci* 1989; 15:88–94.

152. Ruth VJ, Raivio KO: Perinatal brain damage: Predictive value of metabolic acidosis and the Apgar score. *Br Med J* 1988; 297:24–27.

153. Rutter M, Macdonald H, LeCouteur A, Harrington R, Bolton P, Bailey A: Genetic factors in child psychiatric disorders. II. Empirical findings. *J Child Psychol Psychiatry* 1990; 31:39–83.

154. Rutter M, Tizard J, Whitmore K (eds): *Education, Health and Behaviour*. London, Longman, 1970.

155. Salafia CM, Mangam HE, Weigl CA, Foye GJ, Silberman L: Abnormal fetal heart rate patterns and placental inflammation. *Am J Obstet Gynecol* 1989; 160:140–147.

156. Sarnat HB, Sarnat MS: Neonatal encephalopathy following fetal distress, a clinical and electroencephalographic study. *Arch Neurol* 1976; 33:696–705.

157. Scher MS, Dobson V, Carpenter NA, Guthrie RD: Visual and neurologic outcome of infants with periventricular leukomalacia. *Dev Med Child Neurol* 1989; 31:353–365.

158. Schneider NG, Houston JP: Smoking and anxiety; *Psychol Rep* 1970; 26:941–942.

159. Sexson WR, Sexson SB, Rawson JE, Brann AW: The multisystem involvement of the asphyxiated newborn. *Pediatr Res* 1976; 10:432.

160. Shy KK, Luthy DA, Bennett FC, et al: Effects of electron fetal-heart-rate monitoring, as compared with periodic auscultation, on the neurologic development of premature infants. *N Engl J Med* 1990; 322:588–593.

161. Siesjo BK: Cell damage in the brain: A speculative synthesis. *J Cereb Blood Flow Metab* 1981; 1:155–167.

162. Skidmore MD, Rivers A, Hack M: Increased risk of cerebral palsy among very low birth-weight infants with chronic lung disease. *Dev Med Child Neurol* 1990; 32:325–332.

163. Spiro A, Stark L, Tyc V: Common coping strategies employed by children with chronic illness. *Newslet Soc Pediatr Psychol* 1989; 13:3–7.

164. Stanley FJ: Perinatal risk factors in the study of the cerebral palsies. *Clin Dev Med* 1984; 87:98–104.

165. Stanley FJ: The changing face of cerebral palsy? *Dev Med Child Neurol* 1987; 29:263–265.

166. Stevenson J, Graham P: Behavioral deviance in 13-year-old twins: an item analysis. *J Am Acad Child Adolesc Psychiatry* 1988; 27:791–797.

167. Sullivan JL: Iron, plasma antioxidants and oxygen radical disease of prematurity. *Am J Dis Child* 1988; 142:1341–1344.

168. Svenningsen L, Eidal K: Lack of correlation between umbilical arterial pH, retinal hemorrhages and Apgar score in the newborn. *Acta Obstet Gynecol Scand* 1987; 66:639–642.

169. Sykes GS, Molloy PM, Johnson P, Gu W, Ashworth F, Stirrat GM, Turnbull AC: Do Apgar scores indicate asphyxia? *Lancet* 1982; 1:494–496.

170. Tack E, Perlman JM, Hause C, Griffen M, Martin T: Systemic manifestations of perinatal asphyxia in the newborn. *Pediatr Res* 1986; 20:362A.

171. Takashima S, Mito T, Houdou S, Ando Y: Relationship between periventricular hemorrhage, leukomalacia and brainstem lesions in prematurely born infants. *Brain Dev* 1989; 11:121–124.

172. Thomas A, Chess S: The dynamics of psychological development. New York, Brunner/Mazel, 1980.

173. Ting P, Yamaguchi S, Bacher JD, Killens RH, Myers RE: Hypoxic-ischemic cerebral necrosis in midgestational sheep fetuses: Physiopathologic correlations. *Exp Neurol* 1983; 80:227–245.

174. Van de Bor M, Guit GL, Schreuder AM, Wondergem J, Vielvoye GJ: Early detection of delayed myelination in preterm infants. *Pediatrics* 1989; 84:407–411.

175. Via WF Jr, Churchill JA: Relationships of cerebral disorders to faults in dental enamel. *Am J Dis Child* 1957; 94:137–142.

176. Volpe JJ: *Neurology of the Newborn*, ed 2. Philadelphia, WB Saunders Co, 1987.

177. Volpe JJ: Intraventricular hemorrhage and brain injury in the premature infant: Neuropathology, pathogenesis, diagnosis, prognosis and prevention. *Clin Perinatol* 1989; 16:361–412.

178. Volpe JJ, Herscovitch P, Perlman JM, Kreusser KL, Raichle ME: Positron emission tomography in the asphyxiated term newborn: Parasagittal impairment of cerebral blood flow. *Ann Neurol* 1985; 17:287–296.

179. Voorhies TM, Lipper EG, Lee BCP, Vannucci RC, Auld PAM: Occlusive vascular disease in asphyxiated newborn infants. *J Pediatr* 1984; 105:92–96.

180. Walter T, DeAndraca I, Chadud P, Perales CG: Iron deficiency anemia: Adverse effects on infant psychomotor development. *Pediatrics* 1989; 84:7–17.

181. Watanabe K, Kuroyanagi M, Hara K: Neonatal seizures and subsequent epilepsy. *Brain Dev* 1982; 4:341–346.

182. Wechsler Intelligence Scales for Children. New York, Psychological Testing Corp, 1949.

183. Weiss G, Hechtman L, Milroy T, Perlman T: Psychiatric status of hyperactives as adults: A controlled prospective 15-year follow-up of 63 hyperactive children. *J Am Acad Child Adolesc Psychiatry* 1985; 24:211–220.

184. Wender EH: Attention deficit disorders, in Hoekelman RA (ed): *Primary Pediatric Care*. St Louis, CV Mosby Co, 1987, p 672.

185. Willoughby A, Graubard BI, Hocker A, Storr C, Vietze P, Thakaberry JM, Gerry MA, McCarthy M, Gist NF, Mangenheim M, Berendes H, Rhoads GG: Population-based study of the developmental outcome of children exposed to chloride-deficient infant formula. *Pediatrics* 1990; 85:485–490.

186. Wise SP: The primate premotor cortex: Past, present, and preparatory. *Annu Rev Neurosci* 1985; 8:1–19.

187. Woods J, Plessinger M, Clark K: Effects of cocaine on uterine blood flow and fetal oxygenation. *JAMA* 1987; 257:957–961.

188. Yerushalmy J: The relationship of parents' cigarette smoking to outcome of pregnancy: Implications as to the problem of inferring causation from observed associations. *Am J Epidemiol* 1971; 93:443–456.

189. Zametkin AJ, Nordahl TE, Gross M, King AC, Semple WE, Rumsey J, Hamburger S, Cohen RM: Cerebral glucose metabolism in adults with hyperactivity of childhood onset. *N Engl J Med* 1990; 323:1361–1366.

190. Zigler E: Familial mental retardation: A continuing dilemma. *Science* 1967; 155:292–298.

CHAPTER 12

Differing Effects of Male and Female Fetuses on Pregnancy Outcome

---

MATERNAL BLOOD PRESSURE

BLOOD VOLUME EXPANSION

NEONATAL RESPIRATORY DISTRESS
   SYNDROME

CONCLUSIONS

There are several published reports that male fetuses outnumber females in preeclamptic and eclamptic pregnancies.[1,2,11,13] We used data from the Collaborative Perinatal Study (CPS) to try to discover the responsible mechanisms. One possible mechanism might be that male fetuses produce something that predisposes to preeclampsia. Another possibility is that more female than male fetuses die in preeclamptic gestations, leaving males to survive and be identified with preeclampsia and eclampsia. If confirmed, this second possibility would be somewhat of a surprise because females are better able to survive almost all types of stress than males.[7]

MATERNAL BLOOD PRESSURE

Analyses were first undertaken to determine if male fetuses outnumbered females in preeclamptic and eclamptic gestations in the CPS. The results revealed some surprising relationships between the sex of the fetus and maternal gestational blood pressures (Fig 12–1). Male fetuses were strongly associated with preeclampsia (maternal hypertension and proteinuria), but only when gravidas had net pregnancy weight gains greater than 12 kg. Net pregnancy weight gain is the total weight gain of the gravida at the end of pregnancy minus the weight of the fetus and placenta. When net pregnancy weight gains were less than 12 kg, there was a heavy preponderance of female fetuses, particularly when hypertension was severe. These findings raise the possibility that gravidas with proteinuria had a larger extracellular fluid volume increase with male than with female fetuses. This possibility arises because net pregnancy weight gain is in large part a measure of the increase in maternal blood and extravascular fluid volume during pregnancy.

The findings were somewhat different when gravidas did not have proteinuria. Female fetuses predominated in normotensive gestations when net pregnancy weight gains were low (see Fig 12–1). This female predominance progressively disappeared as net pregnancy weight gain increased. The findings reversed when

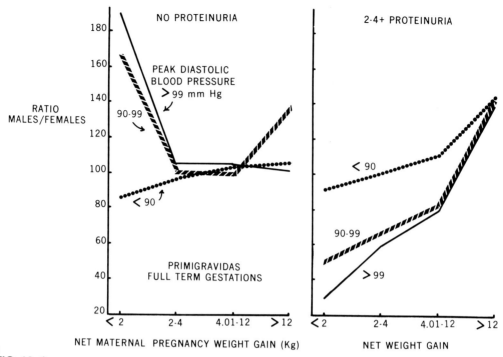

FIG 12-1.
Relationship of blood pressure, proteinuria, and maternal weight gain to the sex ratio of newborns of primigravidas. The sex ratio is the number of males per 100 females.

gravidas were hypertensive. There was a heavy predominance of males with net pregnancy weight gains of less than 2 kg which disappeared with weight gains of 2 to 12 kg. These findings again suggest that the sex of the fetus may have some influence on the size of maternal extracellular fluid volume increase during pregnancy.

All of the aforementioned findings in the pregnancies of primigravidas were present but attenuated in the pregnancies of multigravidas (Fig 12-2).

BLOOD VOLUME EXPANSION

Analyses were next undertaken to try to determine if the sex of the fetus affected maternal blood volume expansion during pregnancy. Maternal hemoglobin values, measured during pregnancy, were analyzed because a persistently high hemoglobin value is a characteristic indication that a mother's blood volume remained low instead of expanding during pregnancy. An increase in plasma volume

usually contributes more to this blood volume expansion than an increase of erythrocytes. The result is an inverse correlation between the blood volume expansion and maternal hemoglobin values; when blood volumes are low, hemoglobin values remain high.[4] Hypertensive women had lower third-trimester hemoglobin values with male than with female fetuses which supports the view that gravidas with female fetuses had lower blood volumes during late gestation than gravidas with male fetuses (Table 12-1).

In a second approach to the same issue, placentas were analyzed for microscopic findings that are characteristic of abnormally low uteroplacental blood flow.[8] A failure of the maternal blood volume to increase progressively during pregnancy is one of the most frequent causes of low uteroplacental blood flow.[3] Trophoblastic syncytial knots in the placenta increase in number as pregnancy advances. An excessive number of such knots is an indication that blood flow from the uterus to the placenta was subnormal for at least sev-

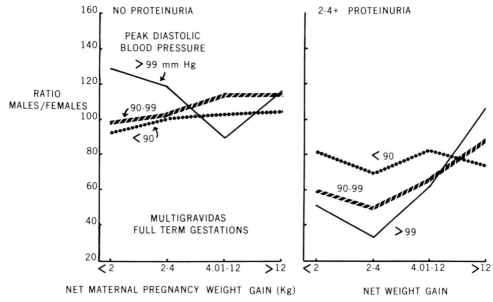

FIG 12–2.
Relationships of blood pressure, proteinuria, and maternal weight gain to the sex ratio of newborns of multigravidas.

eral weeks before delivery.[6,9] In the CPS an excessive number of syncytial knots were more often present in the placentas of girls than of boys (Table 12–2). This difference between the sexes was greater in first than in subsequent pregnancies.

Taken together, all of these findings suggest that maternal blood volume expansion and uteroplacental blood flow are greater with male than with female fetuses. There is still more evidence to support this thesis. A large blood volume expansion enhances blood flow from the uterus to the placenta, which could be the reason why boys born to hypertensive gravidas in the study were less often

stillborn than girls (Table 12–3). Early gestational weight gains were significantly higher in preeclamptic gestations with male than with female fetuses, which may indicate that the greater maternal blood volume expansion with male than with female fetuses started in very early gestation (Table 12–4).

NEONATAL RESPIRATORY DISTRESS SYNDROME

It has long been known that the neonatal respiratory distress syndrome (RDS) is more frequent in males than in females at

TABLE 12–1.

Comparison of Fetal Sex and Maternal Hemoglobin Values by Peak Levels of Maternal Gestational Blood Pressure in Primigravidas

Peak Maternal Diastolic Blood Pressure During Pregnancy (mm Hg)	Lowest Maternal Third-Trimester Hemoglobin Values (g/dL)*	
	Male Fetuses†	Female Fetuses†
<90	10.3 ± 1.0 (2,334)	10.3 ± 1.0 (2,341), $P > 0.1$
90–99	10.2 ± 1.0 (502)	10.4 ± 0.9 (448), $P < 0.01$
>99	9.0 ± 0.9 (77)‡	10.7 ± 1.0 (158), $P < 0.01$‡

*Mean values ± 1 SD.
†Number of cases are in parentheses.
‡$P < .001$ compared with value in <90–mm Hg diastolic pressure category.

TABLE 12–2.

Comparison of Fetal Sex, Maternal Parity, and Presence of Excessive Syncytial Knots in the Placenta

	Percentage of Placentas With Excessive Syncytial Knots*			
	Primigravidas		Multigravidas	
Gestational Age (wk)	Males	Females	Males	Females
26–34	1.4 (6)	4.3 (16), $P < 0.03$	1.2 (9)	2.3 (19), $P > 0.1$
>34	5.4 (158)	8.9 (242), $P < 0.001$	3.4 (171)†	4.5 (228), $P < 0.01$†

*Numbers in parentheses are placentas with excessive syncytial knots.
†$P < 0.001$ compared with same sex and gestational age in primigravida category.

TABLE 12–3.

Sex Ratio (No. of Males per 100 Females) in Perinatal Deaths, in Neonates with the Respiratory Distress Syndrome, and in Survivors

Pregnancy Outcomes	Normotensive Gravida*	Hypertensive Gravida*
Stillbirths	111:100 (185)	73:100 (21), $P < .05$
Neonatal deaths	126:100 (194)	171:1001 (29), $P < .01$
Survivors	102:100 (18,001)	107:100 (3,405), $P < .001$

*Numbers of males are in parentheses.

TABLE 12–4.

Comparison of Fetal Sex, Maternal Early Gestational Blood Pressure, and Pregnancy Weight Gain

Peak Maternal Diastolic Blood Pressure and Proteinuria During Pregnancy	No. of Cases	Diastolic Blood Pressure at 15–17 Weeks' Gestation (mm Hg)	Maternal Weight Gain at 15–17 Weeks' Gestation
Proteinuria absent			
Peak pressure <90 mm Hg			
Male fetuses	946	68 ± 10	2.5 ± 2.7
Female fetuses	991	67 ± 9	2.1 ± 3.0
		$P < .05$	$P < .02$
Proteinuria $2+ – 4+$			
Peak pressure <90 mm Hg			
Male fetuses	73	65 ± 9	2.2 ± 2.6
Female fetuses	77	68 ± 8	1.5 ± 2.3
		$P < .05$	$P < .05$
Peak pressure 90–99 mm Hg			
Male fetuses	22	72 ± 8†	4.3 ± 2.6†
Female fetuses	33	74 ± 8†	0.6 ± 2.4†
		$P > 0.1$	$P < .001$
Peak pressure >99 mm Hg			
Male fetuses	15	74 ± 5†	3.8 ± 4.3†
Female fetuses	13	76 ± 7†	0.6 ± 1.4†
		$P > 0.1$	$P < .005$

*Mean values $\pm$ 1 SD.
†$P < .05$ compared with value in category <90 mm Hg, same sex.

every gestational age. In the CPS this male dominance was limited to the offspring of primigravidas (Fig 12–3). This finding in turn was responsible for a much greater difference in neonatal mortality between the male and female neonates of primigravidas than of multigravidas (Fig 12–4). In preeclamptic gestations full-term females had higher neonatal hemoglobin values than males, whereas this difference was absent in the neonates born of normotensive gestations (Table 12–5). High hemoglobin values in neonates are most often the consequence of disorders that produce chronic fetal hypoxemia.[9]

CONCLUSIONS

All of these findings provide a matrix of evidence that male fetuses affect the intrauterine environment somewhat differently than do female fetuses in preeclamptic gestations (Fig 12–5). These environmental differences produced higher fetal

but lower neonatal mortality rates for preterm born girls than for boys (see Table 12–3). There is indirect evidence that these effects started with early gestational differences in maternal blood volume expansion. Primigravidas had larger pregnancy weight gains and lower late gestational hemoglobin values with male than with female fetuses. The lower hemoglobin values with males likely reflected a larger maternal plasma volume expansion with resulting greater hemodilution in pregnancies with male than with female fetuses. A large blood volume expansion enhances uteroplacental blood flow, which could explain why preterm born boys of primigravidas were less often stillborn than preterm born girls.[5] A subnormal uteroplacental blood flow is known to accelerate fetal lung maturation,[9] which is a plausible explanation for the less frequent neonatal RDS in girls than in boys born to primigravidas. A larger-than-normal blood volume expansion with male than with female fetuses

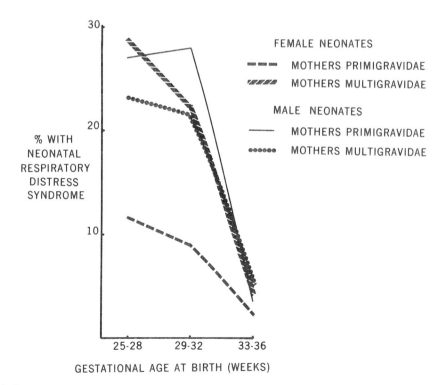

FIG 12–3.
Relationships of maternal parity and the newborn's sex to the frequency of the neonatal respiratory distress syndrome.

could also be part of the reason why hypertension was more frequent in gravidas with male than with female fetuses.

In the present study fetal sex-associated differences in maternal gestational blood pressures and weight gain were present by 15 to 17 weeks of gestation, a time when high levels of gonadotropins and testosterone are circulating in male but not in female fetuses.[10,12] Testosterone can initiate sodium retention, but it is not known if this or some other mechanism might be responsible for the proposed differences in maternal blood volume expansion between male and female fetuses. Whatever the mechanism, findings in the present study provide a plausible unifying explanation for a number of pregnancy, fetal, and neonatal phenomena that up until now have been attributed to genetic dif-

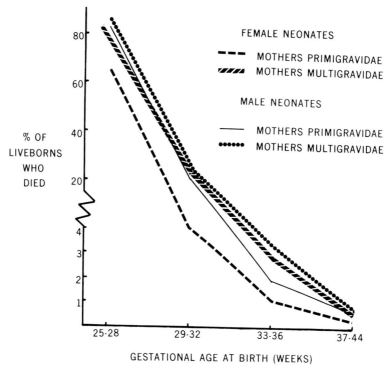

FIG 12–4.
Relationships of maternal parity and newborn's sex to neonatal mortality.

TABLE 12–5.

Comparison of Child's Sex With Neonatal Hemoglobin Values by Levels of Maternal Gestational Blood Pressure and Gestational Proteinuria*

Peak Maternal Diastolic Blood Pressure During Pregnancy (mm Hg)	Mean Hemoglobin Values in Newborn Infants at 48 Hours of Age (g/dL)†	
	Males‡	Females‡
<90 and no proteinuria	18.4 ± 2.5 (2,501)	18.5 ± 2.6 (2,492)
≥90		
No proteinuria	17.9 ± 2.6 (859)§	18.1 ± 2.5 (721), $P < .06$§
Peak proteinuria 1+	18.3 ± 2.5 (376)	18.8 ± 2.7 (361), $P < .05$
Peak proteinuria 2+ – 4+	18.5 ± 2.8 (64)	19.4 ± 2.7 (79), $P < .02$

*Data are from full-term infants whose mothers did not smoke during pregnancy.
†Mean values are ± 1 SD.
‡Numbers of cases are in parentheses.
§ $< .05$ compared with values in <90 and no proteinuria category.

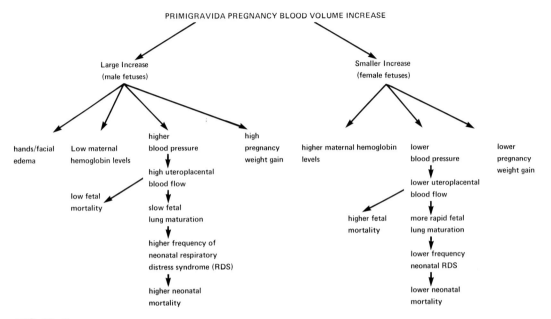

FIG 12–5.
Flow chart showing differing effects of male and female fetuses on the mother and on pregnancy outcome.

ferences between males and females. Included on this list are sex-related differences in the frequencies and outcomes of preeclampsia, stillbirth, neonatal RDS, and neonatal death.

REFERENCES

1. Butner O: Statistik und Klinik der Eklampsie im Grossherzogtum Mecklenburg-Schwerin. *Arch Gynaekol* 1903; 70:322–410.

2. Campbell DM, MacGillivray I, Carr-Hill R, Samphier M: Fetal sex and pre-eclampsia in primigravidae. *Br J Obstet Gynaecol* 1983; 90:26–27.

3. Gallery EDM, Hunyor SN, Gyory AZ: Plasma volume contraction, a significant factor in both pregnancy-associated hypertension (preeclampsia) and in chronic hypertension in pregnancy. *Q J Med* 1979; 48:593–602.

4. Goodlin RC, Dobry CA, Anderson JC, Woods RE, Quaife M: Clinical signs of normal plasma volume expansion during pregnancy. *Am J Obstet Gynecol* 1983; 145:1001–1009.

5. Grunberger W, Leodolter S, Parschalk O: Maternal hypotention: Fetal outcome in treated and untreated cases. *Gynecol Obstet Invest* 1979; 10:32–38.

6. Merrill JA: Common pathological changes of the placenta. *Clin Obstet Gynecol* 1963; 6:96–109.

7. Naeye RL, Burt LS, Wright DL, Blanc WA, Tatter D: Neonatal mortality, the male disadvantage. *Pediatrics* 1971; 48:902–906.

8. Naeye RL, Demers LM: Differing effects of fetal sex on pregnancy and its outcome. *Am J Med Genet* 1987; 3(suppl):67–74.

9. Naeye RL, Tafari N: *Risk Factors in Pregnancy and Diseases of the Fetus and Newborn.* Baltimore, Williams & Wilkins Co, 1983.

10. Reyes FI, Boroditsky RS, Winter JSD, Faiman C: Studies on human sexual development. II. Fetal and maternal serum gonadotropin and sex steroid concentration. *J Clin Endocrinol Metab* 1974; 368:612–617.

11. Saltzmann KD: Do transplacental hormones cause eclampsia? *Lancet* 1955; 2:953–956.

12. Siteri PK, Wilson JD: Testosterone formation and metabolism during male sexual differentiation in the human embryo. *J Clin Endocrinol Metab* 1974; 38:113–125.

13. Toivanen P, Hirvonen T: Sex ratio of newborns: Preponderance of males in toxemia of pregnancy. *Science* 1970; 170:187–188.

CHAPTER 13

Being an Expert Witness: Claims of Birth Injury

The first part of this chapter deals with the nature, origin, and prevention of malpractice claims. The second segment outlines how to identify the cause of death or malfunction that is the focus of the malpractice claim. The final segment of the chapter focuses on the personal experiences of participants in malpractice cases. A discussion of other facets of malpractice claims, such as how the legal system works, standard of care issues, duty and breach of duty questions, and fetal and maternal rights can be found in oth-er publications. An excellent source for this latter information may be found in Eden et al.[1]

NATURE AND ORIGIN OF MALPRACTICE CLAIMS

In the United States perinatal injury usually tops the list for large monetary awards in the settlement of malpractice claims. Most of these claims fall into one of two categories: (1) birth injury to a child's brain, or (2) the wrongful death of a fetus or neonate. After reading the records associated with several hundred of these claims, it seems to me that their origin falls into several categories. The most frequent is the inability of a family to cope with a child's impairments. Many malpractice actions are initiated to obtain funds to purchase services for an impaired child and to buy for parents some time away from the responsibilities imposed by living with a severely handicapped child. Another frequent reason for malpractice claims is poor communication between health system personnel and the parents of impaired or dead children. Some of these parents have had conflicts with medical personnel, but more often they are not satisfied with the information they have received about the cause of a child's impairments or death. A death that is sudden and unexpected is particularly likely to generate malpractice claims. Finally, there are instances in which families have logical reasons to think that health system personnel mismanaged obstetric or medical care.

THE PREVENTION OF MALPRACTICE CLAIMS

What can be done to prevent malpractice claims? Suggestions commonly fall into the following categories: (a) change tort law, (b) improve community services to handicapped children, (c) improve the quality of obstetric and pediatric care, (d) improve physicians' communicating skills with patients and parents, (e) identify all of the events that led to a child's disability or death and explain them in detail to the parents. This last suggestion should be a top priority for health system workers because it is often the most conclusive way to deal with malpractice claims. Identifying all of the events that led to disability or death usually requires the detailed sharing of information between obstetricians, pediatricians, pathologists, radiologists, and often pediatric neurologists. The resulting answers are more likely to satisfy the parents of an impaired or dead child if the information is provided quickly rather than delayed. The pathologist who examines the placenta and performs the autopsy has a particularly important role to play in providing this information.

IDENTIFYING THE ANTENATAL AND NEONATAL EVENTS THAT LED TO A CHILD'S DEATH OR DISABILITY

Perinatal Death

The pathologist can determine the cause of most stillbirths and neonatal deaths if clinical information and the results of a placental examination are available to supplement the findings of a complete autopsy. Identifying the initiating event for such deaths is particularly

important because most of these events take place outside of the control of the health care system. Parents almost always want to know whether something they did or failed to do was responsible for the death of their infant. When they do not receive this information or do not understand it, guilt can cause discord among family members and doubts can arise about the competency of obstetric and pediatric care. To avoid these problems, autopsy and placental findings on stillborn and newborn infants should be rapidly analyzed and reported to the referring physician. This report should then be promptly given to the family, its medical details explained, and the family's questions answered. More than one meeting with the family is often necessary because new questions often arise in the minds of parents after the initial interview. If the family has questions the pathologist needs to answer, the pathologist should talk with the family. Over the years I have talked with many families who had questions about the death or impairments in their child and on occasion I have shown them specific findings under the microscope. Families who have such questions deserve to receive the most complete and accurate answers that health care professionals can supply.

The initiating event that starts the chain of events leading to a child's death will often go unrecognized without the help of the pathologist. Identifying this initiating event is critical because it is usually outside of the control of the health care system. In a 1983 study we were able to identify the presumed initiating disorder for all but 3 of 91 consecutive fetal and neonatal deaths that occurred at our institution.[3] All of the initiating disorders arose outside of the control of the health care system. All but three of the infants who died were born preterm. Forty-eight of these preterm born infants died in the neonatal period of disorders that are characteristic consequences of immaturity. If these deaths had been solely attributed to immaturity, some parents might have wondered if medical intervention could have prevented the preterm birth and subsequent death. By examining placentas and taking all of the clinical information into consideration, we were able to show that none of these preterm births could have been anticipated or prevented. It is almost always more appropriate to attribute such deaths to the disorders that led to preterm birth than to the secondary disorders of immaturity. For example, 53% of the deaths in the 1983 study were linked to acute chorioamnionitis, a disorder that cannot be predicted or prevented.[9] Acute chorioamnionitis invariably starts labor that cannot be stopped by any currently available drugs or other therapy.[10]

Fifteen of the 48 cases of acute chorioamnionitis were associated with premature rupture of the fetal membranes. Studies have shown that about half of such premature membrane ruptures are the result of membrane weakening by preexisting acute chorioamnionitis.[8] Ten of the perinatal deaths (11%) were initiated by placental abruptions. Four of the 10 abruptions were probably initiated by acute chorioamnionitis.[6] Since the inflammatory process involved the areas where the abruptions began, some of the hemorrhages that initiated the abruptions likely originated from blood vessels damaged by the infections.[2,9] Other abruptions in our study were associated with maternal cigarette smoking, a well-known cause of placental abruption. All of these mothers had been advised of the dangers of their smoking during pregnancy. Twelve (13%) of the perinatal deaths in our study were attributed to chronic hypertension or preeclampsia, disorders that characteristically produce low blood flow from the uterus to the placenta.[9] Such disorders are the second most frequent cause of spontaneous preterm birth.[5] Acute chorioamnionitis, the disorders of low uteroplacental blood flow, abruptio placentae, and major congenital malformations were responsible for almost all of the stillbirths in our 1983 study.[3] There is nothing that health care personnel could have done to prevent these disorders or the resulting deaths.

Children With Brain Malfunction

Pathologists can sometimes provide information that makes it possible to identify the origin of motor, cognitive, and behavioral disorders in children. The analytic strategy is much the same as that just described for determining the causes of fetal and neonatal deaths. More than 20 placental, umbilical cord, and fetal membrane disorders are associated with neurologic, cognitive, and behavioral disorders.[4,6–8] More than two-thirds of the litigated brain damage claims relate to cerebral palsy (CP) which the plaintiff has attributed to birth asphyxia or trauma. In Chapter 11 we have identified the origins of over half of such CP cases by integrating placental findings with clinical findings from the pregnancies, deliveries, and the children's neonatal periods. Only 4% of the CP was found due to birth asphyxial disorders, and there was good evidence that no cases of asphyxial CP were missed by the analyses. Birth asphyxial disorders were found not responsible for any of the nonquadriplegic CP in the study. Clinical findings in neonates that are characteristic consequences of birth asphyxia were severalfold more frequent in CP children who had developmental disorders than in children who had been asphyxiated.

CONSULTATIONS, DEPOSITIONS, AND TRIALS

Preparation

Physicians who testify in malpractice cases are not always adequately prepared. Both those testifying to the facts in a case and those who serve as expert witnesses need to inform themselves about every detail of a case before they testify. Those who testify should also have a full knowledge of the medical literature that relates to the issues being disputed in the case. Consultants should be prompt in delivering requested information and opinions through the attorney whose client they are serving. Every detail of the case that might be subject to questioning should be discussed with this attorney before a consultation report is submitted, a deposition is given, or testimony is presented in court. Expert witnesses should not support anything they know is untrue or offer opinions that go beyond their knowledge. It is easy for health care professionals to get caught up in the problems of the plaintiff or the defendants and give biased opinions. Avoid such misrepresentations. If an expert witness distorts or does not give truthful opinions, this will be discovered and eventually known throughout the legal and medical communities. Answering a question with "I do not know" or "That question goes beyond my expertise" is more apt to increase than diminish the credibility of a witness before a jury.

The Setting

The legal process can make the most experienced health care professional uncomfortable. The adversarial atmosphere is often jarring to the sense of fair play and to the self-respect of such professionals. Personal competence is routinely challenged and characterized in ways that can appear irresponsible. The questioning of witnesses and rulings from the bench sometimes seem to obscure rather than reveal the truth. This is unavoidable because the legal system is run by rules that are dictated by law and custom, and not by personal ad hoc judgments about what is good, just, or true.

The Lawyers

Many health system workers view plaintiffs' attorneys as all-knowing and all-capable. In fact they vary greatly in these qualities and some lack the knowledge and skills that are needed to fully develop their clients' cases. Plaintiffs' attorneys frequently have reputations as dynamic performers in court who ask clever questions designed to distort the truth and trap opposing witnesses into awkward or false admissions. In my experience such attorneys are few in number and far more frequent are the attorneys who may know as much about some aspects of stillbirth, neonatal death, and brain damage as do the experts they are questioning. Most attorneys are not particularly dynamic in the courtroom, and their questions quite often reflect genuine confusion and misunderstanding about the issues being discussed. What is most striking about some attorneys in court is their tension and fatigue, particularly when their case is going poorly.

Giving Testimony

There are several points to keep in mind when answering the questions of attorneys during depositions and court appearances. First, answer only the question that is asked and keep your answer short and to the point. The attention of the jury is often lost during long answers. Some attorneys talk at length before they ask a question. If this happens, don't be irritated; be patient. Don't anticipate what an attorney's question will be, and do not try to answer a question before it is asked. Often an attorney's prologue is tangential to the question that is finally asked. If a question is too long, too complex, or too convoluted to be easily understood, state that you do not clearly understand it and ask to have it restated in simpler terms. Another way to respond to such a question is to restate it in your own words and see if the interrogating attorney agrees with your formulation. If an attorney asks a series of questions in tandem without stopping, ask to have them restructured into separate, single questions. No matter how unfair or prejudicial a question may be, stay cool, and never reply with irritation, sarcasm, or condescension. Do not malign the character or integrity of other witnesses who may have offered opinions that differ from your own. Assume that their testimony is as well motivated as your own.

The jury is usually able to weigh the conflicting facts and opinions that it hears and come to a sound conclusion. However, such sound conclusions are less likely if a jury does not clearly understand the testimony of a witness.

The Jury

The needs of the jury are sometimes given inadequate consideration during a trial. Too often jury members must listen to medical testimony which they do not understand. When this happens, the attention of some jurors wanders and others experience irritation because they cannot ask clarifying questions. These problems are compounded when witnesses ignore the jury by speaking only to the interrogating attorney. This is a mistake; witnesses should face the jury and speak directly to them when they give an answer. Attorneys usually try to reinforce testimony they think is important by repeating or summarizing it. These summaries are sometimes confused or misleading and they very often omit important facts and explanations. This happens most often late in the course of trials when attorneys are fatigued. If the opposing attorney uses this tactic, the attorney whose client you are representing will usually object and attempt to make corrections. Less confusion will result if a witness's original testimony is clear, concise, and spoken directly to the jury.

Why are many health system professionals such ineffective witnesses in court? The reasons relate to problems being experienced by the jury as well as to the communication skills of the witness. First, jury members are often tired, confused, and in a questioning frame of mind when a witness begins to testify. In some instances the jury may even be hostile, particularly to a witness for the defense if previous witnesses have painted a negative picture of the defendant. These problems are most apt to be overcome if the witness respects the intelligence of the jury and shows this respect by giving clear, easy-to-understand answers, and by not being condescending. Talk to the jury

the way you would talk to your favorite uncle. This requires that every question be answered by speaking directly to the jury in a friendly manner, even when the question is irritating and you feel like making a caustic reply. Control your irritation so that the jury can focus on the issues at hand rather than on personality conflicts. Always look into the faces of the jury to determine if an answer is being understood. If it is understood, it is less subject to distortion by what attorneys subsequently claim you said. If a witness communicates with a jury effectively, the respect that is visible in the faces of the jury will counterbalance many of the less pleasant experiences of a court appearance.

CONCLUSIONS

Enough scientific information is now available to prevent or resolve without extensive litigation many of the malpractice claims that relate to perinatal death and long-term neurologic abnormalities. Approaching such claims on the basis of scientific evidence is the most satisfactory way to resolve them. Many malpractice claims would probably never come to litigation if parents were always promptly informed about the causes of their child's death or impairments. It is the responsibility of physicians and other health system professionals to discover this information and then supply it to the family, quickly and in a form that can be easily understood.

REFERENCES

1. Eden RD, Boehm FH, Haire M: *Assessment and Care of the Fetus.* Norwalk, Conn, Appleton & Lange, 1990, pp 921–1013.

2. Naeye RL: Coitus and antepartum hemorrhage. *Br J Obst Gynecol* 1981; 88:765–709.

3. Naeye RL: The investigation of perinatal deaths. *N Engl J Med* 1983; 309:611–612.

4. Naeye RL: Umbilical cord length: Clinical significance. *J Pediatr* 1985; 107:278–281.

5. Naeye RL: Pregnancy hypertension, placental evidences of low uteroplacental blood flow and spontaneous preterm delivery. *Hum Pathol* 1989; 20:441–444.

6. Naeye RL: Acute chorioamnionitis, its origins and its clinical consequences, in Bellisario R, Mizejewski GJ (eds): *Transplacental Disorders: Perinatal Detection, Treatment and Management.* New York, Alan R Liss Inc, 1989, pp 10–11.

7. Naeye RL: The clinical significance of absent subchorionic fibrin in the placenta. *Am J Clin Pathol* 1990; 94:196–198.

8. Naeye RL, Peters EC, Bartholomew M, Landis JR: Origins of cerebral palsy. *Am J Dis Child* 1989; 143:1154–1161.

9. Naeye RL, Tafari N: *Risk Factors in Pregnancy and Diseases of the Fetus and Newborn.* Baltimore, Williams & Wilkins Co, 1983.

10. Nazir MA, Pankuch GA, Botti JJ, et al: Antibacterial activity of amniotic fluid in early third trimester: Its association with preterm labor and delivery. *Am J Perinatol* 1987; 4:59–62.

Index

Hypoxia *(cont.)*
  intrapartum *(cont.)*
    organ dysfunction in neonatal period from, 340–341
    periventricular leuko-malacia from, 337–338
    selective neuronal ne-crosis from, 337
    status marmoratus from, 337

I

Immunogobulins, unevenly accelerated placental maturation and, 139–140
Impulsive behavior, 318–320, 320–322
Indomethacin, fetal effects of, 17
Infants
  full-term, cerebral palsy in, 330–333
  preterm, cerebral palsy in, 333–334
Infarction, placental, 143–146
  fetal/neonatal death of twins from, 282–283
  maternal floor, 149, 151–154
Infection(s)
  congenital, fetal growth and, 50–51
  maternal, teratogenicity of, 9
  of placenta
    bacterial, 183–204 *(see also* Bacterial infec-tions of placenta)
    fungal, 204
    mycoplasmal, 183–204 *(see also* Mycoplas-mal infections of pla-centa)
    parasitic, 210–213 *(see also* Parasitic infec-tions of placenta)
    viral, 204–210 *(see also* Viral infections of placenta)
Inflammation
  of decidua, 230–231
  of umbilical cord, acute, 113–114
Ingratiating behavior, 326, 327
Intervillous thrombi, 180–182

Intrauterine death of one twin, 288–289
Intraventricular hemorrhages, placental villous edema and, 177–178
Intrinsic biologic error the-sis of birth defect ori-gin, 7
Iodine deficiency, perinatal mortality and, 37
Ionizing radiation, terato-genicity of, 15–16
IQ values, high, 303–304
Ischemic necrosis, focal or multifocal, from fetal asphyxia, 338
Isoniazid, fetal effects of, 17
Isotretinoin, teratogenicity of, 15

K

Kidneys
  dysfunction of, from in-trapartum asphyxia and hypoxia, 340
  failure of, placenta in, 226–227
Knots, umbilical cord, 102–104

L

Labor, brain damage dur-ing, as risk factor for central nervous system disorders, 296
Langhans' cells, 121
Language, abnormal, 304–305
Laxatives, use of, in preg-nancy, 13
Learning disorders, 303
Leprosy, placenta in, 202, 204
Leukomalacia, periventricu-lar
  from fetal asphyxia, 337–338
  placental villous edema and, 177–178
Listeriosis, placenta in, 199–200
Liver transplantation, pla-centa in, 227
Lobe, placental, succenturi-ate, 131–133
Lung(s), fetal
  growth of, smoking and, 84

maturation of, 38
  smoking and, 84
Lupus anticoagulants, pla-cental disorders and, 148–149
Lupus erythematosus, pla-cental disorders in, 146, 148

M

Macrosomia, fetal, 68
  maternal diabetes and, 64–65
Malaria, placental involve-ment in, 210–211
Malformations
  congenital *(see* Congenital malformations)
  explanation of, 6–10
Malpractice claims
  nature and origins of, 359–360
  prevention of, 360
Marginal insertion of umbil-ical cord, 99–100
Marijuana
  fetal growth and, 70
  teratogenicity of, 13
Maternal disorders during pregnancy, teratogenic, 8–9
Meconium aspiration syn-drome, 259–261
Meconium in amniotic fluid, fetal membrane disor-ders and, 257
Membranes, fetal
  amnionic band syndrome and, 263–266
  amnion nodosum and, 262–263, 264
  disorders of, 248–266
  fetal trauma to, 227–229
  gross edema of, 255
  hemosiderin in, 261–262
  meconium aspiration syndrome and, 259–261
  meconium in amniotic fluid and, 257–259
  necrosis of, 254–255, 256
  premature rupture of, 248–254 *(see also* Premature membrane rupture)
  preparing sections of, for microscopic examina-tion, 248
  squamous metaplasia of amnion and, 262, 263
Mental retardation, 297–302

Torsion of umbilical cord,
104
Toxoplasma gondii, placental infection from,
211–213
Trauma, fetal, to placenta,
umbilical cord, and fetal membranes,
227–229
Tridione, teratogenicity of,
11
Trilobed placentas, 129–131
Trimethadione, teratogenicity of, 11
Triplets
preterm birth of, 273
teratogenicity of, 9
Trypanasomes, placental infection from, 211
Twin(s)
brain dysfunction in,
289–290
disorders of, 277–290
fetal growth of, 70–71,
280–281
fetal/neonatal death of,
causes of, 281–288
abruptio placentae as,
282–283
acute chorioamnionitis
as, 282
congenital malformations as, 283
neonatal respiratory
distress syndrome as,
282–283
placental infarctions as,
282–283
premature membrane
rupture as, 282
twin-to-twin transfusion
syndrome as,
284–288
umbilical cord compression as, 284
frequency of, 277
one, intrauterine death of,
288–289
preterm birth of, 273
teratogenicity of, 9
zygosity of, 277–279
Twin-to-twin transfusion
syndrome,
fetal/neonatal death of
twins from, 284–288

U

Ultrasound
in identification of gross
placental abnormalities, 233–234

pregnancy outcome and,
16–17
Umbilical artery, single,
106–109
Umbilical cord
blood vessels of, thrombosis of, 109–110
compression of,
fetal/neonatal death of
twins from, 284
disorders of, 92–114
embryonic remnants of,
112–113
entangled, 104
fetal trauma to, 227–229
gross edema of, 106,
107
inflammation of, acute,
113–114
knots in, 102–104
length of, abnormal,
92–95
long, maternal placental
floor infarction and,
153
marginal insertion of,
99–100
narrow, 98–99
prolapse of, 105–106
single umbilical artery in,
106–109
tight around neck,
104–105
tissue for microscpic examination of, selecting,
92
torsion and strangulation
of, 104
twisted, 95–98
velamentous insertion of,
100–102
Upset, becoming, in reaction to frustration,
315–316
Uteroplacental blood flow,
chronic low, preterm
birth and, 272

V

Vaccinia, placental involvement in, 208
Valproic acid, teratogenicity
of, 11
Varicella, placental involvement in, 208, 209
Vasoconstriction, unevenly
accelerated placental
maturation and, 140
Velamentous insertion of
umbilical cord,
100–102

Video display terminals,
pregnancy and, 16
Villi, placental
disorders of, 169–183
calcium localized in terminal villi as, 169,
170
chronic villitis as,
169–174
hemorrhagic endovasculitis as, 182–183
from high altitude, 182
intervillous thrombi as,
180–182
placental villous edema
as, 174–179
widespread fibrosis of
terminal villi as,
179–180
edema of (*see* Villous
edema)
evolutionary development
of, 119–122
in placental maturation,
136
terminal
calcium localized in,
169, 170
widespread fibrosis of,
179–180
Villitis, chronic, 169, 174
Villous degenerations, subinfarctive, 172
Villous edema, 174–179
large placenta and,
128–129
Viral infections of placenta,
204–210
cytomegalovirus as,
204–205
hepatitis as, 208–209
herpes simplex as, 207
mumps as, 208
rubella as, 207–208
smallpox as, 208
varicella as, 208
Vitamin A congeners, teratogenicity of, 15
Vitamin D deficiency, perinatal mortality and, 37
Vitamin K antagonists, warfarin embryopathy
from, 10
Vitelline duct remnants of
umbilical cord, 113
Vomiting in pregnancy, fetal growth and, 58

W

Warfarin, teratogenicity of,
10